The Student-Physician

Renée C. Fox
Mary E. W. Goss
Mary Jean Huntington
Patricia L. Kendall
William Martin
Robert K. Merton
Margaret Olencki
CONTRIBUTORS   George G. Reader, M.D.
Natalie Rogoff
Hanan C. Selvin
Wagner Thielens, Jr.

A REPORT FROM THE
BUREAU OF APPLIED SOCIAL RESEARCH
COLUMBIA UNIVERSITY

The Student-Physician

INTRODUCTORY STUDIES IN THE

SOCIOLOGY OF MEDICAL EDUCATION

EDITED BY

Robert K. Merton

George G. Reader, M.D.

Patricia L. Kendall

Published for The Commonwealth Fund

BY HARVARD UNIVERSITY PRESS

Cambridge, Massachusetts

Published for *The Commonwealth Fund*

BY HARVARD UNIVERSITY PRESS

CAMBRIDGE, MASSACHUSETTS

Distributed in Great Britain

BY OXFORD UNIVERSITY PRESS, LONDON

Library of Congress Catalog Card No. 57–12526

Printed in the United States of America

TO
DAVID PRESWICK BARR, M.D.

PREFACE

The continuing growth of the professions in American society has brought with it an extended and deepened interest in the purposes, substance, and organization of professional education; for it is plainly in the professional school that the outlook and values, as well as the skills and knowledge, of practitioners are first shaped by the profession.

This critical interest in professional education appears especially marked in medicine. Understandably, the prime emphasis in current re-examinations of medical education has been upon matters of what is being taught, what should be taught, and how it might most effectively be taught. This is not, however, the emphasis in this volume. There is no intent here to appraise current medical curricula or to advocate changes in them. Instead, the focus is upon the educative process in the medical school, upon the ways in which its social structure, like that of other organizations, largely forms the behavior of its members and so affects the making of the medical man.

In our ongoing studies, the medical school is conceived as a social environment in which the professional culture of medicine is variously transmitted to novices through distinctive social and psychological processes. The school is regarded as a decisive middle term between the native and previously trained capacities of selected individuals and the emergence of the professional self, the identification of these individuals, by themselves and by society, as medical doctors. It is the aim of these studies to find out in detail how this comes about: how the aspirant, with his characteristic anticipations, fears, hopes, and abilities emerges as a socially certified physician, outfitted with a definition of his professional status (what it means to be a doctor), with attitudes toward that status (dispositions to regard some of his roles as indispensable and others as secondary), with a self-image (a conception of how he measures up to the requirements of the physician's status), and with a set of professional values (in terms of which he relates himself as a physician to others in the society). How does it happen, for example, that some students emerge from a medical school with one conception of their roles as physicians, and others with appreciably different conceptions? In short, to what degree and through what processes does the medical school shape the professional self of the student, so that he comes to "think, feel, and act like a doctor?"

There is, in this sociological view of medical education, something more than a passing resemblance to the renewed emphasis in medicine itself upon regarding the patient as a person greatly affected by his social environment, rather than as simply a disease entity or a case of sickness. Just as the patient is recognized as more than a disease entity, so the medical student must be recognized as more than a passive receptacle into which new knowledge is being poured. The physician of today is reminded that a sick person is often an anxious person, that his anxieties and difficulties, as well as his potentials for recovery, may be significantly affected by his social ties, by his situation within the family and workplace and in other groups important to him. In much the same terms, the development of the medical student must be considered in the light of *his* social and psychological environment, of his position within significant groups which makes it more difficult, or less, for him to cope with the stresses of his environment and to acquire the knowledge and values of medicine.

The collection of papers in this volume constitute a first set of reports on continuing studies in the sociology of medical education begun some years ago by the Bureau of Applied Social Research of Columbia University in collaboration with the students and faculties of the schools of medicine of Cornell University, the University of Pennsylvania, and Western Reserve University. They are introductory reports, based upon only a fraction of the materials now in hand. Other studies will be published in the form of short monographs, of the kind briefly described in Appendix B, each of which, though prepared in conjunction with the rest, can nevertheless stand alone as a study of a selected problem. It is our belief that such periodic reports of special studies are better suited to this early stage of development in the sociology of medical education than a single comprehensive book. Until investigation has resulted in serried ranks of special monographs on distinct problems in this field, it would be premature to attempt even a limited synthesis of what is currently known.

That these studies could have been conducted at all is owing to the active participation and collaboration of many. We gratefully acknowledge the collegial help given us by the students, faculties, and administrations of the schools of medicine at Cornell, Pennsylvania, and Western Reserve. In particular, we wish to thank the following who have taken most active part in these studies: at Cornell, Dr. Joseph C. Hinsey, Dr. E. Hugh Luckey; at Pennsylvania, Dr. John McK. Mitchell, Dr. Kenneth E. Appel, Dr. John P. Hubbard, Dr. William B. Kennedy; at Western Reserve, Dr. Joseph T. Wearn, Dr. T. George Bidder, Dr. John L. Caughey, Jr., Dr. Thomas Hale Ham, and Dr. John W. Patterson. The concept of a dualism in the underlying assumptions by which men live we owe to Robert S. Lynd, as this is set forth in his *Knowledge for What?* To the Commonwealth Fund we are greatly indebted for grants which have made these studies possible.

In dedicating this volume to Dr. David Preswick Barr, we join with many others to pay our tribute to his continued vision and leadership in medical education.

R. K. M.

G. G. R.

P. L. K.

CONTENTS

PREFACE   vii

PART I.   THEORETICAL AND HISTORICAL CONTEXT
          OF STUDIES

          Some Preliminaries to a Sociology of
          Medical Education
          Robert K. Merton   3

          The Cornell Comprehensive Care and
          Teaching Program
          George G. Reader, M.D.   81

PART II. CAREER DECISIONS

          Introduction   105

          The Decision to Study Medicine
          Natalie Rogoff   109

          Some Comparisons of Entrants to Medical
          and Law School
          Wagner Thielens, Jr.   131

          Tendencies toward Specialization in
          Medical Training
          Patricia L. Kendall and Hanan C. Selvin   153

Contents

PART III. PROCESSES OF ATTITUDINAL LEARNING

        Introduction   177

        The Development of a Professional Self-Image
        Mary Jean Huntington   179

        Preferences for Types of Patients
        William Martin   189

        Training for Uncertainty
        Renée C. Fox   207

PART IV. TWO STUDIES OF THE CORNELL COMPREHENSIVE
CARE AND TEACHING PROGRAM

        Introduction   245

        Change in the Cornell Comprehensive Care
        and Teaching Program
        Mary E. W. Goss   249

        Range of Patient Contacts in the Comprehensive
        Care and Teaching Program
        Margaret Olencki   271

APPENDICES

        Appendix A.   Socialization: A Terminological
                       Note   287

        Appendix B.   Research in Progress   295

        Appendix C.   Note on Significance Tests   301

        Appendix D.   Questionnaire on Attitudes and
                       Experiences of Medical Students   307

INDEX   355

Part I

Theoretical and Historical Context of Studies

Robert K. Merton

SOME PRELIMINARIES TO A
SOCIOLOGY OF MEDICAL EDUCATION

Every human society has its healers. It has specialists charged with the responsibility for the care and the cure of the sick; a responsibility which is, of course, not always effectively discharged. As Dr. Dana Atchley among others has noted, even without training in scientific medicine "the genuinely talented healer [who] can understand the personality and environment of his patient . . . may be of such value that the patient's life is happily altered while nature is curing the ailment that led him to seek help." Particularly if he is aware of the great extent of his ignorance, so that he does not mistake it for sound knowledge, the healer can do good, even in the absence of scientific knowledge. In this large sense, the practice of healing and of "medicine" is a universal part of the institutional arrangements of all societies.

INSTITUTIONAL SETTING OF MEDICAL EDUCATION

Although some socially patterned provision for the practice of healing and medicine is in this sense universal, it is only in fairly recent times that the empirical craft and art of the healer has been greatly supplemented by the sciences which, in composite, make up the science of human biology.[1] In this vastly enlarged form,

[1] For an eloquent and pointed statement of this, see the address given by David P. Barr, M.D., at the Opening Exercises of Cornell University Medical College, September 12, 1956.

3

the arts and sciences of medicine and health care have become the core of one of the *major* social institutions of our time. When the sociologist takes inventory of the major institutions of American society—for example, the family and the economy; political, religious, military, communications, and recreational institutions —he must include, by virtue of its greatly expanded scope and amplitude, the institution of medicine and health care.

This institution can be sociologically regarded as uniting large numbers of people in the performance of numerous and diversified tasks all aimed at the same central purposes: the prevention of illness, the care and cure of the sick, and, ultimately, the active mobilization of personal resources by those in a state of comparative health and well-being. From the sociological standpoint, also, the organization of medical and associated personnel has as its major and pervasive *social function* (whether or not this be the *intent* of individual practitioners) the provision of means for coping with a major *internal threat* to the effective operation of the economy and the society. The most immediate *personal* impact of illness is, of course, upon the sick and upon those intimately linked with them in close-knit primary groups of family and friends. But the more general social impact is upon wider social systems, as familiar statistics amply attest. A crude measure of the magnitude of the task which still confronts the health institutions of our society is provided by the fact that some 7 million Americans are disabled by illness and infirmities on an average day of the year. These millions are kept from performance of their ordinary social roles and consequently affect the work and lives of many more millions of others. To consider the direct economic consequences alone, illness and disability annually reduce the labor force available to the country by about 6 per cent, resulting in an estimated annual loss of more than $27 billion in national wealth. But the disturbances to the social system occasioned by illness and disability are, of course, not fully registered in these figures; the consequences of illness for many other kinds of groups find no direct reflection in statistics now available.

Other well-known figures testify to the large scope of medicine as one of the major institutions of our society. Some 4 to 5 per cent of consumer expenditures by Americans are now being devoted to medical care and associated services, this amounting to over $11 billion annually. More than 110 million Americans are now enrolled in voluntary health insurance programs. Altogether, the organizations directly concerned with the prevention of illness, the care of the sick, and the maintenance of health now form a vast institutional complex, bringing together into one interdependent whole a great variety of personnel, organizations, and facilities—patients and physicians; nurses; dentists and pharmacists; proliferating numbers and varieties of health technicians; diversified and specialized hospitals; many kinds of centers devoted to medical research; agencies designed to protect the public health; philanthropic organizations aiding research, practice, and education in medicine; large, growing, and highly competitive drug houses; associations to provide health insurance; and professional schools, in and out of universities, to educate health personnel. This great complex confronts the society with the formidable task of finding means for coordinating and consolidating these components into an effective whole.

At the heart of this large, sprawling institutional complex is the medical school and teaching hospital—a center of continuing and cumulative advances in the scientific knowledge upon which so much of medicine is based, a center of advances in the ways of practicing medicine, and, of course, a center concerned with the preparation of those who will take up their roles as physicians. Since it is part and parcel of this larger institutional system, the medical school cannot help being affected by what is taking place elsewhere within the system. The medical school is, in effect, continuously subject to the changing demands and expectations of those in the society.

But to say that medical schools are interdependent with these other parts of the institutional complex is to say that they must take these into account. It is not to suggest that the schools must only adapt themselves to these other parts of the institutional system. It is not the function of medical schools to accommodate themselves to any and all demands made of them. Like other social institutions, but particularly the institutions centered on the various professions, medical schools must have a large measure of autonomy; they must have their own definitions of objectives and procedure, which will not infrequently be at odds with the expectations and demands of particular groups in society. It is an institutional obligation of the medical schools to resist those demands which, upon examination, prove to be incompatible with what the best-informed judgment of medical educators take as the major values and basic knowledge composing medicine at the time; for a professional school without a substantial amount of autonomy becomes a tenuous association of men uncertain of their way.

As sociologists have also noted, however, free societies continue to grant relative autonomy to their component institutions only so long as these responsibly discharge their functions. And this implies unending change in medical schools, as in other social institutions. A society in course of change, a body of knowledge continuously growing in scope and content, a changing composition of the major health problems of the society in part brought about by the antecedent accomplishments of medicine itself— all these press for appropriate changes within medical education as well. Like other institutions, also, medical schools can develop vested sentiments and interests, can continue with established ways of doing things not only when they are still optimum ways but also, on occasion, when they are no longer appropriate to the acknowledged purposes of the institution. The mores of medicine require continued scrutiny in the light of changing needs and opportunities.

Oddly enough, the capacity for such functionally appropriate changes in medicine and medical education can be greatly reinforced by a great emphasis upon the *traditions* of medicine. Ordinarily, tradition is that part of a culture which is resistant to change, persisting for a time even when it is out of sorts with the newly emerging requirements of the society. But this is a wholly formal view, not a substantive one. The social function of tradition depends upon its content. And in medicine, the great tradition is typically that associated with celebrated physicians of the past, with those who have shown a capacity to move forward when most of their colleagues were satisfied to let things remain as they were. The great tradition in medicine is in large part a tradition of commitment to the search for improved, and therefore changing, ways of coping with the problems of the sick. It is in this sense that respect for medical tradition is an enduring part of the culture of medical education. Frequent ceremonies serve to keep alive a sense of the core-values of medicine as these are exemplified in the achievements of those who have gone before. It is in this sense, also, that every truly outstanding physician is in some degree a historian of medicine, taking pride and finding precedent in the values and accomplishments of the great physicians of the past. This helps perpetuate the long-term values of medicine and provides the basis for continuing to put these into practice through newly-appropriate means. Medical schools thus become the guardians of the values basic to the effective practice of medicine.

It is within this broad institutional setting that the medical schools find their place. It is their function to transmit the culture of medicine and to advance that culture. It is their task to shape the novice into the effective practitioner of medicine, to give him the best available knowledge and skills, and to provide him with a professional identity so that he comes to think, act, and feel like a physician. It is their problem to enable the medical man to live up to the expectations of the professional role long after he has left the sustaining value-environment provided by the medical school. This is the context within which psychological and sociological inquiry into medical schools can identify the extent to which this comes about and the ways in which it comes about.

But before examining the character of such inquiries, we should see problems of medical education in historical perspective.

HISTORICAL PERSPECTIVES ON MEDICAL EDUCATION

It requires an active effort of mind to see the contemporary scene in its historical context. And when the effort is made, it is hemmed in by lack of access to that wisdom of hindsight which is one of the principal assets of historians. This is as true of medical education as of other social institutions. It is no easy matter to identify current developments which will have cumulative consequences for the future and to discriminate these from passing enthusiasms, best forgotten before they have run their course. It is difficult to distinguish the resistance to change which aims to maintain intact the core-values of medical education from the resistance which is a product of professional habit, sentiment, and the uncritical wish to let thoroughly alone what superficially seems to be well enough. To detect the rudiments of basic institutional change is even more difficult than to detect the persistence of practices grown anachronistic. As John F. Fulton has remarked in this connection, "important history is often being made in our midst, passing largely unrecognized. . . ."

Sociological studies of medical education are in their bare beginnings, with little by way of direct precedent. But precisely because we sociologists have only lately begun to study the organization and functions of contemporary medical education, it is all the more necessary to have some historical perspective on the subject. There is no need here to sketch even the outlines of that long, checkered history.[2] But some perspective may be gained by examining, in some detail, at least one of the early developments in the history of American medical education, and to consider, more cursorily, some later climactic episodes. For, as we shall see, the first proposal for new forms of social organization designed to transmit the culture of medicine—its knowledge and skills, its values and attitudes—involved what was, in effect, a distinctly sociological orientation toward medical education.

In 1765, Dr. John Morgan, the first American professor of the Theory and Practice of Medicine, delivered his justly celebrated *Discourse upon the Institution of Medical Schools in America.*[3] The thirty-year-old Morgan was eminently qualified to speak on this subject. Half his life had been spent preparing himself for the practice of medicine in ways which virtually recapitulate the various forms of medical instruction then available: six years as apprentice to a physician, four years in military life "principally

[2] No later treatise on the subject has yet taken the place of Theodor Puschmann, *A History of Medical Education from the Most Remote to the Most Recent Times*, translated and edited by Evan H. Hare (London, 1891). See also W. F. Norwood, *History of Medical Education in the United States before the Civil War* (Philadelphia: University of Pennsylvania Press, 1944).

[3] This pioneering document is available in a photo-offset reprinting of the first edition by The Johns Hopkins Press in 1937. Appropriately enough, this printing contains an introduction by Abraham Flexner.

with a view to become more skillful" in his profession, and five years of study in Europe "under the most celebrated masters in every branch of Medicine." It was upon his return from Europe, and in particular from Edinburgh, that Morgan presented his prophetic views at a public commencement of the College of Philadelphia.

Morgan's *Discourse* has long been recognized as a prescient and eloquent statement of a philosophy of medical education. It is that, of course, but it is something more. In its methodical regard for the kinds of social arrangements which, in Morgan's judgment, were required to educate good physicians, it exhibits a remarkable sociological sense of what this entailed. Even a short analytical résumé of the principal ideas in the *Discourse* will serve to identify these problems and to see the continued pertinence of some of them in the present day.

Throughout, it will be seen, Morgan in effect adopted a sociological perspective on medical education, aiming to develop an effective social organization for learning, rather than adopting a psychological perspective directed principally toward identifying the attributes of individuals which qualify them to become good physicians. It was not, of course, that he neglected this important latter consideration. It was only that he saw with singular clarity the respects in which even the ablest men might be less than able physicians if the organized arrangements for their training were defective. Morgan thus affords an object lesson easily overlooked, as we shall see, even in present-day research on medical education. The process of education, he says in effect, can be instructively examined not only in terms of the *psychology* of learning, focused on the processes by which organisms undergo those functional changes classified as learning, but also in terms of the *sociology* of learning, focused on the social and cultural environments which facilitate or hamper learning.

These considerations can be set forward by allowing Morgan to speak largely for himself.

The division of medical practice. Morgan starts from the premise that the education of the physician must take due account of what he regarded as the effective organization of medical practice. In making his case for the division of labor (specialization) in medicine, Morgan importantly anticipated Adam Smith, whose *Wealth of Nations* was to appear only a decade later. The parallel between the two extends even to the detail of drawing upon the then-popular analogy with experience gained in the manufacture of pins, in which, Morgan reminds his readers:

> . . . a variety of hands, no less commonly than five, six, or seven different artists unite their industry. By this means they finish more work in a limited time, and can afford to sell it at a cheaper rate, than they could, if every individual was employed in all the separate branches. But each having a particular province assigned to himself, while all conspire in one uniform plan, they become more skillful and dextrous in their respective parts, and all more usefully subservient to one end. Are the good qualities of accuracy, dispatch, and cheapness, not to speak of the greater perfection of the work, no recommendation to the manner of doing it? [xv]

In drawing this prudent analogy between social arrangements for the lowly manufacture of pins and the lofty practice of medicine, Morgan was well aware that he was departing from the long-established tradition which would not allow that the prestigious scientist or scholar can learn anything from the experience of the artisan. He attacks this sentiment directly:

> Why should the more difficult, but more ingenious and liberal arts, scorn to be taught wisdom from their example? . . . The human body is certainly one of the most compound machines in nature. Medicine is one of the noblest and most difficult of arts, made up of a number of sciences different from each other. The practice of physic requires deliberation, reasoning, judgement, and experience. Surgery calls for different powers and qualifications rarely uniting in one man. Are these then all to be blended with the apothecary, the botanist, and chymist, which ought to be, and are, each of them separate and distinct in their very nature? Whilst we labour amidst such a variety of pursuits, all improvement must be at a stand. Whereas, let each cultivate his respective branch apart, the physician, surgeon, apothecary, &c. the knowledge of medicine will be then daily improved, and it may be practiced with greater accuracy and skill as well as a less expence. [xv–xvi]

All apart from his assumptions of specialized capacities for particular skills, Morgan is quick to see some of the problems of education to which specialization in the medical arts gives rise. An extreme of specialized knowledge will produce the narrow man, untutored except in his own specialty. It will produce only limited competence and special biases, with little basis for a consensus of values among those engaged in their distinct spheres of activity. But this, he points out, need occur only if the formal training of the physician is confined to his specialty. Such an extreme he rules out; a liberal education should precede medical studies. In addition to this general education in the arts and sciences, there must be general education in medicine.

> It is not only expedient, but necessary that a physician should have a general and extensive knowledge of the whole art, and be acquainted with the principles of every branch of his profession. Thus the general of an army should be acquainted with every part of military science, and understand the whole detail of military duty, from that of colonel down to a private centinel. But there is no need that he should act as a pioneer and dig in a trench. Where a proper subordination is wanting, there is a perversion of all practical knowledge. No more then is a physician obliged, from his office, to handle a knife with a surgeon; to cull herbs with the botanist; to distill simples with the chymist; or compound drugs with the apothecary. [xvii]

The point is not, of course, that Morgan was a missionary for a high degree of specialization in medicine more than a century before the specialties rose into prominence. It is, rather, that he thought in terms of new arrangements designed to meet the health requirements of the society and linked these up with his proposals for medical education. Much the same philosophy underlies current efforts to revamp medical education as medicine becomes progressively aware of its enlarged role in society. As the concept of medical care changes, it brings in its wake a changing conception of the forms of medical education most appropriate to the needs of the time.

The division of labor in medical instruction. In Morgan's view, the same principles of division of labor hold both for medical practice and for the effective organization of medical education. The then prevailing pattern of the medical apprentice meant that the novice learned principally from a single busy practitioner, who was neither omnicompetent nor readily available. Fresh from his years of study in Europe, Morgan was prepared to advocate a radically different organization of medical instruction which called for the "united efforts" of diversely accomplished men.

> Never yet has there offered a coalition of able men, who would undertake to give compleat and regular courses of Lectures on the different branches of Medicine; and such an extensive field it is, as requires the united efforts of several co-operating together, to cultivate it with success. As well might a parent take upon himself the private tuition of his son, and to make him master of all the different languages, arts, and sciences, which are generally deemed requisite, previous to his entering upon the higher studies of Law, Physic and Divinity; as that a Physician, engaged in an extensive practice, should undertake to deliver to his apprentices, in a regular manner, the precepts of his art in all its branches. [19–20]

And then, with an organizational foresight not translated into institutional reality for more than a century, Morgan virtually states the case for full-time teachers of medicine. What is more to the present point, in doing so he proceeds on the sociological premise, only worked out in detail since his day, that motivations are characteristically translated into corresponding behavior only when the social context provides for this. The same motives in different institutional settings take different expression: the same conscientious devotion to duty leads soldiers to destroy life and physicians to save it. Correlatively, differing motives in the same institutional setting may take approximately the same expression: egoistic motives for self-advancement, just as altruistic motives, can be harnessed to professionally competent work. What is needed, says Morgan in effect, are new and functionally appropriate social arrangements which will make it readily possible for physicians to achieve professional objectives. As he goes on to say:

> This [instruction of apprentices by busy practitioners] is as impracticable as it is unreasonable to expect. In spite of himself and his inclination to qualify young men in the profession, they must of necessity be left, for the most part, more to their own ingenuity, and precarious application, than a good man could wish. These are difficulties which he would rejoice to have removed; but they are evils which have hitherto been without a remedy. The fatigue, the greatness of expence, and the want of leisure time, which physicians involved in business cannot command, are bars, which those most willing to perfect students cannot get over. [20]

In short, the good will of good men, indispensable as it is for the purpose in hand, is not enough to get the job done. A basic reorganization of the modes of medical instruction is required to enable the motivations of able men to achieve their otherwise frustrated objectives. By direct implication, this focuses attention, not only upon the important matter of selecting men of great capacity both for teaching and for practice, but also upon the equally important matter of developing organizational arrangements in which these capacities are given optimum occasion for development. Morgan observes that the activities of talented men have quite different consequences, depending on whether they are carried out severally or through "united efforts." [28] If organization is not all, as it evidently is not, neither is unorganized talent enough.

Patterned sequences in the medical curriculum. From matters of organization, Morgan turns to matters of curriculum. The particular ordering of curriculum content which he advocated is of course only of historical interest. He would begin with anatomy, followed by "The Materia Medica and Botany," chemistry, the theory of medicine, and would conclude with the study of practice. But what has more enduring significance is his view that it is not only the substance of what is taught that matters, but the sequence in which it is taught.

> The great extent of medical science, which comprehends under it so many different branches, makes it impossible to learn it thoroughly without we follow a certain order. Whilst we neglect this, all our ideas are but crude conceptions, a rope of sand, without any firm connection. Should the student, as chance or whim might direct, sometimes apply himself to one branch, sometimes to another; or read indiscriminately even the best authors on the different parts of Medicine; for want of method, all his knowledge would be superficial; though he might take as much pains as would suffice to make him eminently skillful, had he from the beginning pursued a well concerted plan. What progress could we make in Mathematics, if we did not proceed step by step, and in a certain order? [15]

Again, almost a century intervened before a graded sequence of instruction was regularly introduced into American medical schools. Of more immediate relevance is the further fact that the problem is, by general consent, even now far from solved. Current experiments in medical education aim almost as much at discovering an optimum sequence of instruction as they do at identifying its most effective content. Although he may have thought the solution more nearly at hand than it proved to be, Morgan sensed the strategic problem of discovering what it is best for students to learn contemporaneously, and what sequentially.

The role of the educational "experiment." Morgan was, of course, the advocate and zealous missionary for his idea of a medical school, rather than the detached observer. But he did look upon the proposed undertaking as a trial run, which might have consequences far beyond the immediate case. He saw the advancement of medical education as proceeding from trials such as the one he proposed. The experience gained in the course of the venture would become widely diffused, just as the personnel trained in it would become widely distributed. He held that, in the measure of its demonstrable success, such an experimental institution for medical education would have multiplier-effects.

> Perhaps this Medical institution, the first of its kind in America, though small in its beginning, may receive a constant increase of strength, and annually exert new vigour. It may collect a number of young persons, of more than ordinary abilities; and so improve their knowledge as to spread its reputation to distant parts. By sending these abroad duly qualified, or by exciting an emulation amongst men of parts and literature, it may give birth to other useful institutions of a similar nature, or occasional rise, by its example, to numerous societies of different kinds, calculated to spread the light of knowledge through the whole American continent, wherever inhabited. [58–59]

Sources of resistance to institutional change. Morgan was thoroughly aware that his proposals would meet with objections founded not only on possible defects of his ideas but, beyond these, upon the commitments of his colleagues to competing ways of doing things. Institutional procedures, once functional for their time and place, engage the loyalties of men involved in them. These men, able to point to the undoubted accomplishments of the past and confident that their motives are above suspicion, find proposed new arrangements unsettling and excessively unsure. When the relative merits of competing alternatives are difficult to demonstrate, as they commonly are in establishing or modifying social institutions, the resistance to change is all the more intense. Morgan addresses himself to his Philadelphia colleagues, quietly suggesting that institutional change, however uncomfortable it may be, is in the order of things.

> I doubt not that every practitioner here of education, experience, and integrity, has pursued the plan which, in his opinion, was best suited to the place and people. But as circumstances alter, so does the propriety of particular established customs, which gradually give way to others better suited to those changes which happen in a course of years. May I not hope to meet with the same candour that I show to others, and be admitted to act from the same honest principles, in recommending what I think an improvement of practice, that I allow those who have pursued a plan different from mine? [xx]

Even among those who see merit in the proposal to try a new kind of medical education, there will be some who hold that the society is not ready to sustain the experiment. "It may perhaps be objected, that the colonies are yet in so infant a state that any attempt to establish medical schools is premature." [38] This is a matter of difficult judgment, Morgan agrees, and therefore an argument not without merit. Not all proposals for institutional change are necessarily sound or, if sound in principle, necessarily suited to the social circumstances of the time. Yet, it should be considered that "the longer we follow any faulty system, the more difficult we find the task to break through the shackles of it, even when it enslaves us to our greatest detriment." [40]

As we know, Morgan won his case, at least in part, though he was far from having envisaged what was to follow, if not as a consequence, at least as an aftermath. He was appointed to a chair of the theory and practice of medicine and soon after, William Shippen the younger, Adam Kuhn, and the young Benjamin Rush joined him as colleagues in what was eventually to become the School of Medicine of the University of Pennsylvania.[4] But as is often the case with planned institutional change, the essentials of the plan, as these have been reviewed, were far from

[4] It is not without parochial interest that this school of medicine is one of the three—the others being at Cornell University and at Western Reserve University—which have taken part in the sociological studies of medical education reported in this volume.

being fully incorporated into schools of medicine for generations to come.

Instead, there followed the great nineteenth-century decline in which the appearance of a medical school was taken for the reality. As Flexner and others have noted, the decisive importance of the affiliation of the medical school with the university, which Morgan had emphasized, was lost to view. Medical colleges multiplied as private enterprises. There were, of course, such developments as the reforms which Eliot imposed on Harvard, and a little later, the requirement for a three-year medical course at Pennsylvania. But even so, the gap between the standards which such forward-looking medical educators as Pepper and Osler felt should obtain, and the operating reality, became a source of malaise, if not of despair. When Osler, for example, said in 1889 that "the American 'system' of medical education [had become] a byword amongst the nations," he was only saying in public what many others were saying in private. Yet the perceptive eye of an Osler could detect a "revolution" in the teaching of medicine, even before the delayed opening of the Johns Hopkins medical school, and could bear authoritative witness to the changes which were required.

Like Morgan, Osler had a distinct sense that the profession of medicine must set its house in order, or the environing society would insist on having it done. Like Morgan, also, he had an acute sense of the basic role of organization, as well as of curriculum and personnel, in bringing this silent revolution to pass. With virtual prescience of the Flexner report which was not to come for almost two decades, he could envisage the requirements that there be an "organic union" of the schools of medicine with university seats of learning, a bringing together of student and patient into close contact "not through the cloudy knowledge of the amphitheatre, but by means of the accurate, critical knowledge of the wards," and an adequate recognition of the teacher of science in the medical schools. In that notable address which states this case, he apostrophizes his University of Minnesota audience in historical perspective:

Fellow teachers in medicine, believe me that when fifty or sixty years hence some historian traces the development of the profession in this country, he will dwell on the notable achievements, on the great discoveries, and on the unwearied devotion of its members, but he will pass judgment—yes, severe judgment—on the absence of the sense of responsibility which permitted a criminal laxity in medical education unknown before in our annals. But an awakening has come, and there is sounding the knell of doom for the medical college, responsible neither to the public nor the profession.[5]

What Osler proclaimed to audiences of physicians, whenever the occasion presented itself or could be contrived, was in a sense generally "known." But there was still little in the way of a concerted social force to lessen or close the gap between what was privately known, or known within the profession, and what was imposed upon the attention of the public at large. It was the celebrated Flexner report which served this function.

Following upon the conferences and reports in 1906–07 of the Council on Medical Education of the then recently reorganized American Medical Association—intramural reports which largely identified the substandard condition of many medical schools— Flexner put diplomacy to one side and dramatically publicized the parlous condition of most of the 155 institutions ostensibly providing medical education in the United States and Canada.[6] The distinctive function of the famous Bulletin Number Four was that of bringing into the public eye the extreme departures from generally acknowledged standards of medical education which obtained in the medical schools of the time. There is something to be learned in this connection from Malinowski's observations among the Trobriand Islanders. There, Malinowski reports, organized social action is not taken on behavior which departs widely from a social norm unless there is *public* announcement and

[5] From an address in 1892, printed in Sir William Osler, *Aequanimitas* (Philadelphia: The Blakiston Company, 1945, 3rd edition), pp. 23–41. As is well known, Osler's prophecy has been fulfilled to the letter and, in a sense, according to schedule. Fifty-five years later, the historian of American medicine, Richard H. Shryock, summarized the record in just these terms. Shryock, *American Medical Research: Past and Present* (New York: The Commonwealth Fund, 1947), Chapter IV. (Now published by Harvard University Press, Cambridge, Mass.) See also Shryock's earlier book, *The Development of Modern Medicine* (New York: A. A. Knopf, 1946); and F. H. Garrison, *History of Medicine* (Philadelphia: W. B. Saunders Company, 1929).

[6] Abraham Flexner, *Medical Education in the United States and Canada: A Report to the Carnegie Foundation for the Advancement of Teaching*, Bulletin Number Four (New York, 1910).

demonstration of the deviation. This is not merely a matter of acquainting *individuals* in the group with the facts of the case. Many of these individuals have already had private knowledge of at least the broad outlines of these facts. But they do not press for concerted action until the deviations from norms are made public simultaneously for all. Only then are tensions set in train between the "privately tolerated" and the "publicly acknowledgeable."

The social and psychological mechanisms making for the great impact of the Flexner report would seem to have operated along the same lines. After all, exacting standards and norms prove distinctly inconvenient for some individuals in the society. They militate against the satisfaction of certain wants and interests. When many find these standards excessively burdensome, there is some measure of leniency in applying them, both to oneself and to others. Departures from these standards develop, and these departures are privately tolerated, though not approved. But this continues only so long as individuals can avoid taking a public stand on the issues. Publicity, such as that provided by the Flexner report, enforces public recognition of the deviations, and requires individuals to take such a stand. They must either range themselves with the deviants, thus repudiating the generally accepted standards and thus asserting that they too are outside the framework of norms, or, whatever their private predilections, they must fall into line and support these standards. The publicity afforded by the Flexner report largely closed the gap between private knowledge of departures from accepted standards and public insistence on the standards. It exerted pressure for an overriding single set of high standards for medical education by preventing continued public evasion of the issue. It called forth public reaffirmation of the norms and, in due course, greater conformity to these norms.[7]

From the outset, the sociological study of medical education should be distinguished in purpose, character, and functions from such technical appraisals of medical education as that represented

[7] This is a paraphrase and application of conceptions set forth by Paul F. Lazarsfeld and Robert K. Merton, "Mass Communication, Popular Taste and Organized Social Action," in: Lyman Bryson, ed., *Communication of Ideas* (New York: Harper and Brothers, 1948), pp. 95–118, especially pp. 102–103.

by the celebrated Flexner report. For Flexner's purposes, it was enough to engage in what he later described as a "swift tour of medical schools." As everyone now knows, that swift tour of almost a half a century ago enabled Flexner to discover numerous chambers of educational horrors, principally in the proprietary schools but in some university-affiliated schools as well. Lucrative professorial "chairs" were being sold to the highest bidders, eager to lay their hands on the rich fees accruing to lecturers. Requirements for admission to medical study were negligible. At times, they came to little more than the ability to pay tuition fees. Examinations were often farcical. Some schools lacked laboratories altogether or included make-believe laboratories with little or no apparatus. Members of faculties were ineptly trained and clinical facilities were meagre or altogether absent.

Since these faults were so gross and lay so near the surface, Flexner soon concluded (and history has borne him out) that "in the course of a few hours a reliable estimate could be made respecting the possibilities of teaching modern medicine in almost any of the 155 schools I visited. . . ."[8] It scarcely required prolonged and detailed inquiry to conclude that a physiological laboratory which consisted in its entirety of one small sphygmograph was less than adequately equipped or that schools without access to dispensaries were hardly prepared to provide suitable clinical training. Quick, incisive inventories of glaring deficiencies were enough for the purpose; more detailed and extended study of the educational environments provided by these schools would have been premature and ill advised.

Partly as a result of the Flexner report and of the marked advancement of medical knowledge, this condition of the medical schools soon changed. Proprietary schools eventually disappeared; sectarian schools dwindled in number and improved in character; a growing proportion of medical schools were affiliated with universities. All in all, the last half century of medical education can be set down as one of the most remarkable periods of institutional change in the entire history of modern education. What Morgan, Osler, Welch, and many others planted, Flexner and his

[8] A summary of this experience is found in the memoirs of Abraham Flexner, *I Remember* (New York: Simon and Schuster, 1940), Chapter 9.

associates watered; but several generations of physicians, scientists, and medical educators gave the increase. Medical education entered upon a plane of standards and accomplishments which is perhaps not fully appreciated because it is so largely taken for granted.

But this achievement must also be seen in historical perspective, even though there is too little historical distance from the contemporary scene to provide the sort of wisdom which is peculiar to hindsight. Having consolidated past gains, many medical educators are engaged in trying to establish new, and more demanding, sights for the time ahead. Even should they so wish, they cannot uniformly settle down into a state of complacency; for the medical schools today are not deprived of criticism—from within the profession and from without. Indeed, it is precisely the antecedent advances which cumulate to provide the basis for considering new and further advances in medical education.

In short, it may not be too soon to say, in broad outline if not in precise detail, what is bringing about the current and fairly widespread efforts on the part of the faculties of many medical schools to reexamine, reassess, and, in part, reconstitute the existing organization and content of medical education. What was the revolution of preceding generations has become the accepted pattern for the next. But these changes do not occur, it seems, at a uniform tempo. Great forward strides in one direction—for example, the systematic incorporation of the basic sciences into medical education—elicit, after a time, not so much a counter movement as a correlative movement to bring other advances in medicine, still more or less unconsolidated in education, abreast of the developments which have moved forward most rapidly. It is as though medical educators, successively aware of the unevenness of development, seek to straighten out the lines of advance. Research in the laboratories and clinics has steadily advanced and thereby changed the nature of medical knowledge and, in large degree, the nature of medical practice. Many medical educators have come to believe that these advances call for correlative and continuing experimentation in the form and substance of medical education. But persuaded that change need not mean change for the better, the same educators engaged in reorganizing the educational environment constituted by the medical school wish to have examined, in as methodical and detached a fashion as can now be done, the consequences of these changes for the development of the medical student. It is in this historical setting that sociological studies of medical education have been begun.

CONVERGENCE TOWARD THE SOCIOLOGY
OF MEDICAL EDUCATION

Richard Shryock is one among many who has remarked that prior to the nineteenth century, physicians *observed* their patients; thereafter, they began to *examine* them.[9] In much the same sense, it can be said that, before this midcentury, medical educators took note of how they were teaching students, but have only lately begun to examine the process of their teaching and the educational environment they were creating for students. This recently emerging interest in medical education as a social and psychological process appears to be the result of a convergence of forces at work in medicine and of others at work in sociology.

Sources of Convergence in Medicine

Advancement of medical knowledge. As has been often said, the growth of science itself provides an important source of continuing and periodically intensified scrutiny of the current content and organization of medical education. Every considerable advance in medical knowledge, or in the sciences upon which medicine draws for a large part of its intellectual sustenance, brings in its wake the pressing question of how this new knowledge can be most effectively taught to the student. Moreover, science advances at an increasing rate. Although the scientists responsible for these advances in knowledge do not of course have this impact upon going systems of medical education as their immediate objective, it is nevertheless an observable result. Most sciences have some bearing upon one or another part of medicine and, as these develop, they generally have some repercussions on medical education. Only in the thinkable but preposterous cir-

[9] Richard Harrison Shryock, "The Interplay of Social and Internal Factors in the History of Modern Medicine," *The Scientific Monthly*, 76:221–230, at 226, 1953.

cumstance in which medical education were completely insulated from new developments in the sciences would this unceasing pressure for changes in the curriculum and organization of medical education not obtain.

As Barry Wood points out, for example, the recent advances in psychosomatic medicine have "been based upon as clear scientific evidence as those of any other branch of clinical medicine." These advances at once raise the question of how this new knowledge can most effectively be incorporated into medical education: primarily by training more psychiatrists, by establishing departments of psychosomatic medicine, or, as Dr. Wood advocates, by placing experts in this branch in departments of internal medicine, pediatrics, surgery, and obstetrics in order "to convince undergraduate students that this important field belongs in everyday clinical practice." Whatever the institutional answers to this question, and these will doubtless continue to vary for some time, the principal fact to be noticed here is that these increments in clinical knowledge, like those coming from the laboratory sciences, press for reexamination of the methods, content, and organization of medical instruction. Such reexamination, as we shall soon see, has distinctively sociological aspects which are beginning to gain recognition.

Stresses on time-budget of the curriculum. The results of research in laboratories and clinics are not alone in exerting pressure upon medical educators for an unending series of institutional decisions about the nature of the education they are providing. The time-bound character of the curriculum has this consequence also. As everyone connected with it is acutely aware, the timetable of a medical school is fixed within fairly narrow limits (although a few schools have lately extended the academic year from 36 weeks to as many as 48).[10] Although the time set aside for instruction has been steadily increasing during the past half-century, it is not indefinitely expansible.

This means, of course, that departments and faculty members of

[10] There is evidently a long history of debate on the amount of time required for an "adequate" education in medicine. Galen argued that, in view of the immensity of knowledge required by the physician, no fewer than eleven years were required; Thessalus, on the contrary, held that six months were quite enough.

the medical school in effect compete for the scarce time of the student just as patients compete for the scarce time of the physician. Hours of instruction are carefully computed and parceled out. The introduction of new teaching materials and courses must often be at the expense of other materials and courses. Considered all apart from the particular personalities and motivations of members of the various departments—though these too may play a part in the actual outcome—the relatively fixed number of hours available means continued competition between departments for their due share of time. In this sense, and without any pejorative implication of the word "competition," some degree of competition among faculty members for time in the curriculum is built into the structure of medical education, with its numerous branches of knowledge and application.

The prevailing organization of medical schools as a federation of departments contributes further to this form of competition. As with political states in federative union, so with departments federated in the medical school. Departmental loyalties develop. It requires a strong sense of loyalty to the school as a whole and an appreciable consensus on the nature and purposes of medical education for departments to relinquish willingly, rather than under the duress of their colleagues, long-established or newly-emerging claims to a particular share of time in the curriculum. As with competition generally, there must develop rules of the game—agreed-upon norms or standards for judgment—to govern the process. These norms can then be used to adjudicate competing claims to the limited time of the student, ideally in terms of the assumed functional significance of each kind of knowledge for the effective training of the physician. The curriculum is a public register of the provisional outcome of this process, in about the same sense that prices, the comparative growth of firms, and profits compose a register of the provisional outcome of competition in the market place.

Apart from this similarity, there is, of course, a basic difference between the forms of competition in the medical school and in the market place. However much they may differ in their conception of how this is best to be achieved, the departments of a medical school are expected to be committed to the same shared values of providing optimum medical training for the student. Unlike the competition between business firms, self-aggrandizement is not institutionally legitimized. Nevertheless, the process of competition for time which is built into the structure of the curriculum, as well as the more intensely personal conflicts which sometimes develop between departments and between their members (in medical schools as in other types of organizations) do serve, whatever their other outcomes, to keep many medical educators alerted to new problems and potentialities of medical instruction. It is difficult for them, even if they were so inclined, to rest comfortably on their oars.

The departmental form of organization and the resulting competition thus lead to a fairly continual, greater or less, pressure for examining the current curriculum and modes of instruction. This pressure need not actually result in substantial change. There may develop a balance of forces between departments loath to give up their established claims in the curriculum, with the result that all remains as it was. This is the type of circumstance, presumably, which led the medical dean described by John F. Fulton to exclaim in despair, "It's easier to move a cemetery than to change the curriculum."

Occasionally, the pressures of advancing knowledge produce also the discomforts of change, leading some medical educators to maintain an alert and, under the stress of competition, a sometimes disproportionate concern with change—or lack of change. Individual departments cannot easily remain aloof from this process. There are few schools, it seems, in which the structure of authority is so centralized that change in the form and content of instruction can effectively originate by decree from the administration. Rather, the more typical pattern seems to be one of pulling and hauling among departments, each, naturally enough, persuaded of the importance and legitimacy of its own claims on the time of the student. This places a great premium upon an appreciable consensus among the divisions of a medical school on the purposes, standards, and values of education as a basis for coping with periodic disturbances to the equilibrium of social relationships among them.[11]

[11] To a more limited extent, the same kind of "competition" operates among the departments in the other divisions of a university. But some reflection will show

Rediscovery of the patient as person. Contributing further to an emerging interest in the sociological study of medical education is the renewed emphasis, within medicine, upon the concept of "the patient as a whole person." The lineage of this idea is, of course, ancient. Medical chapter and verse could easily be cited to show that the great physicians in every age have recognized that the patient must be seen as a whole, including, that is to say, his interpersonal relations and his social environment. Not to reach back to the time and practice of Hippocrates, it is well known that this was regarded as a commonplace in the time of John Locke. Or, to move to the more recent past, the implications of this concept were epitomized by Francis Weld Peabody in his classic paper on "The Care of the Patient."

Although the conception of "the patient as a person" is long established and generally acknowledged in medical circles, it is also said to be a conception more honored in the breach than the observance. Many physicians, it is said, continue to regard the patient as a case of sickness rather than as a person. This suggests that there are forces in the situation which make it difficult for some physicians to live up to this conception. It is, therefore, held essential that these forces be counteracted by methods of education designed for the purpose.

In an earlier day, the local physician could have an intimate knowledge and understanding of his patients. The personal relations between the physician and his patients were often sustained and close—though not, perhaps, as often as we now sometimes suppose. To the extent that this was so, "the old-fashioned general practitioner intuitively recognized [the factors making up the patient's environment, factors] which can sometimes be discovered only through intimate acquaintance with the patient and familiarity with his environment, with his life day by day, and with his family history."[12] In short, the structure of the society

---

that these often loosely connected departments experience a great difference in the degree of such competition, if not in kind. There is not much competition, for example, between a department of fine arts and a department of physics.

[12] Similar observations have been made by many physicians with a capacity for considering the practice of medicine as itself a social system, variously relating the physician to his patients and to the community. This particular phrasing is by the physician-biochemist-and-sociologist, L. J. Henderson, *The Study of Man* (Philadelphia: University of Pennsylvania Press, 1941), pp. 12–13. Elton Mayo is

and the organization of medical practice were such that many practitioners would intuitively and almost automatically take into account both the stresses and the potentials for therapeutic support which the environment afforded the patient.

With the growing complexity of the social environment, the increasing specialization of medical practice, and the often diminished association of physicians with their patients outside the sphere of health care, the problem of taking the social context of the patient into account becomes greatly enlarged. Faced with such exigencies, physicians may find themselves backsliding from what they acknowledge to be the appropriate conception of the patient. The patient, in turn, often confronting a physician whom he knows only slightly or not at all, is more apt to become one of those "frightened people" described by Elton Mayo. He finds it more difficult to communicate a sense of his daily life —his relationships within the family and outside, the stresses of his work situation, his difficulties in coping with the demands of his multiple roles in society. The joint changes of the social structure and of the profession of medicine create new difficulties in treating the patient as a person.

These social changes have evidently induced a newly-emphasized concern with the old problem of having the patient regarded as a whole person. The changes are, of course, not confined to the United States. It is symptomatic, for example, that the First World Conference on Medical Education repeatedly returned to this theme. Dr. S. M. K. Mallick, of the Dow Medical College at Karachi maintains that "consideration of the patient as an individual with a peculiar environment and a particular psychic background is largely ignored."[13] Sir Geoffrey Jefferson, the Professor of Neurosurgery at the University of Manchester, ob-

---

another physician-and-sociologist who has developed this hypothesis in some detail: *Some Notes on the Psychology of Pierre Janet* (Cambridge, Mass.: Harvard University Press, 1938), Appendix, pp. 111–126. This importance of continuity of medical care has not infrequently been appreciated by laymen. In Chapter 3 of her *Janet's Repentance*, for example, George Eliot has someone remark that "it's no trifle at her time of life to part with a doctor who knows her constitution." (Needless to say, the juxtaposition of the two Janets in this note is sheer coincidence; they do not even qualify as homonyms.)

[13] The World Medical Association, *Proceedings of the First World Conference on Medical Education* (London: Oxford University Press, 1954), p. 39.

serves: "Patients are people. The student must find out who these people are, get a mental picture of their lives and of the ways they have lived them, discover how they have come to be sick. Call this psychosomatic medicine or sociology if you will; the things that are newest are their names."[14] The Professor of Social Medicine at the University of Amsterdam, Dr. A. Querido, who has a particularly lucid conception of the contemporary role of sociology in relation to medicine, takes it as his task to consider these questions: "How can the social elements which have contributed to the syndrome of illness of a certain patient be integrated in the clinical teaching? And how can the social factors that may benefit the patient's recovery and rehabilitation be properly evaluated?"[15]

But even those physicians who see a distinct and growing place for a sociological orientation in medicine sometimes write as if, though they obviously do not intend to say this, the social environment affected only the socially disadvantaged patient: the poor, the uneducated, the decrepit. In suggesting that the sociological orientation should be included in the curriculum of the medical school, Sir Henry Cohen elects, interestingly enough, to put the case in just these illustrative terms:

> . . . the student must ever have it borne in on him that when a patient comes into hospital he leaves his environment, his occupation, his family, and his friends behind. Yet these might well have played a major part in the genesis and course of his illness. The patient in hospital—clean, well clad, tidy, lying in a comfortable bed and eating three good meals a day—is often a very different being in the squalor, anxieties, and discords of his home and job. The student to-day sees too little of the conditions in which disease thrives —the overcrowded, ill-ventilated, and unheated homes, the undernutrition which results from poverty, the effects of chronic illness in the home, the moral cankers of unemployment, and the like. Our training must ensure that the doctor is not a man of confined vision.[16]

It is true, of course, that the medical student may often encounter patients, on the wards and in the outpatient department, who live in surroundings such as these. But this should not invite

[14] *Ibid.*, p. 406.
[15] *Ibid.*, pp. 671–672.
[16] *Ibid.*, p. 388.

the fallacious though superficially plausible inference that sociological considerations are pertinent only in such instances of gross defects of environment. Well-fed patients living in well-ventilated and well-heated houses may also be subject to less conspicuous but no less stressful conditions of environment, in their homes, at work, and in the other groups of which they are a part.

Some physicians apparently have another image of sociology, in which it is pictured as a means of equipping medical students with the indispensable professional qualities of sympathy and tact. In more invidious terms, this sometimes appears in the opinion that a sociological orientation toward the patient leads the student to replace a scientific point of view by gross sentimentality.

That both these distorted images of sociology bear no resemblance to the reality is the gist of the following observations by Professor Querido:

> There is no reason why the social data should not be of the same scientific value as those from the laboratory or x-ray department. The time is gone when we had to content ourselves with information on the composition of the family, number of rooms, rent, sleeping arrangements, and the questionable presence of a bath, when asking about the social conditions of our patient. We know now that in order to understand the patient we must learn about his family relations, ties, and tensions, his work, friends, aspirations, hopes, and frustrations, about his development, his attitude to his place in society, his habits, his compensating and escape mechanisms.[17]

Though far less frequent than it evidently once was, another image of sociology still occasionally intrudes itself among physicians. This is the conception that sociology advocates "the socialization of medicine." It is reported, for example, that an "inspiring address" before the House of Delegates of the American Medical Association concluded with the remark that: "Sociologists, economists and political scientists have made strenuous efforts to bring medicine under the domination of . . . [nonprofessional] groups through the mechanism of legislative enactment."[18] In this respect, sociology finds itself in much the same

[17] *Ibid.*, p. 672.

[18] Reported by Morris Fishbein, *A History of the American Medical Association, 1847 to 1947* (Philadelphia: W. B. Saunders Company, 1947), p. 483.

situation as "social medicine." As Dr. Hubbard has observed: "The average citizen—and many a physician too—doesn't really know what he means by socialized medicine, but he is sure it is bad. And social medicine doesn't sound very different."[19]

But such misconceptions of the nature of sociology are being dissipated by actual collaboration between physicians, medical educators, and sociologists. Indeed, it is being suggested that, in *one* of its principal aspects, medicine can itself be usefully conceived as a social science. This was a frequent assertion by the middle of the nineteenth century,[20] but it was then more nearly a figure of speech than the designation of an actual state of fact. By 1936, however, L. J. Henderson could write, in an exacting and responsible sense, of "The Practice of Medicine as Applied Sociology."[21] And by 1955, the Dean of the Faculty of Medicine of Columbia University could state that medicine "must be recognized as a social as well as a biological science. It is imperative today that medical instruction recognize and deal with the social, economic, emotional, and other environmental elements in illness, health, and incapacity because the concern of the present-day physician must be with society as well as with medicine, with human beings in their environment and with their multitude of anxieties and emotions as well as with their pathology."[22]

The emergence of new perspectives, in medicine as in other disciplines, often generates conflicts of outlook, and these, in turn, easily lead to extravagances of opinion. For extended periods, the sciences which later proved to be basic to medicine—chemistry in

[19] *Proceedings of the First World Conference on Medical Education,* p. 747. When Auguste Comte invented that "convenient barbarism," the word *sociology,* he could scarcely foresee the connotations which would be foisted upon it. As we shall see in a later part of this paper, the confusion is worse confounded by the fact that the word "socialization" is a technical term in sociology and psychology which is far removed from its meaning in such phrases as "the socialization of medicine."

[20] As indicated, for example, by Henry E. Sigerist, *Medicine and Human Welfare* (New Haven: Yale University Press, 1941), p. 101.

[21] I am indebted to Dr. George G. Reader for having called my attention to this paper in the *Transactions of the Association of American Physicians,* 51:8–22, 1936.

[22] Willard C. Rappleye, *Report of the Dean of the Faculty of Medicine* (New York: Columbia-Presbyterian Medical Center, 1955), p. 19. Dean Rappleye goes on to say that "these considerations need not and should not substitute for a thorough education in the basic disciplines, but rather should supplement and vitalize it."

the eighteenth century and even physiology in the next—were
rudely rejected as plainly being of no value to medicine at all.
At other times, they provided occasion for excessive enthusiastic
hopes that they would clear up, once and for all, the still-unsolved
problems of medicine. As Shryock describes the early eighteenth-
century orientation toward therapeutics:

> Since no practical benefits seemed to result from the pursuit of
> pure medical science, questions about the utility of research were
> naturally raised and were difficult to answer. Of what avail was it
> after all "to know that the pancreas has a duct?" It is easy to observe
> that science, in the long run, was bound to enrich practice, but this
> was not obvious at the time. In any case this thought would have af-
> forded small comfort to the sick, who could hardly wait a century
> or more for cures.[23]

Quite apart from historical analogies, which are properly sus-
pect, there is, perhaps, an object lesson here for the contemporary
role of sociology in the field of medicine. Difficult and uncomfortable as this policy is, it might be well to steer a course between the
enthusiasts who optimistically make large, and still unjustified,
claims for what sociology can contribute to the training of practitioners and to the practice of medicine, and the cynics who, impatient to see immediate results and persuaded that large gains
from sociology have not accrued, insist that it is bootless to
pursue this line of inquiry at all. It is not necessary to reproduce,
in this field, the long history of cleavage, if not downright hos-
tility, between the clinicians and the laboratory scientists.

The fact is that uncritical enthusiasm and uncritical opposition
work to reinforce one another, to the detriment of both medicine
and social science. There is no need to claim, too soon and without
the warrant of sufficient evidence, that social science is *now*
prepared to make large contributions to the improvement of
medical practice. Such excessive claims are probably not unrelated to the refusal, on the part of some medical educators and
practitioners, to allow *any* place to the social sciences. The more
fixed and unthinking the opposition to any utilization of social
science in medicine, the greater the tendency, on the part of some,

[23] Shryock, *The Development of Modern Medicine*, p. 21, and see the whole of
Chapters 2 and 3.

to make exaggerated claims for social science, if only by way of rebuttal.

But such an excess of sentiments, both pro and con, seems to be dwindling. Instead, there has developed among many medical educators an attitude of guarded and critical receptivity to sociology, an attitude of benevolent skepticism.[24] This is reflected, for example, in the judgment of Dr. Howard C. Taylor, Jr. when he observes:

> The failure to associate medicine with sociology is perhaps the most obvious oversight in medical education . . . the physician [is] largely unprepared, unfamiliar even with the vocabulary of the sociologist, and without the basic knowledge of social principles enabling him to act or to recommend in this field.
> . . . the [medical] student could with benefit receive some instruction in formal sociology. Such work would provide a framework for the student's now considerable but unorganized observational data on social ideas.[25]

It is a moot point whether didactic instruction in sociology would presently best suit the need of medical students to acquire the perspectives of sociology. It may well be that a further extended period of inquiry in medical sociology is first required before such instruction can become truly useful. However this may be, none of the views we have examined proposes, of course, that the medical student become a sociologist and psychologist as well as a physician. In the education of the medical student, it would presumably be with these fields as it has long been with the other sciences basic to medicine. At best, he can be taught to grasp the fundamental principles rather than the full range of specific details of these disciplines, to acquire the objective frame of reference of psychology and sociology for understanding human behavior. Complete neglect of these subjects, on the other hand, means that physicians will tend to practice in terms of

[24] See Mary E. W. Goss and George G. Reader, "Collaboration between Sociologist and Physician." *Social Problems*, 4:82–89, July 1956.

[25] Howard C. Taylor, Jr., in: Mahlon Ashford, ed., *Trends in Medical Education.* (New York: The Commonwealth Fund, 1949), p. 103. (Now published by Harvard University Press, Cambridge, Mass.) See other comments to the same effect by F. W. Jackson, Thomas A. C. Rennie, and Thomas D. Dublin, *ibid.*, pp. 227, 260, 290–291.

an uninformed, perfunctory, and amateurish psychology and sociology.

The historical fact is, however, that medicine is at heart a polygamist becoming wedded to as many of the sciences and practical arts as prove their worth. Nor has medicine lacked for would-be mates, the most recent and vocal of these being the psychological and social sciences. If these have at times seemed importunate and impatient, this may be because they feel themselves to have been left, for too long, to cool their heels in the vestibule. And if at other times, they have acted shy and perhaps overly diffident, this may be because it is a source of wonder to them that they are being considered at all. Moreover, as is often the case with polygamy, the first set of wives—say, the biological and chemical sciences—are reluctant at first to approve yet another addition to the ménage. But there is still hope. As the burden of work plainly becomes more than can be managed by the present members of the household, they become ready for new accessions to help carry the load of what needs to be done.

To the extent that medical educators have come to adopt a favorable view of the place of sociology *in* medical education, they have also come some distance toward developing an interest in sociological studies *of* medical education. Thus far, we have considered three sets of circumstances which appear to have contributed to the emerging interest of medical educators in education as a social process: the continuing advancement of medical knowledge which must somehow be incorporated into the curriculum, the structurally determined competition for time between departments in the medical school, and the growing recognition of the social sciences as having a place in medicine. Yet this interest might well have continued to be confined to episodic, uncontrolled, and casual impressions on the part of medical educators of how one or another form of medical education is working out, just as the greater part of opinion about the workings of higher education in general is based on this kind of casual empiricism. Still other elements in the situation have served to convert this continuing *concern* with the problems of educating the medical student into provisional but *methodical inquiries* into the processes and results of distinct forms of medical education. One of these elements is the historically developed aversion of medicine to sheer empiricism.

Reduction of empiricism. Medicine, in company with most of the other sciences, has experienced through the centuries an irregular alternation between periods of raw empiricism and periods of extreme rationalism. But the secular tendency, particularly in recent generations, has been toward repudiating these misleading alternatives. There has been a steady move toward reducing what Conant has called the "degree of empiricism" in medicine and in the sciences upon which it draws. In this commitment to the scientific point of view, there is an insistent pressure to transform the empiricist "let's try it and see" kind of experimentation, little informed by prior theoretical formulations, into the kind of controlled observation and experiment which is guided by an explicit conceptual scheme. Like the sciences generally, medicine is engaged in a continuing effort to reduce the degree of empiricism in its body of knowledge by increasing the systematic empirical verification of logically connected sets of ideas.

For a long time, it was tacitly assumed that this outlook is appropriate for medicine but not for the study of medical education. More recently, the same scientific outlook is being transferred to this latter sphere. Committed to a belief in the eventual superiority of systematic inquiry over casual empiricism, some medical educators, together with associates in psychology and sociology, are turning to methodical study of the educational process, rather than relying upon casual impressions.

Innovations in medical education. This interest in finding out as methodically as present methods of inquiry permit the actual course and outcome of differing forms of medical education is, understandably enough, particularly marked in those schools which Dr. George Packer Berry has described as developing "provocative experiments . . . aimed at making revisions in our teaching programs which are consistent with a growing understanding of the whole patient rather than just a part of the patient." To be sure, most medical schools are constantly engaged in revising their curricula. But it is especially when these involve changes of some considerable magnitude that there develops a marked interest in systematic observation of how these changes are actually working out. Naturally enough, the faculties of these medical schools seek, so far as is now possible, to apply scientific method to the study of the workings and consequences of these new arrangements, if only because they have been committed to that method in the development of medical knowledge itself.

When the faculty of the School of Medicine of Cornell University construed its Comprehensive Care and Teaching Program as "an experiment in medical education," they set about almost at once to collaborate with sociologists in a continuing study of the operation and educational results of that program.[26] This work was begun in the spring of 1952. Shortly thereafter, members of the medical faculties of Cornell and of Colorado, also engaged in developing a program of teaching the comprehensive care of patients, met with sociologists from Columbia University and psychologists from Colorado to advance plans for studies of these innovations. Similarly, from the start of its basic reconstruction of curriculum, the School of Medicine at Western Reserve University has considered it an integral part of the undertaking to provide for systematic study of the new program. And for much the same reasons, the School of Medicine of the University of Pennsylvania undertook, some two years later, to collaborate with a group of sociologists in a study of the processes of learning among their undergraduate students.[27] It is the continuing studies at Cornell, Western Reserve, and Pennsylvania which are in varying degree drawn upon in this first volume of preliminary reports.

[26] For a short account of how the experimental attitude toward this program led to this study, see the following paper in this volume by Dr. George G. Reader.

[27] For an account of the emergence of the programs of research at Cornell, Colorado and Western Reserve, see George G. Reader, Fred Kern, Jr., and Thomas Hale Ham, "Research in Medical Education: A Preliminary Report," presented October 11, 1954, to the Conference of Professors of Preventive Medicine. See also the "Reports on Experiments in Medical Education" by Joseph T. Wearn, T. Hale Ham, John W. Patterson, and John L. Caughey, Jr.; by Fred Kern, Jr. and Kenneth R. Hammond; and by George G. Reader, *J. Med. Educ.*, *31*:516–552, August 1956.

Although each of these schools is engaged in its own program of research, provision is made for periodic pooling and comparison of experience. The Columbia University Bureau of Applied Social Research is collaborating closely with the groups at Cornell, Western Reserve, and Pennsylvania.

The rationale and character of these studies have, in effect, been stated by those charged with the recent survey of medical education. In their summing up, Deitrick and Berson state the case in these terms:

> To the majority of medical schools, the curriculum is a matter of vital concern. Shifts and changes are constantly being made in the content and duration of the whole and of its separate parts. New programs are frequently tried, and it is claimed that they are experiments. Where, however, is there evidence of a planned, scientific approach, in which the results are measured by their effect upon the student and in comparison with carefully established controls? Little or no evidence is to be found throughout the country of real experiments in medical education, even though experimentation and research are part of the armamentarium of medicine. Even when circumstances bring about a situation that would permit of a real experiment, with ready-made controls, the experiment is not carried out. . . . The faculty should ask itself how effective a new program or a change in the curriculum really is. There is a real need for such experiments in medical education and in the study and testing of teaching methods. Too much reliance is placed on tradition and authority.[28]

For the most part, the continuing studies upon which the papers in this volume are based do not meet the strict requirements of experimental inquiry to which Deitrick and Berson refer. On occasion, these requirements are fairly well approximated, as in the study of the Cornell Comprehensive Care and Teaching Program. Generally, however, the studies are more nearly like methodical studies in natural history and ecology, than like laboratory experiments. But studies of this kind are at a far remove from casual impressions and, it is believed, provide a basis for sound estimates of processes through which the student develops into a physician. Inquiries of this kind can serve also as a useful prelude to more rigorous experimental study.

Doubtless, much else has brought about the current interest in processes of medical education. But in short retrospect, the sources of interest among medical educators in the sociological study of these processes seem to have been principally these five:

1. The great and possibly accelerated advances of medical

[28] John E. Deitrick and Robert C. Berson, *Medical Schools in the United States at Mid-Century* (New York: McGraw-Hill Book Company, 1953), pp. 323–324.

knowledge which raise new problems of how to make this knowledge an effective part of the equipment of medical students;

2. Stresses on the allocation of the limited time available in the curriculum which lead to continued review of the bases for one rather than another arrangement;

3. Renewed recognition of the importance of the social environment both in the genesis and the control of illness together with growing recognition of the role of the social sciences in providing an understanding of that environment;

4. A commitment to scientific method which calls for replacing howsoever skilled empiricism by the beginnings of more systematic and rational analysis of the process of education; and

5. As a precipitating factor, substantial innovations in medical education which require systematic comparisons of the objectives of these innovations with their actual outcome.

Sources of Convergence in Sociology

Consideration should also be given to independent developments in the field of sociology which have been leading to a substantial interest in the study of medical education.

The sociology of the professions. First among these is the marked growth of the sociology of occupations.[29] For reasons which need not concern us here, studies of the social organization of occupations and of occupational roles which were sporadically undertaken during the last generation,[30] have more recently accumulated into a steady and growing stream. Occupations in general and the professions in particular have come to be recognized as one of the more significant nuclei in the organization of society. A great share of men's waking hours is devoted to their occupational activities; the economic supports for group survival

[29] For a recent short overview, see Ernest O. Smigel, "Trends in Occupational Sociology in the United States: A Survey of Postwar Research." *American Sociological Review,* 19:398–404, August 1954; see also Theodore Caplow, *The Sociology of Work* (Minneapolis: University of Minnesota Press, 1954).

[30] Robert E. Park did much to initiate the sociological study of occupations at the University of Chicago in the 1920's. This was developed further by his colleague, Everett C. Hughes, who turned his attention in part to studies of professions. At Harvard University, Talcott Parsons contributed theoretical formulations which did much to enlarge interest in the sociological study of the professions. And during the past decade, studies in this field have been carried forward at Columbia University.

are provided through the pooled work of socially interrelated occupations; men's aspirations, interests, and sentiments are largely organized and stamped with the mark of their occupations.

As part of the newly-emphasized focus on this field of inquiry, there was established, in 1950, a Columbia University Seminar on the Professions. Composed of twenty-three members representing eight professions—medicine, law, architecture, engineering, social work, the ministry, nursing, and education—the Seminar devoted itself to developing a framework for investigation and instruction on the place of the major professions in American society.[31] One of the conclusions to which the Seminar came in the course of its deliberations held that, although the professional school plainly constitutes the major formative influence upon the development of the professional man, there is very little systematic knowledge about the social and psychological environments provided by schools in the various professions and about the ways in which the processes and results of learning are related to these environments.

On the basis of these considerations, it was felt that sociological study of the medical school would afford a prototype for comparable studies in the other professions. All inquiries into the comparative prestige of the professions in American society have uniformly found that medicine commands the greatest measure of public esteem. There is evidence also that the other professions frequently look to medicine as a model, albeit not as a model immune from criticism, for the directions their own development might effectively take. If systematic studies of the medical school should prove their worth, it seems likely that other professions would follow suit.[32]

Lending further particular interest to the sociological (as distinct from the psychological) study of medical schools[33] is the

[31] The work of the Seminar was greatly facilitated by a grant from the Russell Sage Foundation. A volume based on the proceedings of the Seminar is nearing completion: William J. Goode, Robert K. Merton, and Mary Jean Huntington, *The Professions in American Society.*

[32] As will be seen from the paper by Wagner Thielens in this volume, a similar study of a law school is now in progress.

[33] The following part of this paper distinguishes the distinctively psychological and distinctively sociological approaches to medical education and attempts to indicate their connections.

relative complexity of the social structure of these schools. Medical students must relate themselves to many and diverse groups in the course of their training; more so than students in any of the other professions (except, possibly, for social workers and nurses). They not only enter into relations with fellow-students and with faculty—these relationships they share with students in the other professions. They also enter into relationships with patients and with a varied professional and technical staff, in the hospital and outside it—with nurses, social workers, medical practitioners, physical therapists, pharmacists, and administrative personnel. Schools of law and of engineering, for instance, have no parallel to these complex patterns of relationships with diverse individuals and groups during the course of training. Such networks of relationships, it is assumed, constitute important parts of the social environment of learning by the medical student, and therefore call for systematic study.

Collaboration of social science and health professions. We have noted that there appears to have developed, in modern medicine, a distinct interest in examining the actual and potential connections between the medical and the social sciences. A very considerable growth of interest in such collaboration has also become evident among social scientists.[34] (A recent census by Robert Straus has identified some 175 individuals at work in medical sociology; even a decade ago, a comparable census would have probably found only a small fraction of this number.)

Just as laboratory and clinical research has had and continues to have an essential part in radically reshaping medical practice and teaching throughout the first part of the century, so the social and psychological sciences, in their own necessarily limited fashion, bid fair to provide perspectives and knowledge during the second part of the century. This is regarded, not as a prophecy or a mission, but as a summary description of tendencies now much in evidence and promising to become accumulatively more marked. As disciplined inquiry moves forward on the social, and

[34] For a recent account of this convergence of interest, see Leo W. Simmons and Harold G. Wolff, *Social Science in Medicine* (New York: Russell Sage Foundation, 1954). The Health Information Foundation has been issuing an inventory of *Social and Economic Research in Health* which bears witness to a growing volume of sociological research in this field, year by year.

not only the economic, contexts of illness and medical care, there is developing a body of knowledge which can be drawn upon in the clinical training of medical students. Even now, sociologists and psychologists have here and there been attached to the staffs of medical schools to develop further the use of social science in helping to prepare the physician for his role in society.

The sociological study of organization. It is a short step from this interest in the sociological study of illness and medical care to an interest in the sociological study of the medical school itself, for this links up with a long-standing tradition of sociological study of social institutions and formal organization. During the past generation, this tradition has taken on a new vitality as empirical research based on systematic field observations rather than only on available documentary evidence has begun to be developed.[35] In large part, these have been studies of industrial and business organizations, government departments, trade unions, and hospitals.[36] But the methods of inquiry and some of the

[35] This new phase in the empirical study of organization was largely generated by the work of Elton Mayo and his associates of the Harvard Business School. See, for example, Elton Mayo, *The Human Problems of an Industrial Civilization* (New York: The Macmillan Company, 1933), and for the major report on these studies, Fritz J. Roethlisberger and William Dickson, *Management and the Worker* (Cambridge, Mass.: Harvard University Press, 1939). The accumulation of subsequent studies is by now considerable; for critical reviews of these, see George C. Homans, *The Human Group* (New York: Harcourt, Brace and Company, 1950); William Foote Whyte, "Small Groups and Large Organizations," and Conrad M. Arensberg, "Behavior and Organization: Industrial Studies," in: John H. Rohrer and Muzafer Sherif, eds., *Social Psychology at the Crossroads* (New York: Harper and Brothers, 1951). For theoretical statements, see Talcott Parsons, "Sociological Approach to the Theory of Organization," *Administrative Science Quarterly*, June and September 1956; Herbert A. Simon, *Administrative Behavior* (New York: The Macmillan Company, 1947).

[36] Again, only a few among these many studies can be cited here: Philip Selznick, *TVA and the Grass Roots* (Berkeley: University of California Press, 1949); Alvin W. Gouldner, *Patterns of Industrial Bureaucracy* (Glencoe, Ill.: The Free Press, 1954); Peter M. Blau, *The Dynamics of Bureaucracy* (Glencoe, Ill.: The Free Press, 1955); S. M. Lipset, M. Trow, and J. Coleman, *Union Democracy* (Glencoe, Ill.: The Free Press, 1956); R. G. Francis and R. C. Stone, *Service and Procedure in Bureaucracy* (Minneapolis: University of Minnesota Press, 1956); A. H. Stanton and M. S. Schwartz, *The Mental Hospital: A Study of Institutional Participation in Psychiatric Illness and Treatment* (New York: Basic Books, Inc., 1954). (In view of the greatly differing connotations of "bureaucracy" apparently current in medical and in sociological circles, it should be remarked that for the social scientist, "bureaucracy" is a technical term designating a formal, hierarchic organization of statuses, each with its sphere of competence and responsibility. In the social science vocabulary of organization, "bureaucracy" is not a pejorative.)

fundamental concepts are equally appropriate for study of the social organization of the medical school in its bearing upon the behavior and learning of those involved in it.

These developments, which are here barely mentioned rather than described in detail, have occurred only during the past generation or so. Before then, it would not have been possible to conduct systematic empirical studies of the medical school as a social environment. The social sciences were distinctly not ready. Psychology, sociology, and social anthropology had first to develop additional skills and knowledge before they could consider, even programmatically, the pertinence of their disciplines for medical training and practice. This is not to say, of course, that these social sciences are now in full maturity and need only to be routinely applied. They are still in an early stage of effective utilization. But they have reached a point, in the judgment of many persons who are both critical and informed, where they can be utilized to advance our understanding of illness, of medical training, and of medical care. A growing sense of these potentialities, among medical educators and social scientists, has led to field studies of the social environment which the medical school provides for its students.[37]

The process of socialization. Social scientists have long had an enduring interest in studying the process of "socialization."[38] By this is meant the process through which individuals are inducted

[37] In addition to the studies at Cornell, Pennsylvania, and Western Reserve, on which this volume is based, and the studies begun at Colorado at about the same time, numerous related studies are being planned or initiated. For example, Professors Everett C. Hughes and David Riesman, of the University of Chicago, are directing a study of the University of Kansas Medical School, and Dr. Bernard Kutner, of the department of preventive and environmental medicine, is engaged in a similar inquiry at the Albert Einstein College of Medicine of Yeshiva University. Other more or less comparable investigations are being planned or carried forward at Yale, Iowa, and Buffalo; there have been expressions of interest in undertaking studies, comparable in part or whole to our own, in the schools of medicine at Albany, Duke, Kansas, North Carolina, Pittsburgh, Stanford, Tufts, Tulane, Utah, Vanderbilt, Virginia, and Wisconsin.

[38] As was implied earlier in this paper, it is advisable to acknowledge the historical fact that the word "socialization" has quite a different and long-standing connotation in medical circles. This fact cannot be exorcized; it must, instead, be taken into account if we are not to become needlessly involved in semantic confusions and controversies. With this in mind, I have prepared a detailed terminological note on the concept of socialization in the hope of forestalling such bootless conflicts of meaning. This note will be found in Appendix A.

into their culture. It involves the acquisition of attitudes and values, of skills and behavior patterns making up social roles established in the social structure. For a considerable time, studies of socialization were largely confined to the early years in the life cycle of the individual; more recently, increasing attention has been directed to the process as it continues, at varying rates, throughout the life cycle. This has given rise to theoretical and empirical analyses of "adult socialization."[39]

From this standpoint, medical students are engaged in learning the professional role of the physician by so combining its component knowledge and skills, attitudes, and values, as to be motivated and able to perform this role in a professionally and socially acceptable fashion. Adult socialization includes more than what is ordinarily described as education and training. Most conspicuous in the process of medical learning is, of course, the acquisition of a considerable store of knowledge and skills which to some extent occurs even among the least of these students. Beyond this, it is useful to think of the processes of role acquisition in two broad classes: direct learning through didactic teaching of one kind or another, and indirect learning, in which attitudes, values, and behavior patterns are acquired as byproducts of contact with instructors and peers, with patients, and with members of the health team. It would seem particularly useful to attend systematically to the less conspicuous and more easily neglected processes of indirect learning. For as with all educational institutions, it is natural for those far removed from the details of life and work in the medical school to assume that the great bulk, and the most significant part, of what the student carries away with him is learned through formal instruction—an assumption which many members of medical faculties reject as remote from the actual facts of the case. It is clear that not all which is taught in medical school is actually learned by students and that not all which is learned is taught there, if by teaching

---

[39] Talcott Parsons, *The Social System* (Glencoe, Ill.: The Free Press, 1951), Chapter VI and, in particular, the remarks on adult socialization on pp. 207–208; John Dollard, "Culture, Society, Impulse, and Socialization," *Am. J. of Sociol.*, 45: 50–63, 1939; Irwin L. Child, "Socialization," in: Gardner Lindzey, ed., *Handbook of Social Psychology* (Cambridge, Mass.: Addison-Wesley Publishing Company, 1954) which includes an extensive bibliography.

is meant didactic forms of instruction. Students learn not only
from precept, or even from deliberate example; they also learn—
and it may often be, most enduringly learn—from sustained involvement in that society of medical staff, fellow-students, and
patients which makes up the medical school as a social organization.

In our ongoing studies,[40] therefore, we include more than a
sidelong glance at the informal and unpremeditated ways in which
students come to acquire the attitudes and values by which some
of them will presumably live as medical men. We have provisionally assumed that in the course of their social interaction
with others in the school, of exchanging experiences and ideas
with peers, and of observing and evaluating the behavior of their
instructors (rather than merely listening to their precepts), students acquire the values which will be basic to their professional
way of life. The ways in which these students are shaped, both
by intent and by unplanned circumstances of their school environment, constitute a major part of the process of socialization.

It should be parenthetically said that although the technical
skills and knowledge of medicine are, of course, central to the
role of the physician, these are not considered, except incidentally,
in this first set of research reports. Instead, the focus here is
temporarily upon the attitude and value components of the physician's role. As is periodically indicated in this volume, however,
later studies will deal with the relations between the attitudinal
and cognitive components of the medical role.

Methods of social research. The past generation has also witnessed distinct advances in the methods of collecting and analyzing sociological facts which have made empirical studies of
organization possible. Detailed accounts of these methods of sociology are available in several recent books,[41] but an abridged sum-

[40] A series of monographs on selected problems of this kind is now in process.
These are briefly described in Appendix B.

[41] Among these, see William J. Goode and Paul K. Hatt, *Methods in Social
Research* (New York: McGraw-Hill Book Company, 1952); Paul F. Lazarsfeld
and Morris Rosenberg, eds., *The Language of Social Research: A Reader in the
Methodology of Social Research* (Glencoe, Ill.: The Free Press, 1955); Leon
Festinger and Daniel Katz, eds., *Research Methods in the Behavioral Sciences*
(New York: The Dryden Press, 1953); Marie Jahoda, Morton Deutsch, and Stuart
W. Cook, *Research Methods in Social Relations* (New York: The Dryden Press,
1951), 2 volumes; John Madge, *The Tools of Social Science* (London: Longmans,

mary may serve to indicate the principal ones adopted in the studies on which the present volume is based.[42]

FIRST-HAND OBSERVATION. In many respects, the procedures of field observation, as used in sociology, have been the least subject to change. These are much like the procedures adopted by the social anthropologist for observing "social processes under natural conditions." Although primarily qualitative in nature, direct observation of repeated and delimited situations—for example, among preceptoral groups of students—provides data on social interaction which can be quantified.

Particularly in the early part of the present investigation, and to some extent throughout its course, field observers have been conducting what is tantamount to a social anthropological study of the medical school and of associated sectors of the teaching hospital. The field workers[43] have observed the behavior of students, faculty, patients, and associated staff in the natural, that is to say, the social setting. They have made observations in lecture halls and laboratories; have, upon invitation, accompanied physicians and students on rounds to note the social interaction there; have spent time observing the kinds of relationships which develop between student and patient, and between student and teacher. These many hours of observation have been recorded in several thousand pages of field notes, making up a detailed account of recurrent patterns of students' experience. Some examples of the types of situations under observation are these: occasions which have proved especially stressful to students; the latent (as distinct from the expressly didactic) teaching of physician-patient relationships by faculty members who serve as role models for students; the emotional tone or social atmosphere of students at work in laboratories; the patterns of faculty-student interaction and of interaction among students themselves.

Green and Company, 1953). For comparison with how matters stood a generation ago, see Sidney and Beatrice Webb, *Methods of Social Study* (London: Longmans, Green and Company, 1932).

[42] Further brief discussion of these will be found in other papers in this volume; a detailed account is scheduled for later publication.

[43] At Cornell, Mary E. W. Goss and Dr. Renée Fox, and at Pennsylvania, Dr. Samuel Bloom have been engaged in observational studies; at Western Reserve, Dr. Milton J. Horowitz has been independently observing preceptoral groups in particular.

For example, early in our study, observation was focused upon the teams of four students at work in the anatomy laboratory. Since students select their partners, we can learn from the composition of these teams the characteristics which students look for in their first work partners. We can then compare these with independent evidence on the relationships later established among students, to see how these change and how these are connected with the formation of attitudes. From the sociological perspectives of the observer, it is sometimes possible to see implications of recurrent situations in the school which might go unnoticed by others. For instance, when observing the behavior of students at their first autopsy, he notes how the group operates to sustain certain reactions and to curb others, even though such "regulatory social processes" are ordinarily not perceived as such by those directly involved in them.

One of the principal purposes of direct observation of this kind is to identify those aspects of the social environment which provisionally seem to have most direct bearing on processes of attitudinal and cognitive learning. So far as possible, tentative hypotheses deriving from the observations then become a basis for deciding upon the more systematic data to be collected through other methods. This illustrates a major characteristic of the array of procedures used in the sociological study of so complex an institution as a medical school: no one set of data collected through a particular procedure (say, through direct observation) stands alone; it is, instead, typically interwoven with data, on the same subject, collected through other procedures (say, interviews and standardized questionnaires). This serves to reduce, if not to eliminate, the shortcomings of any one procedure by providing collateral evidence to test the implications drawn from a single body of data.[44]

SOCIOLOGICAL DIARIES AND FOCUSED INTERVIEWS. Direct observation permits us to take note only of what students and faculty do and say in particular situations. It does not necessarily furnish a sufficient basis for inferring how they perceive and evaluate the situa-

[44] This short review of method does not consider the procedures for crosschecking and dovetailing the various kinds of experience. This will be examined in detail in the later report on methods, to which I have referred.

tion, for discovering what it means to them. Private definitions of the meaning of a social situation are not always evidenced in outward and visible behavior. As one further basis for tentatively identifying at least part of the range of reactions to the same situation, at first four, and later, two students in each of four years of training have kept detailed journals. These journals describe, often in formidable detail, daily routines of experience, reactions to these experiences, and developing attitudes toward fellow-students, faculty, patients, family, and friends.

These records of the subjective meanings of the events in which this small number of students has been involved do not, of course, indicate the entire range of meanings which students at large have assigned to the events in the school. But they do afford supplementary information which would otherwise have been largely lost to view. Moreover, these typically detailed and lively reports of responses to the environment provide tentative leads to the processes through which students develop their values, learn new orientations, gain recognition of the limits to their own individual competence and to the competence of current medical knowledge itself. Some of these leads in turn become the basis for developing hypotheses about the diversity of responses among students to what is ostensibly the "same" environment of learning.

As a short example of how the same episode involved contrasting definitions of the situation, consider these independent accounts by student-diarists in the same class:

> *Student A:* Monday, we got back our chem. exams. As I supposed, I did flunk it. The marks in general were good; most folks about me got high 80's and 90's. *I guess some of us are just naturally born stupid and careless.*
> *Student B:* Well, we got back our chemistry tests today. I didn't do as well as I should have, but I passed with a very high C . . . I really knew about a B's worth of material. . . . I seemed to see a lot of 100's and 90's floating around the lab, but what can you do about that? *So many of the fellows were chemistry majors and/or took elementary biochemistry in undergraduate school.*

In one respect, these divergent reactions are in accord with the working assumptions of sociology that the meaning assigned to evaluations of one's performance will be *relative* to what the person perceives to be (or knows to be) the entire range of evaluations of those he regards as his peers. Self-images do not develop within a social vacuum; they are affected by comparisons with the performance of others who thus unwittingly compose the framework for self-appraisal. But this first approximation leaves untouched the further question of how it happens that the one student concludes from his comparative failure that he may not have the capacities needed for satisfactory performance whereas the other finds reassurance in contrasting the extent of his earlier preparation with that of his peers. Repeated evidence of such diverse definitions of situations which are outwardly much the same has furnished a basis for our exploring more systematically the roots of such divergences. Just as first-hand observation has suggested hypotheses for further inquiry, so have the volumes of diary materials.

The uses of these diaries have been enlarged by the use of interviews with students focused upon some of the implications of what they have recorded.[45] Weekly installments of the diaries are carefully studied by the field worker as a source of tentative hypotheses about distinctive aspects of the social environment and their significance for processes of attitudinal and cognitive learning. The hypotheses are then explored through intensive interviews with the student-diarists which center on experiences, responses, and concerns only briefly touched upon in the original entries.

On the basis of the observational and documentary materials, as well as of lecture notes and syllabi, Dr. Renée Fox is preparing what might be described as "a sociological calendar of the medical school." This is a detailed chronological account of the important attitudinal and cognitive learning that takes place in the classroom and outside of it, so far as it is possible to piece this together from such diverse materials. When completed, this sociological calendar will provide a provisional overview of the major sequences of learning thus far identified and may be of interest to

---

[45] This procedure was developed by the field-workers themselves, largely on the initiative of Dr. Renée Fox. For a statement of procedures adapted to this purpose, see R. K. Merton, Marjorie Fiske, and Patricia L. Kendall, *The Focused Interview* (Glencoe, Ill.: The Free Press, 1956).

the medical educator as well as to the sociologist concerned with the processes of acquiring attitudes and values.

The field observations, student journals, and focused interviews have provided our studies with hypotheses which would otherwise have been overlooked entirely and which, as a matter of record, we did not consider in the early stages of the inquiry. It should perhaps be repeated that in a sociological study such as this one, sound interpretations require the conjoining of data independently obtained by the use of differing methods of inquiry. No single set of materials is regarded as sufficient in itself.

THE PANEL TECHNIQUE. During the past generation, social scientists have been developing a longitudinal design for the study of short-term changes in attitudes, values and behavior which has come to be known as the "panel technique."[46] Essentially, this involves the use of repeated observations, interviews, or questionnaires, for the same individuals over a period of time.

This is not the occasion for discussing the technical details of the panel procedure. Its major advantages can, however, be quickly summarized. It has the advantage of enabling the investigator to identify the individuals who have changed (or have remained constant) with respect to a wide variety of attitudes and behavior, instead of relying, as is necessary with other kinds of interviews, upon the often faulty and systematically biased memories of the individual. Ready comparisons can be made of the orientations expressed by individuals at successive times in the course of the inquiry. By appropriate analysis, it is also possible to learn which types of students—differing, for example, with respect to their social relations within (or outside) the school— are most likely to develop certain kinds of value-orientations. Finally, it is only through the use of the panel procedure that it becomes possible to study, for a comparatively large number of persons, the mutual interplay of different attitudes.

Use of the panel technique has provided us with our most systematic data, consisting of annual (or, in the case of the Cornell Comprehensive Care and Teaching Program, more frequent) soundings of students' attitudes, experiences, social relations, ex-

---

[46] See Lazarsfeld and Rosenberg, *op. cit.*, pp. 231–259; also the forthcoming monograph by P. F. Lazarsfeld and Jiri Nehnevajsa, *The Empirical Study of Short-Range Change.*

pectations, and values. These are obtained through the use of standardized questionnaires,[47] the content of which is largely designed on the basis of observations in the course of field work and on interviews with students. The periodically collected data enable us to relate such developments in students' outlook to various evaluations of their performance by the faculty through the four years of undergraduate training in medicine.[48] Reliable estimates of such patterns of development require repeatedly collected data about the *same* students. Such estimates cannot be soundly based upon comparisons of the attitudes or performance of students in different classes, if each of these classes has provided only a single set of measures at one point in time.

SOCIOMETRIC PROCEDURES. The past twenty-five years have also witnessed the advancement of techniques for charting the interpersonal alignments that emerge within social groups and organizations. These techniques, in composite, have come to be designated sociometry.[49] As a large body of research attests, this has proved to be a powerful tool for systematically identifying the structure of interpersonal relations in groups. The very simplicity of the basic procedures probably contributes to their demonstrable utility. In brief, the now numerous sociometric techniques all depart from the same fundamental idea of having each member of a group "privately specify a number of other persons in the group with whom he would like to engage in some particular activity,"[50]

[47] A description of the procedures adopted to develop these questionnaires, the time schedule for their recurrent use, and a sample of the questions will be found in Appendix D.

[48] Our studies have so far been confined to the undergraduate years, but it is evident that they should ultimately be extended to relate the great amount of information now available about these students to their subsequent performance as interns, residents, and practitioners.

[49] This set of techniques was originated by J. L. Moreno and first comprehensively reported in his treatise, *Who Shall Survive?* (Washington, D.C.: Nervous and Mental Disease Monograph, No. 58, 1934; new and enlarged edition, Beacon, N.Y.: Beacon House, Inc., 1953). It has since been greatly developed by Moreno and his associates, and by a considerable number of psychologists and sociologists. For an extensive bibliography, see the new edition of Moreno's book; for a recent compact summary of inquiry making use of this set of procedures, see Gardner Lindzey and Edgar F. Borgatta, "Sociometric Measurement," in: Gardner Lindzey, *Handbook of Social Psychology*, Chapter 11.

[50] Lindzey and Borgatta, *op. cit.*, p. 407, go on to point out that the procedure also provides for specifying persons with whom each individual would prefer not to associate in one or more activities.

or, by an obvious extension, with whom he has already elected to enter into some interpersonal relation (as, for example, a close friendship).

Procedures of statistical analysis of these choices, both reciprocated and not, have been developed to represent the preferred structure of interpersonal relations in the group, which can, by similar methods, be compared with the actual structure. It has been found, for example, that the greater the discrepancy between the social relations which are prescribed by the formal organization of the group and those which would obtain if the complex of private preferences were carried out, the more the social conflict and tension within the group.

Such sociometric techniques have been adopted to establish the facts of the case about interpersonal relations among medical students. Inquiries are now under way to discover how distinctive patterns of interpersonal relations foster or curb the acquisition of medical skills, knowledge, and values. Some tentative findings indicate, for example, that in one school a small minority of students believes that the physician ought to exercise firm authoritarian control over patients in the course of therapy. Analysis of data on friendships among students finds that the students who hold to this view, which departs from the attitude most commonly held in the school, are chosen by others as friends far less frequently than would be expected on the assumption that this attitude played no part. Current study is being given to the possibility that such "deviant" attitudes tend to persist because those holding these attitudes are thus insulated from intimate association with students holding the more prevalent attitude.[51]

From all indications, sociometric data help appreciably to trace out some of the connections between unpremeditated and undesigned structures of social relations on the one hand, and the acquisition of knowledge and values on the other.

DOCUMENTARY RECORDS. Until sociologists began to collect systematic data on their own initiative—and, on any substantial scale,

[51] This is part of a monographic study by William Nicholls dealing with the connections between attitudinal learning and social relations among medical students.

this is a matter of little more than a generation[52]—they were compelled to rely very largely on the official statistics collected by governmental and other agencies, and on historical materials. As a result, particularly so far as quantitative facts were concerned, the sociologist worked with makeshift data which often had only a tangential or fortuitous relevance to the theoretical problems with which he was concerned. This left a wide margin for error, as the statistics in hand were crudely reorganized in an effort to make them somewhat pertinent to sociological hypotheses. It meant also that research had to wait upon the incidental and, at times, almost accidental availability of relevant data. As the foregoing pages have suggested, this condition has greatly changed. Sociologists now take it as a matter of course that they will themselves try to collect the data which they require.

In the study of social organization and institutions, however, there is no occasion for a *total* shift from the exclusive use of pre-collected data assembled by the institutional agencies of society, to the exclusive use of field data assembled by the sociologist. Instead, the two should be and can be systematically related.

Like other organizations, medical schools assemble a great deal of factual and evaluative information about their personnel. Some of this can be effectively utilized in the sociological study of these schools and connected with the data collected by sociologists themselves. It is not merely that the schools provide *readily accessible* estimates of the quality of performance by students as these are registered in grades. The accessibility of such materials is a distinct gain which the sociologist gratefully acknowledges. But more importantly, these grades have the further significance that they are part and parcel of the institution itself. They are part of a system of evaluation which constitutes an important part of the environment for students. Grading systems vary in many ways:

---

[52] This will be recognized as a general statement which holds in the large, but not in every detail. There were, of course, important exceptions to this in the nineteenth century. Most notable, no doubt, is the detailed field work, more than a century ago, by Frédéric Le Play, particularly as recorded in his extraordinary book, *Les Ouvriers Européens* (1855). The monumental survey by Charles Booth, *Life and Labour of the People of London*, reported in 17 volumes between 1889 and 1903, will also come to mind. The point is, however, that these are in part notable precisely because they were such distinct exceptions.

in stringency or leniency, in the frequency with which students are formally evaluated ("tests," "examinations," and "quizzes"), in the types of examinations, in the observability of these ratings (by having them communicated privately to each student or by posting them so that they can become known to the class as a whole). Preliminary evidence indicates that such institutional variations in practices of evaluating students appreciably affect the nature of the environment as this is experienced by students.[53]

Official records of the medical school thus have a double pertinence for the sociologist. As part of the institution itself, the types of information and evaluation collected by the schools and the ways in which they are collected constitute part of the environment for their personnel, both students and faculty. As a type of information about student performance, this can be collated with field data to relate cognitive learning to social and attitudinal learning. It is possible, for example, to relate the data on changes of attitudes and orientations of students to those measures of performance which the school provides in the form of grades in each year, cumulative averages, scores on the Medical College Admissions Test, evaluations by members of the Admissions Committee, and qualities of students reported in letters of recommendation.

Just as the various kinds of field data are interrelated to arrive at provisional conclusions, so these, in turn, are related with the documentary data provided by the schools.

This short review may perhaps be enough to suggest how recent developments in methods of social research have made possible the systematic and empirical study of social institutions and organizations. When coupled with the other sources of interest in the professions generally and in the medical profession in particular, these advances in method have contributed, in their way, to the growing interest of sociologists in studying the medical school.

In the large, then, at least five coordinate developments in so-

---

[53] For example, see the brief report on the new arrangements at Western Reserve with regard to the number of graded examinations, and the connections of these with the climate of competitiveness among students. R. K. Merton, Samuel Bloom, and Natalie Rogoff, "Studies in the Sociology of Medical Education," *J. Med. Educ.*, 31:552–565, at 557, 1956.

ciology have brought about concerted beginnings of sociological research on medical education:

1.   The marked and cumulating interest in the sociology of professions which includes, as a major component, studies of professional schools;

2.   The growing utilization of social science as composing part of the scientific basis for the provision of health care in contemporary society;

3.   The considerable recent growth in the empirical study of complex social organizations, among which schools constitute an important special class;

4.   The similar growth of interest in the process of adult socialization in general which, in application to the field of medicine, is concerned with the processes by which the neophyte is transformed into one or another kind of medical man; and

5.   The recent advances in methods and techniques of social inquiry which make it possible to examine these subjects and problems by means of systematic inquiry.

The social historian of the future, looking back on this convergence of independent developments in medicine and in social science toward methodical investigation of the processes of medical education, will doubtless record countervailing tendencies which limit the character of these studies. He will perhaps note, as John Morgan did for his own time, that in medicine, as in other institutional spheres, trial innovations meet with resistance. If he is wise, he will also note, however, that not every disturbing innovation necessarily means improvement; that change is not invariably for the better. He will be interested, then, to see to what extent the prevailing responses to these developments were matters of prejudgment, pro or con, and to what extent matters of critical judgment suspended until enough of the evidence was in hand. The historian may also find some parallelism between the reception of the social and psychological sciences by physicians in the mid-twentieth century and that accorded the laboratory sciences basic or ancillary to medicine in earlier centuries. But, in the main, as would appear from the review set out in these pages, he may conclude that reasonably adequate support, both in medical and in social science circles, was given to the beginnings of a scientific rather than empirical study of medical education.

PSYCHOLOGICAL AND SOCIOLOGICAL PERSPECTIVES
ON MEDICAL EDUCATION

As we have noted, social-science studies of medical education should be distinguished from technical evaluations designed to appraise the content and organization of curricula in terms of standards which are so nearly a matter of consensus in the medical profession that they are no longer under debate. There have been periodic evaluations of curricula, facilities, and staff—the renowned Flexner report being neither the first nor the last of these. Current research on medical education by social scientists, however, tends to be of a different kind. Some of it is designed to search out the extent to which medical schools achieve their announced purposes and to identify the circumstances which facilitate or curb the achievement of these purposes. This provides part of the evidence for evaluation by medical men. But other types of social-science inquiry do not have such directly "practical" objectives.

The two main strands of methodical research on medical education have been psychological and sociological. We have intimated—for example, in reviewing Morgan's *Discourse*—that these represent distinctive points of view. To say that they differ is not, of course, to say that they are at odds or are mutually inconsistent. On the contrary, we start from the supposition and shall try to show that they are mutually supporting and complementary, meeting in a middle ground which has been described as social psychology (or, by some, as psycho-sociology).

In order to see how psychological and sociological studies of medical education relate to one another, it is necessary to identify their distinctive approaches, the questions which they characteristically raise, and the types of concepts in terms of which they organize their inquiries. For this purpose, we first examine briefly the general theoretical orientations of psychology and sociology, recognizing that each of these fields includes a wide diversity of specific sets of ideas. We then enumerate and compare a few problems involved in the systematic study of medical schools which have been or can be studied from the standpoints of both psychology and of sociology.

General Orientations of Psychology and of Sociology[54]

Any attempt to set out the theoretical relations between psychology and sociology is subject to at least three misunderstandings. First, the reader will often assume that an effort is being made to establish the boundaries of inquiry which should obtain for each of the two disciplines; that it is an effort to advocate or to legislate jurisdictional boundaries. Second, it will often be taken to claim that each of the two fields of inquiry is homogeneous, with no significant divergences of theoretical outlook, focus on problems, and ways of work. Third, and most extravagantly, it will sometimes be inferred that the effort is concerned with appraising the comparative merits of the two fields, claiming a greater or less capacity of one or the other to identify and to account for regularities of human behavior. Not only are these three assumptions patently untrue in the present instance; they would be irrelevant, even if they were true.

The aim here is both more modest and less invidious than these misunderstandings would allow. Psychologists and sociologists have begun inquiries into medical education. For many, and not only for medical educators, the distinctive concerns, problems, theories, and methods of these two fields are not easily distinguished. Since both are concerned with enlarging our understanding of that great complex whole which is medical education, the distinctions between the theoretical orientations of each are easily blurred. It is the aim of this short discussion to identify these distinctive orientations in order to suggest how they can be consolidated into a single body of knowledge. There is nothing here of jurisdictional *rights;* there is recognition of the evident fact that a variety of theoretical approaches is presently to be found in both fields; and, above all, there is no implication that one or the other has greater value for an understanding of medical education.

<hr/>

[54] For a more detailed and extended statement, see the two essays on the theoretical relations between sociology and psychology by Talcott Parsons and Theodore M. Newcomb in: John Gillin, ed., *For a Science of Social Man: Convergences in Anthropology, Psychology, and Sociology* (New York: The Macmillan Company, 1954), pp. 67–101 and 227–256.

However much they differ in other respects, the various approaches in psychology agree on having a primary focus on the individual. Gestalt theory, field theory, psychoanalysis, behaviorism of various types—to mention only a few theoretical orientations in psychological theory—have major differences among them, but they all attempt to account for certain aspects of the behavior of individuals. This general assertion, loose and subject to modification in detail though it is, will probably gain ready assent, not only because it is an approximate truth but because it has so often been made before. For our present purposes, however, it may be more useful to itemize some of the types of specific questions about human behavior which stem from one and the other type of orientation. Even a small sample of more specific questions will serve to translate the general formulations into more widely understandable terms. Psychologists ask, for example:

—How is the personality of the individual to be conceived, what are its principal attributes, and how are these related?

—Which qualities of individuals enable them to perform certain tasks more or less well? The field of psychometrics, among others, is concerned with identifying and measuring these attributes.

—Which psychological processes within the individual result in one or another characteristic form of behavior, or in one or another type of personality? Are there, for example, self-regulating processes on the psychological plane as there are for the individual conceived as a biological organism?

—What are the regularities of sequence in the development of the individual self—what, for example, are the phases of psychological maturation?

—How do organisms in general, and human beings in particular, learn?

—What individuals perceive is evidently not determined wholly by the "objective" characteristics of what is "out there" to be perceived. What, then, are the determinants of perception?

—The behavior of individuals can be usefully conceived as affected by various dispositions. What properties and processes of the individual affect his motivations?

That this short list is far from exhausting the classes of questions of interest to psychologists is too evident to require discussion. But

it may serve, nevertheless, to suggest that the distinctive orientation is that of identifying properties and processes of the individual which can be thought of as affecting the ways in which
he is likely to perceive, think, act, and feel. The central theoretical emphasis is upon individuals although, to be sure, it is
recognized and generally taken into account that the properties
and processes attributable to individuals will have different behavioral consequences depending upon the situations in which
the individuals find themselves. The pervasive concern is with
finding effective means of characterizing the individual and his
behavior, and the interest in his environment obtains only so
far as it helps lead to this result.

In the same general terms, also subject to correction in matters
of detail, the correlative sociological orientation is directed toward
characterizing the attributes, processes, structure, and functions
of the social and cultural *environments* in which individuals are
involved. In formal terms, the parallelism is fairly regular. What
the psychologist seeks to discover systematically about the individual, provisionally abstracted from his environment, the sociologist seeks to discover systematically about the environments,
abstracted temporarily from the particular individuals who find
themselves in them. Just as psychologists seek to identify the significant attributes of the individual, so sociologists seek to identify
significant attributes of social and cultural environments. And
again, a short listing of characteristic questions raised by sociologists may serve to amplify and to communicate what is meant
by the general statement. Sociologists ask, for example:

—How is social organization to be conceived, what are its principal
attributes, and how are these connected?

—Which properties and structures of social organization enable individuals to operate with greater or less effectiveness within their
social setting?

—What processes in a social organization foster or curb the achievement of the goals of individuals within them, enabling these to be
realized with greater or less stress?

—What are the regularities in the sequences of social status to be
assumed by individuals within the organization or society? What are
the effects of discontinuities and continuities in these sequences of
status?

—The culture of society incorporates the values men in that society live by. How does the structure of the society facilitate or hamper the efforts of men, variously located in that structure, to act in terms of these cultural values?

This specimen list of sociological questions, like the list of psychological questions, only touches upon some of the general problems characteristic of the field of inquiry. But taken in conjunction, the two lists may serve to indicate that however much these distinctive problems differ, they are, nevertheless, complementary. In the main, psychology treats of the qualities *of the individual,* of the processes through which he perceives his environment and learns to cope with it, of the motives governing his behavior, of his development and growth as a function of both learning and maturation. Throughout, the analytical focus is upon the individual, with his social surroundings being regarded as a given which it is not within the theoretical competence of the psychologist to analyze. In the main, sociology treats *of the social environment,* the conditions under which one or another form of social organization comes about, the attributes of organization and their interrelations, the development of social values and norms, their functions in governing the socially patterned behavior of individuals, and the forces making for changes in social structure. Here, the analytical focus is upon the structure of the environment, with the attributes and psychological processes of individuals being regarded as given, and not within the theoretical competence of the sociologist to analyze. And, as has been said, the middle ground in which an effort is made to relate the variability of individuals and the variability of the social environment constitutes the field of social psychology or of psychosociology.

Psychological and Sociological Research on Selected Problems in Medical Education

By and large, social science research in the field of medical education has until recently been marked by three conspicuous characteristics. First, it has been largely confined to psychological studies of medical students and has largely neglected studies of the relations of students to the rest of the personnel in the medical school (medical faculty, associated paramedical personnel, patients). Second, studies of medical students have been largely devoted to the task of identifying those qualities of applicants which will help serve as a basis for admitting some rather than others and for empirical predictions of academic performance in medical school among those who are admitted. An appreciably smaller body of inquiries has been devoted to the responses of students to distinctive parts of the environment provided by the medical school. Third, these studies have been characterized by a strongly empiricist bent, that is, they are primarily designed to find out correlations between measurable qualities or traits of individual students and subsequent academic performance in medical school, primarily as measured by grades. They have ordinarily not been analytical, designed to account for the correlations between individual traits and performance which have been found to obtain.

This triple emphasis—upon the student, upon his individual qualities, and upon empirical correlations of these with his later performance in school—was perhaps to be expected in the early stages of inquiry. Since it was almost entirely psychologists who had first undertaken these studies, it is only natural that they should have focused upon the qualities of individual students. Furthermore, the long-standing concern of medical schools with finding sound criteria for optimum policies of selection from among the numerous applicants only reinforced the tendency to try to discover the properties of applicants which best qualify them for medical study (and, it is provisionally assumed, for later medical practice). Finally, the interest in identifying these attributes of individuals naturally leads to the search for correlations between these attributes and later academic performance.

Now that various kinds of social scientists have greatly extended their interest in research on medical education, it can safely be supposed that the character of these inquiries will become broadened and more diversified. Even a short review may serve to indicate a wider range of problems of medical education amenable to social science inquiry, and to indicate the ways in which collateral problems are approached from distinctively psychological and sociological standpoints.

Research on selection and academic performance. We can draw upon two recent reviews of the hundred or so studies concerned with identifying the attributes of students which make for academic success in medical school.[55] These reviews find that a great diversity of individual qualities and prior performance of students has been included in these studies: high school and college grades; aptitudes as measured by a variety of tests (including the Medical College Admission Test, Moss Aptitude Test, Minnesota Aptitude Test); intelligence (as measured by ACE, AGCT, CAVD, PMA, Kulhman, Otis, Stanford-Binet, and Terman Concept Formation tests, among others);[56] achievement (as registered in tests of arithmetic, classification inventory, zoology, general chemistry, etc.); reading (in terms of speed, accuracy, etc.); study habits; occupational interests (especially as indexed by the Strong vocational interest blank); personality (as indicated in the MMPI, TAT, Allport-Vernon, Bernreuter, Humm-Wadsworth, Rorschach, and Szondi tests); various assessments of attitudes and behavior (based on interviews), and such status attributes of prospective students as age, father's occupation, marital condition, and community of residence.

The general design of these numerous psychological studies is much the same, although they differ considerably in matters of detail. The design of inquiry characteristically consists of (a) the measurement of qualities of prospective students by use of one or more standardized tests, or of selected experiences and academic performance before they have entered upon their medical studies, and (b) the computation of correlations between these measures and measures of subsequent academic performance. The predictive value of these diverse measures has varied greatly. Gottheil and Michael conclude their critical review, for example, by saying:

[55] Donald E. Super and Paul Bachrach, *Review of the Literature on Choice and Success in Scientific Careers,* Scientific Careers Project, Teachers College, Columbia University, Working Paper No. 1, November 16, 1956 (hectographed), Chapter IV being devoted to "The Physician"; Edward Gottheil and Carmen Miller Michael, "Predictor Variables Employed in Research on the Selection of Medical Students," *J. Med. Educ.,* 32:131–147, February 1957. These two comprehensive reviews, independently conducted and covering much the same ground, come to much the same general conclusions.

[56] Since these numerous tests are more definitely indicated in the two review papers, this list identifies them only by title.

. . . the results . . . have not appeared to be highly impressive. Many psychological tests have been applied. . . . In general, these have not improved upon or even equalled the efficiency of premedical grades in predicting medical grades. Nevertheless in those instances when attempts were made to assess, weight, and combine the various factors necessary for achieving satisfactory grades (such factors as ability, interest, personality, and achievement), the results were more encouraging. Multiple correlation coefficients have been reported ranging from 0.52 to 0.66 with an average of 0.58. . . . Thus despite the many limitations of the criteria and predictor variables used in the selection of medical students, it would appear that predictions may actually be considerably more efficient than they have been generally thought to be.[57]

Super and Bachrach come to much the same conclusion, but emphasize the following point:

Studies of intellective factors have reached a plateau, with correlations between intelligence and achievement in medical school clustering in the .40's and .50's. Progress seems likely to be made in the affective areas rather than the intellective, for intelligence is not likely to account for more of the variation in achievement. A real need therefore exists for good measures of motivation and of personality factors. . . . Again, socio-economic, cultural, and experience factors other than type of school course are largely overlooked in the investigations under review, although key persons have been superficially studied (why they become key figures and how key figures function in that capacity has not been considered).[58]

The dean of British experimental psychologists, Sir Frederick Bartlett, himself engaged in studies bearing upon the selection of medical students, summarizes the experience with intelligence and aptitude tests in these general statements:

(a) Negative prognosis is safer than positive; or, more specifically, lack of success in intelligence and aptitude tests is a safer index of failure in life situations requiring intelligence and corresponding aptitudes than is success in the tests an index to success.
(b) It is safer to predict moderate, or routine, success from test results than to foresee outstanding success.
(c) Intelligence-test prognosis has a wider range than that of apti-

---

[57] Gottheil and Michael, *op. cit.,* p. 141.
[58] Super and Bachrach, *op. cit.,* Chapter IV, p. 12.

tude tests, but even the former cannot be made to cover all types of "problematic" situations.

(d) Aptitude tests provide a less safe basis for prognosis, whether of failure or of success on all points, than intelligence tests.[59]

As these observations imply, there is also something of historical irony if not indeed of paradox in the fact that the more efficient these tests prove to be in culling out probable failures among prospective students and the more widely these tests are actually used as a basis for selecting students, the less apt they are to predict varying degrees of academic success among the selected group of students which is admitted. As has been repeatedly indicated and as Gottheil and Michael have emphatically noted, "the magnitude of reported correlation coefficients [between preadmission test scores and grades in medical school] has frequently been decreased by the effect of restriction in the range of cases" available for study in the school.[60] These and other artifacts of the current use of tests probably lessen their capacity to differentiate sensitively between gradations of accomplishment as these are registered in academic grades or ranking in medical school.

Understandably, then, research on medical education has focused very largely on this matter of the personal qualities—intellective, affective, social—of the *individual student*. After all, it seems almost self-evident that the trained capacities of the individual will determine how effective a medical student he becomes and presumably (though little enough is known of this in any systematic fashion) how effective a physician he will be. Moreover, research of this kind provides a basis for definite action: it can affect procedures of selection, and medicine, like all the other professions, is necessarily concerned with the problem of sifting and recruiting the most suitable personnel. For these

[59] Sir Frederick Bartlett, "Use and Value of Intelligence and Aptitude Tests," *Proceedings of the First World Conference on Medical Education*, pp. 198–206, at p. 200.

[60] Gottheil and Michael, *op. cit.*, p. 141. In addition, as Sir Frederick Bartlett notes (*op. cit.*, p. 205), in England "it seems to be the case that the distribution of successes in the final medical examinations is so widely different from that which is normally secured in any known intelligence test that it seems as if one can say straight off that there could never be any significant statistical relation between the two. It may, of course, be the case that if we succeed in finding any satisfactory criterion of professional efficiency we shall find that our initial tests come out rather better as compared with that."

various reasons, research has largely centered on the qualities or attributes of individuals which seem to make for success in medical school. There is still the difficult problem of establishing sound criteria of "successful performance," and all those who have engaged in research on this subject have recognized that this remains *terra incognita*. We have much to learn, for example, about the extent to which grades in medical school are related to the quality of later performance in the role of physician. In turn, the criteria of the "good physician" have yet to be formulated in a form sufficiently precise and valid for use in systematic inquiry.

Technical problems of measurement such as these set certain limitations upon the prediction of subsequent performance on the basis of psychological knowledge about the individual student. Beyond these technical problems, however, there are theoretical problems which have to do with the conceptual framework adopted in these inquiries. Assuming the presently contrary-to-fact premise that the technical problems have been resolved and that reasonably satisfactory criteria and measures of the quality of performance, as student and as physician, have been established, there still remains the distinctively sociological matter that behavior is not merely a result of the individual's personal qualities but a resultant of these in interaction with the patterned situations in which the individual behaves.[61] It is these contexts of social situation which greatly affect the extent to which the capacities of individuals are

[61] This distinctly sociological component of the problem has of course been periodically recognized by psychologically oriented investigators, even when it has not been methodically incorporated into the design of the study. For example, consider this clear formulation of the theoretical issue: "A chronic problem in all studies of the prediction of human behavior . . . lies in the uncertainty about the situation into which prediction is to be made. Particularly is this true of life circumstances in which knowledge of all the conditions and the precise demands they make on individuals varying in personality is usually unavailable. In large measure this accounts for the limited efficiency of our prognostic psychiatric indices." Harold Basowitz, Harold Persky, S. J. Korchin, and R. R. Grinker, *Anxiety and Stress: An Interdisciplinary Study of a Life Situation* (New York: McGraw-Hill Book Co., 1955), p. 285. David C. McClelland makes a correlative observation: "Often a particular [performance] test is processed by machine scoring and yields only a collection of standard scores which are not of very much assistance in trying to characterize an individual's behavior. Neither the problems with which the person was faced nor the particular kinds of successes or failures he made are evident to the observer: all he has is the outcome of a complex, unanalyzed behavior process." *Personality* (New York: William Sloane Associates, 1951), p. 168.

actually realized. It is notable, however, that until recently intensive study of the social environment of learning by medical students has been largely neglected, while study of the psychological attributes of medical students has been progressively intensified.

Technical limits upon the predictive value of various tests of individual qualities and personality therefore need to be distinguished from theoretical limits upon the efficacy of such predictions. Learning to be a physician, like complex learning of other kinds, is not only a function of intelligence and aptitude, of motivations and self-images; it is also a function of the social environments in which learning and performance take place. Concretely, this sociological view holds that medical students of the same measured degree of intelligence and aptitude vary with respect to their status and social relations with others in the school, and, as a result, in the extent to which they acquire the attitudes and values, the skills and knowledge of medicine. This sociological framework calls for systematic study of the socially patterned situations occurring in the medical school. On this conception, we would expect to find, as we do, substantial differences in the extent and effectiveness of medical learning among students of approximately the same intelligence and aptitude. Learning and performance vary not only as the individual qualities of students vary but also as their social environments vary, with their distinctive climates of value and their distinctive organization of relations among students, between students and faculty, and between students and patients.

Though sound evidence on this is still lacking, it can be tentatively assumed that there are appreciable differences (as well as similarities) between the social environments afforded by different medical schools. This is, at least, an impression often reported by medical educators who have moved from one school to another. What is perhaps less immediately evident but, from the sociological standpoint, equally significant, is that the social environment constituted by each medical school varies for the individual students and groups of students within it. It is only at first appearance that this runs to the contrary. In the large, students in a particular medical school have presumably been exposed to much the same members of the faculty, to the same textbooks, the same laboratory and clinical experience, the same values—in short, the same environment. This is true in a first and gross approximation. But on further and more exacting inquiry, this "same" environment is found to be internally differentiated. It comprises a number of distinct environments for various types of students. Some students, for example, are more socially isolated than others. Some enter as lone individuals, others as part of a social network of friends. There is preliminary evidence to suggest that the requirements of the medical school are experienced as less stressful by the students who are incorporated into networks of personal relations than by those who are relatively isolated. The extent to which students can realize their native potentialities may thus be appreciably affected by their social status within the school. As another example, recent findings by William Nicholls in the course of our present studies indicate that the environments constituted by medical fraternities in one school differ greatly for their members. The fraternities are composed of students of differing types (as these have been previously and, of course, confidentially rated by the committee on admissions). A student of high academic potential, as measured by antecedent tests, who finds himself in a fraternity including many of like kind, will to this extent presumably be in a different social environment, subject to differing social stress and support, than a student in another type of fraternity, in which men of this capacity are in the distinct minority.

Moreover, the criteria and procedures for selection of medical students have distinct sociological implication. They have the consequence of helping to shape the interpersonal environment which the school provides for each of its students. For, as the criteria of admission vary, manifestly the composition of the student body will vary. If the admissions committee in one school, for example, assigns prime importance to purely intellective qualities of students, the composition of students in that school will of course be skewed toward the upper reaches of intelligence. As a result, students of any particular degree of intelligence will find themselves in a distinctly different kind of environment of peers than would these same students in a school having a differing set of criteria for selection.

Next to nothing is now known about the ways in which such differences in the composition of the student body present individual students with significantly differing environments and affect the social processes of their learning. One type of student body, for example, may induce a large measure of competitive stress; another type may result in a more relaxed atmosphere for learning. But whatever the consequences of these differences, and these remain to be identified, it can be seen that the criteria and procedures for admission not only have the manifest function of selecting individuals more or less suited to the role of the physician, but also the indirect and latent function of producing a distinctive social environment for each student. In other words, procedures and criteria of selection not only involve the psychological consideration of the personal qualities of each individual student, but also the sociological consideration of the composition of the total student body.

However further inquiry may find all this to be, these few observations may be enough to indicate the distinctive but complementary standpoints of psychology and of sociology in examining this one matter of connections between the personal qualities of incoming students and their later academic performance. As things now stand with regard to this type of problem:

—The psychologist tries, in effect, to identify and to measure the personal qualities of incoming students which are significantly related to their performance in medical school;

—The sociologist tries, in effect, to identify the various positions and social relationships in which students with particular kinds of personal qualities are involved, in order to see how these are related to academic performance of students having the same qualities but occupying differing positions in the social system constituted by the medical school.

Motivations of medical students, and sources of stress and support in the medical school environment. All organizations confront the functional problem of encouraging their members to fulfill their roles, of reinforcing their motivations to do so, and yet of avoiding that "excess" of motivation which subjects members to "undue stress." This connection between motivation and potentiality for stress is widely recognized. The medical student, for example, who has no great involvement in his work may do poorly, but he is also more likely to be exempt from acute distress over his poor performance. There is, so to say, an optimum zone of intensity of motivation. Below the lower limit of this hypothetical zone, the student will not be sufficiently motivated to live up to the requirements of his role; beyond its upper limit, he will invest each new situation he faces with undue significance and experience even fairly routine situations as stressful. The medical school thus faces the formidable problem of providing a "sufficiency" of incentives to medical students for fulfilling their roles without enlarging and intensifying these incentives to the point where they tend to produce that excess of anxiety and preoccupation with role performance which keeps students from realizing their potentialities.

Students vary, of course, in the intensity of their fear of failure, in their capacity to tolerate stress, in their characteristic responses to anxiety. Apart from such individual variability, however, there is variability in the extent to which medical schools, and particular divisions of a medical school, confront students with stressful situations. There are also, we believe, differences in the structure of social relations in which students are involved, which serve to reduce or to increase the frequency of anxiety states. Under some social conditions, anxious students work upon one another to intensify anxieties; under others, the anxieties of individually disturbed students are more readily contained by social mechanisms operating within the group. To the extent that this is so, the cognitive performance of students will be affected not only by the extent to which they are individually prone to anxiety, but also by the group structure which can operate to cushion or to intensify the impact of stressful situations in the school.

Like the problems of recruitment, the problems of motivation, anxiety, and stress have their distinctively psychological and sociological aspects. This has long been recognized, in varying degree, by many medical educators. Indeed, some of the innovations of curriculum and organization in the medical schools under review are addressed to these very problems.

The design of the numerous psychological studies of motivation, stress, and anxiety[62] has been adapted to the study of medical students. Much of this research is devoted to the systematic changes of behavior under acute stress, commonly toward a disruption of organized action or toward rigidity and inflexibility of behavior. Another part of this type of inquiry is concerned with finding out how students with differing types of personalities respond to varying degrees of stress. Here, the pre-eminent problem is that of individual variability in the definition of what is considered threatening and in the type of responses to stress situations.

As has been indicated, the collateral questions, from the sociological standpoint, deal with the characteristics of the environment which make for greater or less frequency of varying degrees of stress and support. Here the primary interest is not with personality differences in the vulnerability to stress, but in the social arrangements which produce varying patterns of exposure to stress. A prime objective is to identify those aspects of the environing social structure which produce more or less stressful situations rather uniformly for all students and those which differentially expose some, rather than other, groups of students to these stresses.

One may begin, for example, with the evident fact that the immediate future of a medical student is largely contingent upon the appraisals of his performance by the faculty. This generally serves to deepen the affective concern of students with teachers. They are motivated to *know* what is expected of them by the faculty and to *know* in what measure they are meeting these expectations. This, of course, is one source of anxieties about grades in courses. When the pattern of periodically reporting their grades to students is curtailed or eliminated, there apparently develops a marked concern to find substitute bases for answering

---

[62] As some among many pertinent reports, see H. G. Wolff, *Stress and Disease* (Springfield: C. C. Thomas, 1953); Basowitz *et al.*, *op. cit.*; Leo Postman and J. S. Bruner, "Perception under Stress," *Psychological Review*, 55:314–323, 1948; O. Diethelm and M. R. Jones, "Influence of Anxiety on Attention, Learning, Retention and Thinking," *Archives of Neurology and Psychiatry*, 58:325–336, 1947; D. P. Ausubel, H. M. Schiff, and M. Goldman, "Qualitative Characteristics in the Learning Process Associated with Anxiety," *Journal of Abnormal and Social Psychology*, 48:537–547, 1953; E. L. Cowen, "The Influence of Varying Degrees of Psychological Stress on Problem-Solving Rigidity," *Journal of Abnormal and Social Psychology*, 47:512–519, 1952.

the institutionally-generated question: "how am I making out?" Students tend to search out clues which will indicate the instructor's judgment of their performance. The most casual remarks by instructors are imbued with deep evaluative significance. Changes in the system of evaluating students thus seem to have consequences, of largely unknown extent and kind, for the extent and intensity of stresses induced by the environment.

There are, in short, sociological as well as psychological dimensions of motivation, stress, and anxiety. These need to be examined jointly if we are to advance toward a full understanding of human behavior.

Career decisions of medical students. What is considered occupational choice from the standpoint of the individual becomes the process of recruitment from the standpoint of the profession and the allocation of personnel in various occupational statuses from the standpoint of the society. What the individual defines as a promising opportunity afforded by the labor market, the profession defines as an "acute shortage" (say, of doctors or engineers or nurses), and the society defines as an imbalance of occupational distribution. These all patently refer to the same facts from the different perspectives of the individual, the occupational group, and the society. The functional problem of articulating these three systems so that the flow and distribution of occupational choices are such as to meet the aspirations of individuals, the requirements of the profession, and an optimum balance among the occupations is one which is still poorly understood. But again, to state the problem is at least to specify the nature of our ignorance and to suggest interrelations between psychological and sociological analysis.

As a case which exhibits the complementary nature of these two modes of analysis, we can briefly consider the matter of career decisions of medical students. Each kind of inquiry involves distinctive kinds of questions. The psychologist will ask, for example, what types of students, as distinguished by personality tests, tend to elect the general practice of medicine, or one or another specialty. There is as yet little firm evidence of a connection between personality and the choice of different kinds of medical careers. But this has not prevented the emergence of a distinct student lore about the type of personality required for each kind of specialized practice. To some unknown extent, this lore itself seems to enter into the process of arriving at a decision. Some students engage in a fairly continual process of trying to match up their own personalities with the alleged personality requirements of various specialties. In contrast to general practice, some students are convinced, surgery and radiology require relatively little ability to reason. "It takes a certain personality to become a surgeon," says one student. "You have to be dashing and aggressive and full of energy. I've talked to a lot of doctors about this and they all say this is true. Why, just look at all the surgeons you know; I can think of only one exception to this rule and I've worked with a lot of them." Pediatrics, says another, requires "the non-aggressive, non-assertive, kind, understanding, yet strong, type. This is generally agreed upon." As for "x-ray men, eye, throat, and ear doctors," reports a third, they are "all of the businessman type running their practice very much like a business with rigid hours and fees." As these few of many such statements imply, students engage in appraising the skills, knowledge, performance, and personalities of faculty members, not only as individuals, but as representatives of a particular specialty. There develops more or less of a consensus among students about the types of psychological qualities required by the different kinds of practice. It remains to be seen whether these images of the various medical roles affect the career choices which students actually make.

In effect, the psychologist attempts to discover the actual truth of what these students assume to be known: he tries to find out whether there is a distinct association between personality, the psychological requirements of each kind of professional role, and the choice of a particular field of practice. The sociologist asks, correlatively, how it is that students of the same personality type elect differing kinds of practice and students of differing personality types elect the same kind. From the standpoint of sociology, each decision—to go no further back than the decision to enter upon medicine as a lifework and the later decision to enter a particular specialty—is in part contingent upon the reactions of others with whom the individual is socially related. As each in this sequence of decisions is being entertained, it is reinforced or countered by others, and this reacts upon the stability of the decision and satisfaction with it. Successive decisions progressively commit the student to pursuing one or another career, narrowing the range of subsequent alternatives. Each decision will meet with greater or less social support, depending upon the values of the medical school in which the student finds himself, the position he occupies in the eyes of the faculty and of his peers, the constellation and values of the family from which he comes.[63] These provide social contexts which operate to make the student's "personal decisions" variously contingent upon his group affiliations, the culture and structure of these groups, and his position within them. And once having entered a specialty, he may find his social personality conforming to the demands of the particular professional role: decisive students may not only elect to enter the field of surgery but, whatever their previous bent, once having begun the practice of the specialty, their personalities may be further shaped by the requirements of the specialized role.

The social process of career decisions involves far more, of course, than the end result of entering a particular field of medical practice. The social context affects the degree of stress attending these decisions. It has been found, for example, that students perceive the various medical specialties as differing in prestige and status.[64] Internists and surgeons are commonly assigned higher standing than, say, obstetricians and psychiatrists. Within such a climate of evaluation, the student who proposes to become a psychiatrist seems, from the preliminary data in hand, to be subject to greater stress than his fellow-students who plan to enter the more highly approved fields of internal medicine or surgery. It may be, of course, that these climates of evaluation vary substantially among medical schools. In that event, the student who decides to specialize in psychiatry in one school, where great value is attached to this field, will be in a substantially different social and psychological situation than the *same kind* of student

[63] The three papers comprising Part II of this volume deal with selected aspects of the social contexts of such decisions.

[64] Merton, Bloom, and Rogoff, *op. cit.*, pp. 563–564.

making this decision in another school in which psychiatry is often derogated. This may serve, if only by way of tentative illustration, to suggest that the same career decisions will have differing psychological significance depending upon the social context.

Once again, the psychological and sociological approaches to a particular problem prove to be complementary. Moreover, each approach can be taken a considerable distance before the two are brought together. In this illustrative case, it will then become possible to establish the probability that various kinds of career decisions will be made by medical students of differing types of personality in various kinds of social environments.

The spectrum of medical values and norms. One last illustration may serve to bring out a further distinctive focus in the sociology of medical education, without comparing this focus with that of psychology. This is the value-environment afforded by medical schools.

The profession of medicine, like other occupations, has its own normative subculture, a body of shared and transmitted ideas, values and standards toward which members of the profession are expected to orient their behavior. The norms and standards define technically and morally allowable patterns of behavior, indicating what is prescribed, preferred, permitted, or proscribed. The subculture, then, refers to more than habitual behavior; its norms codify the values of the profession. This extends even to the details of language judged appropriate by the profession; like other occupations, medicine has its own distinctive vocabulary, and like the vocabularies of other occupations, this one is often described derisively as jargon by outsiders and described appreciatively as technical terminology by insiders.[65] The medical subculture covers a wide range—from matters of language to matters of relations to patients, colleagues, and the community —and it is the function of the medical school to transmit this subculture to successive generations of neophytes.

The composition of values involved in the medical subculture

[65] Being human, physicians in their status as outsiders often regard the distinctive vocabularies of other professions—say, the profession of law—as largely composed of superfluous jargon. It seems to be fairly uniform that one group's language is another group's jargon.

probably varies somewhat in detail and in emphasis among medical schools but there nevertheless appears to be a substantial consensus. Impressions based upon field observation suggest that appreciably the same values and norms obtain with varying emphasis in the medical schools of Cornell, Pennsylvania, and Western Reserve, and that these, in turn, are similar to the values and norms codified in a report of a committee of the Association of American Medical Colleges.[66]

The system of values and norms can be thought of as being organized or patterned in at least two major respects. First, for each norm there tends to be at least one coordinate norm, which is, if not inconsistent with the other, at least sufficiently different as to make it difficult for the student and the physician to live up to them both. Alan Gregg, for example, speaks of the "readjustment" that takes place "between the detachment of the nascent scientist and the none too mature compassion of the beginner in therapy."[67] From this perspective, medical education can be conceived as facing the task of enabling students to learn *how to blend* incompatible or potentially incompatible norms into a functionally consistent whole.[68] Indeed, the process of learning to be a physician can be conceived as largely the learning of blending seeming or actual incompatibles into consistent and stable patterns of professional behavior.

Second, the values and norms are defined by the profession in terms of how they are to be put into effect. They come to be defined as requirements of the physician's role. And since many physicians will find themselves in situations where it is difficult to live up to these role requirements, it becomes the more impor-

[66] "The Objectives of Undergraduate Medical Education," *J. Med. Educ.*, 28:57–59, March 1953.

[67] Alan Gregg, "Our Anabasis," *The Pharos of Alpha Omega Alpha*, 18:14–25, at p. 22, February 1955. This short, brilliant examination of the life of the medical student is virtually a paradigm for our own studies. From the standpoint of these studies it could scarcely have appeared at a more opportune time, for by its selection of matters in point, it reassured us in our occasionally wavering belief that we were indeed studying the salient problems in the role of the medical student.

[68] Various aspects of this process are now being studied. A first report is provided by Gene N. Levine, "The Good Physician: A Study of Physician-Patient Interaction," Working Paper Number 3, Evaluation Studies of the Cornell Comprehensive Care and Teaching Program, Bureau of Applied Social Research, 1957.

tant that they thoroughly acquire the values which are to regulate their behavior.

For convenience, the following abbreviated list of values and norms in the practice of medicine will be itemized in three broad classes: those governing the physician's self-image, his relations to his patients, and his relations to colleagues and to the community.

VALUES GOVERNING THE PHYSICIAN'S SELF-IMAGE

1. The physician should continue his self-education throughout his career in order to keep pace with the rapidly advancing frontiers of medical knowledge.

But: he also has a primary obligation to make as much time as possible available for the care of his patients.

2. The student-physician should be interested in enlarging his medical responsibilities as he advances through medical school.

But: he must not prematurely take a measure of responsibility for which he is not adequately prepared (or, at least, is not legally qualified to undertake).

3. The physician must maintain a self-critical attitude and be disciplined in the scientific appraisal of evidence.

But: he must be decisive and not postpone decisions beyond what the situation requires, even when the scientific evidence is inadequate.

4. The physician must have a sense of autonomy; he must take the burden of responsibility and act as the situation, in his best judgment, requires.

But: autonomy must not be allowed to become complacency or smug self-assurance; autonomy must be coupled with a due sense of humility.

5. The physician must have the kind of detailed knowledge which often requires specialized education.

But: he must not become a narrowly specialized man; he should be a well-rounded and broadly-educated man.

6. The physician should have a strong moral character with abiding commitments to basic moral values.

But: he must avoid passing moral judgments on patients.

7. The physician should attach great value to doing what he

can to advance medical knowledge; such accomplishments deserve full recognition.

But: he should not express a competitive spirit toward his fellows.

VALUES GOVERNING THE PHYSICIAN-PATIENT RELATIONSHIP

8.   The physician must be emotionally detached in his attitudes toward patients, keeping "his emotions on ice" and not becoming "overly identified" with patients.

But: he must avoid becoming callous through excessive detachment, and should have compassionate concern for the patient.

9.   The physician must not prefer one type of patient over another, and must curb hostilities toward patients (even those who prove to be uncooperative or who do not respond to his therapeutic efforts).

But: the most rewarding experience for the physician is the effective solution of a patient's health problems.

10.   The physician must gain and maintain the confidence of the patient.

But: he must avoid the mere bedside manner which can quickly degenerate into expedient and self-interested salesmanship.

11.   The physician must recognize that diagnosis is often provisional.

But: he must have the merited confidence of the patient who wants "to know what is *really* wrong" with him.

12.   The physician must provide adequate and unhurried medical care for each patient.

But: he should not allow any patient to usurp so much of his limited time as to have this be at the expense of other patients.

13.   The physician should come to know patients as persons and give substantial attention to their psychological and social circumstances.

But: this too should not be so time consuming a matter as to interfere with the provision of suitable care for other patients.

14.   The physician should institute all the scientific tests needed to reach a sound diagnosis.

But: he should be discriminating in the use of these tests, since these are often costly and may impose a sizable financial burden on patients.

15.   The physician has a right to expect a "reasonable fee," depending upon the care he has given and the economic circumstances of the patient.

But: he must not "soak the rich" in order to "provide for the poor."

16.   The physician should see to it that medical care is available for his patients whenever it is required.

But: he, too, has a right to a "normal life" which he shares with his family.

VALUES GOVERNING THE RELATION TO COLLEAGUES AND THE COMMUNITY

17.   The physician must respect the reputation of his colleagues, not holding them up to obloquy or ridicule before associates or patients.

But: he is obligated to see to it that high standards of practice are maintained by others in the profession as well as by himself.

18.   The physician must collaborate with others of the medical team rather than dominate them (nurses, social workers, technicians).

But: he has final responsibility for the team and must see to it that his associates meet high standards.

19.   The physician should call in consultants, whenever needed.

But: he should be persuaded that these are really required, and not add unnecessarily to the costs of medical care.

20.   The physician, as a responsible professional man, should take due part in the civic life of his community.

But: he should not get involved in political squabbles or spend too much time in activities unrelated to his profession.

21.   The physician must do all he can to prevent, and not only to help cure, illness.

But: society more largely rewards medical men for the therapy they effect as practitioners and only secondarily rewards those engaged in the prevention of illness, particularly since prevention is not as readily visible to patients who do not know that they remain healthy because of preventive measures.

The list of values and norms is of course far from exhaustive, but it may be sufficient to illustrate the principal point. It is not that each pair of values, or of a value and a practical exigency, are necessarily at odds; they are only potentially so. The ability to blend these potential opposites into a stable pattern of professional behavior must be learned and it seems from the data in hand that this is one of the most difficult tasks confronting the medical student.

Contrary to widespread opinion, the effective acquisition of these values by medical students is not a matter only of "medical ethics," which attaches significance to these values in their own right. They can also be considered, quite neutrally and without reference to their undoubted ethical status, in terms of their instrumental significance for the effective provision of health care. They are not necessarily absolute values, prized for their own sake; they are, presumably, values which serve as effective means to a socially important end. Just as cognitive standards of knowledge and skill in medicine have a manifest function in facilitating sound medical practice, so the moral standards have the same, though often less readily recognized, function. In other words, we are concerned here with the sociological rather than the ethical examination of the role of values in the professionalization of the medical student.

As centers of research, medical schools put students more fully in touch with the frontiers of medical knowledge than many, if not most, of them are apt to be in their later years of practice. This is widely recognized. What seems to have received less notice is the correlative fact that medical students are also being systematically exposed to professional values and norms which are probably "higher"—that is, more exacting and rigorously disinterested—than those found in the run of medical practice.[69] Medical schools are socially defined as the guardians of these values and norms. The schools thus have the double function of transmitting to students the *cognitive* standards of knowledge and skill

[69] This is, of course, only the statement of an impression, but one which has often been reported within the medical profession. It must remain an impression merely until there are systematic comparisons of practice in medical schools and among medical practitioners at large.

and the *moral* standards of values and norms. Both sets of standards are essential to the proficient practice of medicine.

The functional significance of these values and norms is greatly reinforced by the social organization of medical practice. Students may be imbued with values and standards which can be more or less readily lived up to in the special environment of the teaching hospital, where the "right way of doing things" is strongly supported by precept, example, and recognition. But once they have entered upon their own practice, some of these physicians will find themselves working under conditions which are far less conducive to ready conformity with these norms. Many of them will be independent practitioners, in a situation structurally different from that of the medical school. There, students and faculty alike are, in effect, under the continued scrutiny of other medical experts, who set great store by critical appraisal of what is being done. This need not be wholly a matter of plan or of acknowledgement, but the structural pattern is so plain as to be generally acknowledged: peers and superiors in the teaching hospital continually serve in what amounts to the role of monitors of medical practice.[70]

In contrast, the physician in his private office is largely subject to the controls only of the values and norms he has acquired and made his own. The medically uninformed patient is not in a position to pass sound judgment upon the normative adequacy of what the physician does. Medically informed colleagues are not in a position to know what is being done. These structural facts, therefore, put a special premium on having these values and norms instilled in the student during the course of professional

[70] The general matter of varying organizational bases for the "observability" of role performance is basic to an understanding of social structure. Some organizations—the medical school and hospital are cases in point—are so arranged that, apart from intent, the behavior of each member is largely subject to observability by others, with continuing appraisals of that behavior. Other structures—and much of private medical practice is a case in point—are such that there is relatively little visibility of this kind. Sociologically, this is a variable of social structure, independent of the further fact that individuals may be motivated to conform with the requirements of a social role, even when they are structurally insulated from direct observation and appraisal. On the concept of observability, see R. K. Merton, *Social Theory and Social Structure* (Glencoe, Ill.: The Free Press, 1957, rev. ed.), Ch. IX.

socialization in the medical school. If this is not thoroughly achieved under the optimum conditions provided by the medical school, it is unlikely that it will occur under the often less favorable circumstances of private practice.

Further reinforcing the functional significance of value-assimilation for effective medical practice is the sociological fact—known and experienced by physicians everywhere—that the expectations of some patients may in effect invite physicians to depart from the standards of good medical care. After all, the sick person does not necessarily live up to the strict etymology of the word "patient." He is not necessarily long-suffering and forbearing, or "calmly expectant, quietly awaiting the course of events." On the contrary, the etymology of the term and the psychology of the patient are often poles apart.

Suffering people are disposed to want a nostrum, in the realm of health as in the realms of politics and, sometimes, of religion. It requires cultural training in self-discipline to accept the fact, when it is a fact, that a prompt solution to one's troubles is not possible. Not all cultures and societies provide that training. That is one reason why magical beliefs and practices flourish. When sick people have not formed the disciplined attitudes required by the social role of the patient, they may unwittingly exert considerable psychological pressure upon the physician to promise more than he responsibly should promise or even to engage in what one practitioner describes as "senseless and reprehensible treatment." Many patients will thus insist on being relieved of suffering, as soon as possible, and preferably immediately. They urge the physician to do, not as he ought, but as they would have him do. In time, some physicians finds themselves motivated to acquiesce in the expectations of patients who, having made a firm self-diagnosis, insist on one or another type of treatment. As one troubled practitioner put his dilemma, "If I don't do the operation she wants, it would not be [only] a matter of losing her, but all she might refer."[71]

Since numerous kinds of pressures may be exerted upon private practitioners to depart from what they know to be the most

[71] W. R. Cooke, "The Practical Application of Psychology in Gynecic Practice," *Nebraska Medical Journal*, 25:371, December 1950.

appropriate kind of medical care, it becomes functionally imperative that they acquire, in medical school, those values and norms which will make them less vulnerable to such deviations. It is in this direct sociological sense that the acquisition of appropriate attitudes and values is as central as the acquisition of knowledge and skills to training for the provision of satisfactory medical care.

George G. Reader, M.D.

THE CORNELL COMPREHENSIVE
CARE AND TEACHING PROGRAM

ORIGIN AND PLAN

Comprehensive medical care has been defined as the preservation of health and the prevention as well as the cure of disease.[1] It means medical supervision which is sufficiently thorough and which continues sufficiently long to bring the patient through convalescence and rehabilitation to an optimal state of health and productivity. Because of the difficulties of coordinating all the diverse elements necessary for accurate diagnosis and proper treatment, comprehensive care for more than an occasional patient is an ideal that is rarely achieved. It was with the hope that more patients might receive optimal care and that senior medical students might learn better how to give it that Cornell University Medical College and the New York Hospital established the Comprehensive Care and Teaching Program in July of 1951.

Much thought and planning preceded the initiation of the Program, a large number of people over many years contributing to the ideas that eventually were incorporated into it. For example, Dr. David Barr, Professor of Medicine at Cornell and Physician-in-Chief of the New York Hospital, wrote in 1946:

> If experiments are to be devised to indicate future trends in the practice of medicine as well as to meet popular demand, they should

[1] George G. Reader, "Comprehensive Medical Care." *J. Med. Educ.*, 28:34, July 1953.

be so arranged as to offer comprehensive care, including health supervision and preventive as well as curative treatment. Segmental care as represented by diagnostic clinics or clinics for case-finding in a special disease will not suffice. The discontinuous care and patchwork now represented by hospitalization without adequate follow-up will furnish only a partial solution. Treatment should be focused not only on the care of the acutely ill or injured person, but should also include management of convalescence and rehabilitation.[2]

And Dr. Connie Guion, Director of the General Medical Clinic of the New York Hospital and Professor of Clinical Medicine at Cornell, became even more specific in an address in 1951:

I suggest that we set up a clinic, not a medical clinic and not a surgical clinic but a clinic in which the patient whom we accept would be assigned to a member of the staff and a student, who would serve together as the family physician. They would take a careful history, perform a complete physical examination and order the laboratory work indicated. When the survey was finished they would call any consultant required to make a final diagnosis and outline the treatment needed. Hospitalization would be recommended only when ambulant care was not possible. In case of hospitalization, the family "student doctor" would be required to follow the case to its conclusion. In case ambulant care was not wise and hospitalization unnecessary, provision for home care would be made.[3]

Since hospitalization for most people is only an incident, albeit a major one, in the course of an illness, ambulatory patients are usually the most appropriate subjects for the teaching of comprehensive patient care. The proper locus of patient-care teaching in the hospital, therefore, is the outpatient department. But here a difficulty is found in the lower standards of performance compared with those of the hospital wards.

Originally hospitals merely provided a place where the sick person could lie down and have shelter and food; but with the gradual evolution of medicine, hospital bed patients began to serve as convenient subjects for scientific study and observation. Dispensaries, on the other hand, which were at first stations separate from the hospitals where the sick poor could receive symptomatic treatment, have tended to remain much the same when

[2] David P. Barr, "The Next Ten Years in Medicine." *New York Med.*, 2:14, July 1946.

[3] Connie M. Guion, "Medicine on the Wing." *Cornell Univ. Med. Coll. Alumni Quarterly*, May 1951.

later joined to them. Care of ambulatory patients has remained for the most part discontinuous and symptomatic, the greater effort being expended on the bed patient. Younger and less well-qualified members of a hospital staff are traditionally assigned to the outpatient service, where they may labor for years before being permitted to attend on the wards. Opportunity to participate in the care of bed patients is the sought-after prize. Physicians devoting full time to study of ambulatory patients and to teaching the care of them have been a rarity, and the busy practitioners who usually provide the required services are invariably faced with hordes of patients whose needs greatly exceed the time available to them.

There are notable exceptions to this, of course, and expert clinical investigation has been done in some hospitals on selected groups of ambulant patients. Great diagnostic and treatment centers, such as the Mayo Clinic, have grown up; and these provide excellent short-term care. But even in many of the major teaching hospitals with the best outpatient services, the care of the ambulant patient is still much inferior to that of the bed patient.

At the New York Hospital–Cornell Medical Center, the Out-Patient Department has long been devoted to high standards of patient care and has provided a peculiarly fertile soil for the growth of the comprehensive ideal. Since 1946, a pilot clinic for broader medical service has been an active section of the Medical Out-Patient Department.[4] Developed with the support of the Commonwealth Fund, it has aimed at training young internists for clinical service, teaching, and research that would take account of the patient's life situation.[5] Toward a similar end, Dr. Samuel Levine, Professor of Pediatrics and Pediatrician-in-Chief, has for many years carried on a highly successful graduate training program for pediatricians in the Pediatric Out-Patient Department.[6]

In spite of the excellence of the New York Hospital Out-Patient Department service, certain deficiencies were apparent, especially

[4] Under the direction of Harold G. Wolff, M.D., Stewart G. Wolf, M.D., and William J. Grace, M.D.

[5] *The Commonwealth Fund Annual Report, 1949* (New York: The Commonwealth Fund, 1949), p. 4.

[6] Barbara M. Korsch and Samuel Z. Levine, "Graduate Teaching of Pediatricians in a Children's Outpatient Department." *Pediatrics, 14*:171, August 1954.

when ambulatory service was contrasted with patient care on the wards. Follow-up of patients in most clinics was discontinuous; patients would often be seen by different physicians on each visit and rarely would there be time for careful re-evaluation. Treatment, accordingly, tended to be a patchwork even when diagnostic study was thorough and painstaking. Because of the absence of full-time physicians, supervision was necessarily lacking, in contrast to the ward where the interns' work traditionally was checked by the assistant resident and his in turn by residents and attending physicians. Furthermore, consultants from other specialties were not readily available in the clinics, and a patient might have to attend several different ones in order for his problems to receive proper consideration. The patient load in the clinic was difficult to control, too, because of the press of urgent patients, so that the appointment system was regularly disrupted.

Students working with ambulant patients obtained experience primarily in the technique of the history and physical examination and learned something of the attitudes and points of view of a variety of practicing specialists. Each patient contact usually represented merely another demonstration of a clinical entity or disordered portion of the anatomy. During his fourth year at Cornell the student would spend two months in the medical clinics, and for another period of four months would divide his time between pediatric and psychiatric clinics and part-time electives. The remainder of his last year he spent in an inpatient clerkship in Surgery, a combined inpatient-outpatient clerkship in Obstetrics and Gynecology, and in two months of elective work. Little continuity in contact with patients was possible, and the student rarely had the opportunity to check the correctness of his diagnoses or to observe the success or failure of a plan of treatment. There was little chance of his becoming systematically concerned with the total life problems of the patient.

Formulation of Aims

Changes in organization of patient care at the New York Hospital appeared necessary; but before recommending any, those[7] charged

[7] George G. Reader, M.D., George A. Wolf, M.D., Barbara Korsch, M.D., and others.

with planning for more comprehensive patient care set down a list of principles:

1. On each hospital visit the ambulant patient should come to the same familiar place and see the same familiar and friendly faces.
2. The same physician should see the patient at every visit and by appointment.
3. All patients should be considered as candidates for total care, including attention to social and emotional needs.
4. Patients should be seen as part of a family constellation, with well members of the family receiving preventive care as far as that is possible.
5. Hospital services should be extended into the home when appropriate, not only so that the patient's environment may be better visualized but also that hospital beds may be saved for the more acutely ill.[8]

Likewise, before altering the teaching program, a statement entitled "Aims and Methods of Clinical Teaching at Cornell University Medical College: A Consensus,"[9] was formulated as a result of discussion with a large number of clinical teachers.

Although details of the changes finally made and the steps involved have been described in previous publications,[10, 11] it seems appropriate to reiterate here the measures applied and describe how they implement the broad objectives of teaching comprehensive medicine.

Specification of Plans in Terms of Objectives

Continuity of care is a cardinal principle of comprehensive care; and in order to obtain it for the student without disrupting his experience in Surgery and Obstetrics, the periods in Medicine, Pediatrics, and Psychiatry were combined. This allows the student two clinic sessions a week in the Medical Clinic for 22 weeks and two sessions a week in Pediatrics and Psychiatry for 11 weeks each. He thus follows his patient over a number of months,[12] dur-

[8] George G. Reader, "Organization and Development of a Comprehensive Care Program." *Amer. J. of Public Health*, 44:760, June 1954.

[9] George G. Reader, "Aims and Methods of Clinical Teaching at Cornell Medical College: A Consensus." *J. Med. Educ.*, 30:466, August 1955.

[10] George G. Reader, "Comprehensive Medical Care," *loc. cit.*

[11] George G. Reader, "Organization and Development of a Comprehensive Care Program," *loc. cit.*

[12] See Margaret Olencki, "Range of Patient Contacts in the Comprehensive Care and Teaching Program," in this volume, pp. 273–276.

ing which hospitalization may represent one episode in the illness. As the patient periodically revisits his student–physician, the latter inevitably becomes concerned with some of the patient's life problems and begins to see them in proper perspective.

Breadth of experience with large numbers of patients having a variety of problems is another objective of the Program.[13] In addition to patients in the Medical and Pediatric Clinics, those in a number of different specialty clinics are made available to each student on an elective basis. Provision is also made for selected patients to be given family care and home care, the essentials of which will be presently described (see page 89).

Discrimination in the application of therapeutic measures is as important as continuity of care. Some patients are not ready to accept all forms of available assistance and must be brought to an understanding of the usefulness of the help that is offered. Others may be so demanding as to make it impossible to fulfill completely what they feel to be their needs. How much to try to do, how fast to try to go, must be determined for each patient. This the student can learn only through regular contact with the same patient over several weeks or months.

Coordination of personnel and facilities in the interest of the patient is necessary if comprehensive care is to be delivered efficiently. This means that time and effort must be allocated to administration and planning, with appropriate delegation of responsibility within the group involved in patient care. The team of doctor, nurse, and social worker is the basic unit for providing comprehensive care and in the Comprehensive Care and Teaching Program, a medical student, student nurse, and social worker work together with the patient. Physicians, specialists, staff nurses, administrators, and casework supervisors are all available to contribute their knowledge and skills as needed to the members of the basic team.

The physician is legally and otherwise responsible for directing the care of the patient. As the director of a symphony orchestra may call upon a violinist for a solo, however, so may the physician yield the stage to the social worker, nurse, or other specialist at some phase of the patient's course. Like the conductor, the physi-

[13] See *ibid.*, pp. 276–279 and Table 31.

cian must know the potentialities of each performer even though he himself may not play all the instruments. If mutual respect and understanding are present among the members of the group giving patient care, it matters little who is taking the lead at any given time. But if these are lacking or if the physician fails to learn how to call on all those who can help him, comprehensive patient care is impossible.

Quick and accurate communication is essential to coordinated effort, for much information must be transmitted, not only to make possible proper operating decisions, but also to allow common values and ideals to be formulated by the group as a whole. Accordingly, daily meetings on individual patients may be necessary. For this purpose the student schedule is kept as flexible as possible, responsibility for patients being considered to have priority over all other assignments. Regular conferences about patients are held twice a week. One is an informal discussion of management problems by students and staff; the other, the Comprehensive Care Conference, a formal presentation by one student and discussion, often by several experts, of a patient illustrating some principle of management. In addition, there are staff meetings each week to consider intake of Family Care and Home Care patients and to supervise patient care through chart review. Each Wednesday, at a luncheon meeting, student representatives and staff members consider together common problems of teaching and administration. Monthly meetings for instructors and staff allow for regular review and further planning. An Advisory Committee composed of all clinical department heads, the professor of preventive medicine, director of social service, superintendent of the hospital, deans of the medical and nursing schools, and director of the Center meets semiannually to hear reports and consider policy, but in the interim, staff members communicate informally as necessary with their own chiefs, all of whom are represented on the Advisory Committee.

Responsibility for patients is the most effective way for the student to learn wisdom in patient management and gain the ability to think through a clinical problem. It also motivates him to read about the clinical entities he encounters so that he may better help the patient, thus stimulating more intensive study of scientific medicine. The length of the student's contact with the same patients is believed to be the most important determinant of development of a sense of responsibility;[14] but his professional sense can also be enhanced by the way he is treated by instructors and other clinic personnel. In the Comprehensive Care and Teaching Program it is a matter of policy to address the student as "Doctor" and to consider him as a junior colleague of the staff physicians. In the directions for the Course in Comprehensive Medicine there is the statement:

> Relationship of instructor to student will be analogous to that of consultant to physician, although for legal reasons, the instructor must take ultimate responsibility for patient management and must countersign all student notes on the chart.[15]

Time for proper contemplation of the patient's needs, for review of problems with instructors and for study of the literature is essential to a proper atmosphere in which to learn. In the Comprehensive Care and Teaching Program the disruptive effect of patients who have medically urgent problems is countered by assigning one physician to deal with them. He provides care appropriate to their present complaint and refers them for more complete study at a later date. The appointment system is thus protected without endangering the patient through delay.

Furthermore, each student examines a new patient at every clinic session[16] unless he is scheduled to see more than two revisit patients. In this way he is assured of sufficient time for discussion with his instructors if he is a reasonably efficient worker. He can also block off extra time for special consideration of more complex problems if that is necessary. Two mornings or afternoons a week, in addition to regular clinic assignments, are free for study, library work, or seeing patients. The preceptor for each group of ten students also uses this time for seminars on subjects of particular interest to his student group.

Enough personnel—doctors, nurses, social workers, and others—to provide effective service and to have sufficient time over for teaching is also essential to avoid the superficiality induced by

[14] See *ibid.*, Table 30 and discussion pp. 274–275.

[15] Mimeographed instructions to students, "Course in Comprehensive Medicine."

[16] See Margaret Olencki, *op. cit.*, Table 29.

haste. Four full-time internists have supplemented the part-time teachers in the Medical Clinic who carry the major day-to-day responsibility for supervising students; and two full-time pediatricians have served similarly in the Pediatric Clinic. Every effort is made to maintain a one-to-one ratio of teachers to students each clinic session. A social worker and a public health nurse are available full-time for teaching and coordinating patient care activities; and consultants in Surgery, Obstetrics and Gynecology, Psychiatry and Rehabilitation are also available when required.[17]

Family care implies that one physician provides medical services to several members of a family. He is thus better able to appreciate the impact of one member's illness on the rest of the family and to understand how family relationships affect the onset and course of disease. At Cornell, the students see a large proportion of the patients who go through the General Medical and General Pediatric Clinics,[18] and there is some danger that the ideals of comprehensive medicine may be seriously diluted by the press of large numbers. Hence, patients are selected for Family Care partly to serve as models for more complete care. As the student takes on more members of the family as patients and really begins to function as a family physician, he then learns something of the particular advantages of this kind of relationship. For this purpose, each student is assigned at least one family to care for during the semester.

Home care of patients is an integral part of comprehensive care, since patients may be ill at home and unable to come to the doctor. If continuity is to be maintained, the possibility of visiting the patient at home is as important as following him in the hospital ward or clinic. Furthermore, home care introduces the physician or student to the complexities of the patient's usual environment. It places the hospital in proper perspective, as one of a number of available therapeutic modalities. At one time a patient may require hospital care, and at another time home care may be more appropriate. A patient with a fatal illness may wish to die at home, and if the hospital offers no special hope, that wish should be respected. Comforting the family, preparing them for inevita-

[17] See *ibid.*, Table 32.
[18] See *ibid.*, pp. 277–278.

ble loss, and supporting them at the time it happens constitute an important learning experience. The aim of Home Care in the Comprehensive Care and Teaching Program is to give each student at least one patient to care for at home in either an acute or chronic illness, or terminally. Thus far home care has been provided to a wide range of patients and for periods varying from a few visits to months of continuous care.

Teaching of Comprehensive Care has not been without its problems.[19] Aside from the considerable amount of administrative effort required to achieve coordination and keep the activities of the Program moving toward their assigned goals, the students have at times perceived this learning experience as a discontinuity in their preparation for internships, where a higher value is often placed on straight academic knowledge than on the doctor–patient relationship that is required in practice on ambulatory patients. It has been necessary to modify teaching plans from time to time to relieve students' tensions and to support them through the frustrations which a broad view of patient problems may sometimes induce. An important by-product of social science research for purposes of evaluation has been the help it has provided in indicating the need for changes, as will be noted later (page 99).

HISTORY OF THE EVALUATION RESEARCH[20]

The Comprehensive Care and Teaching Program was designated as an experiment in medical education when planning first began:

> The enterprise as outlined must be regarded as an experiment in medical education. No one can say as yet how much of the concept of comprehensive medicine and of preventive medicine for the individual and his family is practically attainable or economically feasible. It is, however, only by trial that these questions can be answered.[21]

Those planning for the teaching of comprehensive medical care at Cornell therefore took into account the possibilities of docu-

[19] George G. Reader, "Some of the Problems and Satisfactions of Teaching Comprehensive Medicine." *J. Med. Educ.*, 31:544–552, 1956.

[20] This section was written in collaboration with Mary E. W. Goss, who was assigned the responsibility for developing the original version of the attitude questionnaire used in the research.

[21] David P. Barr, "The Teaching of Preventive Medicine." *J. Med. Educ.*, 28:49, March 1953.

menting changes brought about by the new program and of testing the hypothesis that students can learn more complete patient management without sacrificing their understanding of scientific medicine.

Several purposes might be served by studying objectively the extent to which anticipated results had been achieved. First, the Program could be improved as a result of information thus obtained. In point of fact, the responses of the students revealed by the research were cause for encouragement but at the same time served as a warning to the teaching staff of the difficulties of altering the students' ideas in the desired direction. Second, other medical educators might find the observations illuminating. Visitors from all over the world come to observe the Program, and nearly all have expressed some interest in objective appraisal of the methods used. And third, techniques might be developed that would measure attributes of the young physician associated with the art, and not only the science, of medicine. For it was clear to the planners of the Comprehensive Care and Teaching Program that little alteration in acquisition of traditional factual knowledge was to be expected or intended.

In 1950, before the Program was initiated, an identical final examination in medicine of objective type was administered to the third- and fourth-year students. The distribution curves of grades could almost be superimposed. In fact, a number of third-year students ranked higher than the highest fourth-year students. This was taken as suggestive, although not conclusive, evidence that students during the fourth year probably did not much increase their factual knowledge. Their instructors were certain, however, that they matured significantly. The objective type of examination on factual material simply did not measure what kind of learning had taken place.

Furthermore, in reviewing the fundamental purposes of medical education in the course of planning the Comprehensive Care and Teaching Program, it became evident that acquisition of facts is only a part of the medical student's job; the development of appropriate values and attitudes is also necessary. Accordingly, the curricular change itself was specifically designed to provide not only for more effective mastery of medical knowledge but also, as previously indicated, an environment where the growth of attitudes and values appropriate to a good physician might best be promoted.

Once it became evident that changes in attitudes and values were important elements to measure, considerable effort was still required to find investigators skilled in the use of suitable techniques. A large number of psychologists, sociologists, and educators were queried unsuccessfully before it was learned that the Bureau of Applied Social Research of Columbia University was suitably equipped to consult in setting up the experiment. The Bureau had developed, to a high degree of quality and effectiveness, the study of attitude change in response to mass communications media and in other situations, and it seemed possible that these techniques could be applied to the educational process. More important was the interest of sociologists at Columbia concerned with the study of the professions, who looked upon the collaborative effort as an opportunity to use the Comprehensive Care and Teaching Program and Cornell Medical College as a laboratory in which observations on the development of the medical man might be made. This would be no mere service, then, but a joint research effort to solve fundamental problems of importance to both medical education and sociology.

Accordingly, in March 1952 Professor Merton of the Bureau arranged for several sociologists to begin an intensive study of the Comprehensive Care and Teaching Program. At the outset it was apparent that the greatest benefits to medical education and sociology might be in terms of broad insights into the forces molding the young physician rather than as a specific record of the exact causes of opinion change occasioned by various aspects of the Comprehensive Care and Teaching Program.

> To view the educational process in its entirety one must study the student as a whole just as the doctor must study the patient as a whole. . . . In certain respects, the training of a physician is an evolutionary procedure during the course of which the student passes from a lay to a professional person. An illumination of the factors or forces that are involved in this process is basic educational research. Such research is a prerequisite for the understanding of the effectiveness of any particular educational innovation.[22]

[22] *The Commonwealth Fund Annual Report, 1954* (New York: The Commonwealth Fund, 1954), p. 13.

Philosophy of the Research

The study group set itself to identify the relevant aspects of the medical educational experience in the light of the interests and ideals of the medical faculty at Cornell, where, as has been noted, the patient as a person is considered the appropriate focus of medical care and teaching. Also, the student is recognized as coequal in many respects with the teacher in the learning process, and medical education itself is looked upon as a matter of providing opportunities for mature young adults to learn rather than as merely a drill in medical knowledge. The investigators directed their attention particularly to the acquisition by students of the attitudes of mature medical practitioners and of the behavior which exemplifies these attitudes. This required investigation of the objectives of medical training specific enough to allow construction of hypotheses that might be tested. In the present state of knowledge of the ideal in the art of medicine, research in this field is extraordinarily difficult and in part must be empirical.

Friendly critics and the investigators themselves have voiced certain reservations about educational research many times. It is well known, for example, that any change in routine may result in greater interest and productivity by the subjects, as in the famous Hawthorne[23] experiments which showed that in the context of focused experimentation on a small group of workers a return to the original conditions increased their productivity as much as any of the innovations. Analogously, medical students participating in a curricular change may react to the teachers' enthusiasm or to the mere deviation from traditional routine itself.

Another fundamental question is whether any rearrangement of courses or teaching exercises is as important as the quality of the teachers involved. It is argued that good teachers are the only important elements in the learning situation. This seems a narrow view of a complex process, but is a question that must be answered, nonetheless. Fortunately there are indications that carrying investigation of the medical education process far enough will help to clarify both these questions. Further, even though it may not be possible to relate curriculum changes to development of specific

[23] T. N. Whitehead, *The Industrial Worker* (Cambridge, Mass.: Harvard University Press, 1938).

attitudes in students, enough information should become available about medical education to make planning for it a somewhat more rational procedure.

Methods

No single research technique or instrument can be expected to yield data relevant to all aspects of a potentially far-reaching educational experience. For example, it was recognized that a standard form filled out daily by students might constitute an appropriate approach to documentation of certain portions of students' clinical experience—such as number of patients seen, types of disease entities observed, number of revisits, and number of consultations and conferences. But such a day-to-day approach would be unsuitable for acquiring information concerning the long-term development of students' attitudes toward patients. Likewise, personal interviews could produce valuable data regarding the extent of students' ability to verbalize the ideals of comprehensive care. But if the actual behavior of student–physicians with patients in the examining room were the center of inquiry, interviewing techniques would be less useful than direct observation of student–patient relationships.

In planning the study of possible effects of the Comprehensive Care and Teaching Program these considerations were taken into account. Before specific research techniques were adopted, tentative decisions were made regarding the focus of the initial exploratory study. When the research group was ready to begin its study there were only a few weeks remaining before the beginning of the academic year and of the new teaching program. In this experiment controls are difficult to apply and it was of urgent importance to obtain an estimate of students' attitudes before they entered the Program so that at least a before-and-after comparison would be possible. For that reason priority was assigned to investigation of the Program's potential impact on students' attitudes and standards relevant to the provision of patient care that would serve as a baseline for further studies. This was to be accompanied by the collection of basic factual data concerning the range and depth of students' clinical experience while in the Program.

Once these broad decisions were made, it became apparent that thorough study of such matters would require considerable time and effort. For, though the main objectives of the research were clear, virtually no standardized tools for acquiring the desired information existed. There were available no already-prepared questionnaires, interview schedules, or observation forms which were appropriate for dealing with the problems which had been posed. Thus it was necessary to construct some quickly so that data collection could begin. Moreover, in addition to improving the tools and methods utilized in gathering information, experience in comparable studies had shown that not a little time would be required for processing and interpreting the findings.

Before describing instruments and methods in detail, an important fact concerning the whole research effort should be emphasized. In this trial phase of the endeavor, none of the data gathered served as a basis for grading students. Thus traditional means of evaluating individual students' progress were maintained. Formal examinations on subject matter and careful faculty observation of students' performance in the clinics remained the basis for grading.

Bearing these considerations in mind, the Program administrators, in collaboration with investigators from the Bureau at Columbia, delineated a concrete—though tentative—research plan. Within the framework of a semiexperimental design, this plan entailed the repeated use of a questionnaire for study of the possible impact of the Comprehensive Care experience upon students' attitudes. It also called for the development of behavior-reporting forms which would furnish both qualitative and quantitative evidence of the nature of students' clinical activities while enrolled in the Course in Comprehensive Medicine. Finally, in order to aid in the construction and interpretation of such forms, as well as to serve as an independent source of information, a staff member of the Bureau was assigned to observe Program events as they occurred.[24]

The Questionnaire

Attitudes are probably best determined by a skilled interviewer, but this method is not easily applicable to large numbers of peo-

---

[24] For a report on some findings growing out of these observations, see Mary E. W. Goss, "Change in the Cornell Comprehensive Care and Teaching Program," in this volume, p. 249 ff.

ple. A self-administered questionnaire was, therefore, the instrument of choice in attempting to document students' attitudes and values.

Construction of questions was accomplished by obtaining suggestions from various interested faculty members as well as by formulating, with the help of the Comprehensive Care and Teaching Program staff, questions that would touch specifically on objectives of the Program. Sociologists interested in the process of professional education, as well as written materials dealing with the aims and methods of medical education, were also consulted. These questions were then incorporated into an interview guide and pretested with ten fourth-year students. Interviews were tape-recorded, transcribed, and analyzed to determine the potential usefulness of the questions employed. Those items which survived this examination, as well as others which emerged from the interview, were then included in the questionnaire.

The questionnaire itself was pretested with several staff members before administration to students. Nevertheless, as the questionnaire was put into use, some items turned out to be ambiguously worded, non-discriminating, or otherwise difficult to interpret. Such questions were dropped or revised. Further, as initial omissions became apparent, new items were added to subsequent versions. A substantial number of items were, however, retained in their initial form.

The questionnaire contained items dealing with students' orientation toward patients, their conceptions of the nature of adequate medical care, their opinions of the value of training in comprehensive care (based first upon what they had heard about it, and later upon their actual experiences in the Program), and various background characteristics such as age, college attended, and marital status.

In order to know whether participation in the Comprehensive Care and Teaching Program had an impact upon students' attitudes and standards, a before-and-after research model was employed, as previously noted. Specifically, all fourth-year students in the class of 1953 were asked to fill out essentially similar versions of the specially designed questionnaire three times during the course of the year. As Figure 1 shows, the first time oc-

FIGURE 1. Time Sequence of Questionnaire Administration in Relationship to Courses Taken by Fourth-Year Students

	GROUP A (43 Students)	GROUP B (41 Students)
May 1952	QUESTIONNAIRE	
	Course in Comprehensive Medicine	Courses in Surgery, Obstetrics and Gynecology, and Elective
December 1952	QUESTIONNAIRE	
	Courses in Surgery, Obstetrics and Gynecology, and Elective	Course in Comprehensive Medicine
May 1953	QUESTIONNAIRE	

curred in May 1952, at the end of the students' third year, when no member of the class had yet taken part in the Program. The second administration of the questionnaire took place in the middle of the students' fourth year, December 1952, when half of the class had just finished the course and the other half was just beginning it. Finally, in May 1953, when the entire class had been exposed to the Program, the questionnaire was administered to the group for the last time.[25]

The May 1952 answers serve as a baseline against which later expressions of attitude can be compared to see if change or development have taken place. Replies to the December questionnaires, when considered in conjunction with the first set, allow comparison of the development of students who were "exposed" (Group A) to the Program with that of students who were "un-

[25] As indicated in the foregoing paper, this process of asking the same group of people the same questions at different crucial points in time is known in social research as the *panel* method. It is particularly suited to the study of changes in attitudes and opinions because, among other things, it does not rely on the sometimes faulty memory of respondents concerning whether or not they have changed. Rather, it enables change or stability to be objectively ascertained by comparison of answers given by the same individuals at selected time intervals. For a complete outline and time schedule of questionnaire waves thus far collected in the three medical schools under study, see Appendix D of this volume.

exposed" (Group B).[26] And the third set—May 1953—permits another kind of "exposed-unexposed" comparison: between the attitudes expressed by the entire class of 1953, all of whom had the
course, and the class of 1952, none of whom had the course. (Although not noted in Figure 1, the class of 1952 filled out questionnaires once, just prior to graduation in 1952, on the basis of their
experience in the traditional curriculum.)

Students took between forty-five minutes and an hour and a
half to complete the questionnaire. Although a small minority
obviously resented the task, this group was outnumbered by another which enthusiastically welcomed the opportunity to express
personal opinions and beliefs. The majority of students seemed
willing to cooperate. This impression is borne out by the very low
proportion of "flip" answers which they gave, as well as by the
generally low percentage of unanswered questions. Since the individual identities of students were kept confidential by the Bureau, such facts suggest not only willingness, but seriousness of
purpose as well.

Other Methods of Inquiry

As has been noted, other methods of investigation in addition to
the questionnaire were employed. These have included, to date,
a study of the operation of the Comprehensive Care and Teaching Program, participant observation of the students' experience
with the Program, a systematic assay of faculty opinion to determine the intellectual and attitudinal climate in which learning
takes place, an investigation of experience in the first three years
of medical school by means of the aforementioned questionnaires
and of weekly interviews of student diarists, and a documentation
of daily student activities in the Program through a self-administered report form. Some of these investigations are detailed in
other chapters of this volume.

These various procedures are capable of being woven together

[26] These "exposed" and "unexposed" groups as of December 1952 cannot, un-
fortunately, be considered "experimental" and "control" units, although they represent an approximation thereto. A true control group would have had to consist of
students who were studying fourth-year Medicine, Pediatrics, and Psychiatry under
the old curriculum, simultaneously with a matched experimental group taking the
new course in Comprehensive Medicine.

to provide checks on information from different sources in order to modify and improve the separate techniques. Data from observation of students and from student diarists have been used, for example, to provide new items for the questionnaire. Likewise, questionnaire responses have been tested by observation and reporting of students' daily activities.

The research has been based on the firm belief that proper standards for a good physician, both in terms of appropriate attitudes and in terms of minimal factual knowledge, are at present far from specific and uniformly agreed upon. No one now knows what constitutes a good physician in objective definable terms, and the concept is unlikely to be amenable to explicit definition. More must be learned about the role of the physician in society, the kinds of problems that doctors are called upon to solve, and the varieties of problems that patients present. A second fundamental tenet, as previously noted, is the idea that medical education is not something to be imposed upon students, but requires, rather, an environment that promotes the formation of attitudes most likely to facilitate the student's best use of his professional skills. These beliefs have colored both the administration of the Comprehensive Care and Teaching Program and the studies of its effectiveness.

The very presence of a research orientation causes those medical educators responsible for innovations in the curriculum to state their objectives as clearly as possible, and carrying forward the research necessitates continual redefinition of objectives. In addition, the research has provided the program administrators with data that have improved their ability to make decisions. First, it has provided information not otherwise available on which sounder judgments may be based, as in indicating the value of Family Care for enhancing the comprehensive viewpoint. Second, it has given new insights into ways of solving problems, for example, the way group decisions act in setting and maintaining standards. The medical educators in this way have acquired a certain degree of critical objectivity which has then been applied both to the educational process and to the studies themselves. The sensitization of faculty members to aspects of students' capacity and performance not previously taken into explicit account has been another by-product of the investigations; and as a result, the regular evaluation of students should eventually be placed on a sounder basis.

As the final test of the effectiveness of the training process, students must be followed through their internships and out into practice. This, to be meaningful, may require the use of control groups from other medical schools where no recent changes have been made in the curriculum, and would lead back into studies on medical practice itself. It will then be necessary to know much more than is known at present about standards by which to judge medical practice and medical practitioners in the community at large.

All this has, however, already provided one exceedingly important result: the Comprehensive Care and Teaching Program has become a living experiment.

Data relating to individual students have always remained confidential, but general information from the research has aided the administrators of the program in making their decisions, and various aspects of the program have thus been subject to constant modification. Likewise, the social scientists carrying on the research have been able to communicate directly with the staff members of the Program in order to learn the underlying assumptions on which new plans are based before they are put into effect. The perspective of both medical educators and sociologists has in this way been enlarged so that not only has the training process for physicians been subject to more insightful scrutiny, but also the implications of this training in defining the role of the physician in society have become more apparent. Both staff members and researchers have visualized the Comprehensive Care and Teaching Program against the backdrop of the total process of medical education and at the same time have attempted to relate it to the more pressing problems of medical care on the American scene today.

In planning a teaching program in patient care, various alternatives might be considered. For example, one might be to provide help for the student only as requested—some psychiatric guidance when a patient's emotional life intrudes, a surgeon to advise where to operate and when. Another might be to organize a group of physicians, specialist consultants, nurses, and social workers, who would think through together the best kind of care to give patients. A new set of values and standards would thus arise, borrowing from the several disciplines represented and from the special human values each individual member might contribute. Students would be absorbed into this group and would acquire a new value system along with new knowledge. This latter has been the endeavor of the Comprehensive Care and Teaching Program. Staff members have grown and developed themselves through the group interaction, and a community has been established into which new members are accepted; physicians, patients, students, and others are altered to some degree by the experience and in turn contribute to gradual change in the community itself. A living, growing, corporate organism is thus created which is capable of adapting itself to the requirements of its surroundings and of carrying forward an ever higher and more clearly delineated standard of patient care and of medical teaching.

Part II

Career Decisions

INTRODUCTION

The papers in this section deal with the behavior of prospective physicians (and, by way of comparison, prospective lawyers) as they make certain crucial choices that will affect the character of their professional lives: first, selecting their occupation itself, and, in the last paper, choosing between an internship that will prepare them for one of the medical specialties and an internship that is frequently followed by general practice.

Running through the papers are a number of common themes that stem in large part from previous related research. Of these, the following are perhaps the most significant.

1. An interest in the social and psychological processes of decision-making that are observable in disparate social situations. Despite their differences in certain respects, some of the underlying mechanisms noted in studies of how people decide on what to buy or what candidate to vote for are also noted in the way people choose their occupation or the kind of internship they will pursue.[1] For example, political studies have shown that (voting) intentions are most likely to be carried out if they correspond to the modal

[1] Two recent works provide excellent formulations of the research on decision-making. See Bernard Berelson, Paul F. Lazarsfeld, and William McPhee, *Voting* (Chicago: University of Chicago Press, 1954), especially Chapter 13, for a discussion that is extremely pertinent to career decisions. *Personal Influence*, by Elihu Katz and Paul F. Lazarsfeld (Glencoe, Ill.: The Free Press, 1955) highlights the role of persons in one's immediate environment who may play an important part in shaping decisions.

choice of the social group to which one belongs. Working-class Catholics who state at the beginning of a campaign that they intend to vote for the Democratic candidate are more likely to go through with their plans than persons of like status who have Republican intentions. A similar tendency is discussed by Kendall and Selvin with regard to internship plans among high-ranking and lower-ranking medical students. In both contexts, the major advice-giving agencies appear to provide more social support for modal choices than for "deviant" choices.

2. Comparisons of the way decisions are arrived at in different institutional contexts, e.g., medicine versus law, often shed light on the institutions themselves. For example, prospective law students decide on their professions at a later age and somewhat more tentatively than do medical students. Thielens relates this disparity to the greater difficulty people have in forming a clear idea of what a lawyer does, to the less rigorous academic prerequisites for admission to law school, and to the more widely accepted pattern of studying law but not practicing it.

3. The consequences for the profession of the "sifting and sorting" that stems from these decisions are of especial interest. Kendall and Selvin show, for instance, that Cornell medical students who rank high in academic performance are more likely to select a specialized internship than lower-ranking students. If this tendency applies to other schools as well, it would suggest a concentration of the most able students in the specialties, and higher prestige and other rewards accruing to specialists.

All three papers examine decision-making as a process that may in fact require years for its culmination. The paper by Rogoff, for example, makes the distinction between first arousal of interest in medicine as a career and final commitment to it; the two events may be separated in time by a decade or more. Kendall and Selvin are able to trace individual cases of change in internship intentions, since the same students were asked about their plans and preferences at different stages in their medical training. This method of repeated observations—the panel method—is not only uniquely suited to research on how people make up their minds, but was actually brought to its present stage of development through its application to the study of decision-making.

The data are derived primarily from the questionnaires administered to medical students at various stages of training. Rogoff and Thielens analyze the responses of students who were just about to begin their first-year studies, while Kendall and Selvin report information on students in each of the four years. Techniques of questionnaire construction, administration, processing, and analysis are by now highly standardized and codified, and no attempt will be made here to describe them. Such a statement would inevitably prove cryptic for the non-professional, and superfluous for the social scientist. Some of the standard reference works in this field have been noted previously in this volume.[2]

[2] See footnote 41, page 42.

Natalie Rogoff

THE DECISION TO STUDY MEDICINE

INTRODUCTION

One of the more enduring questions in the sociology of occupations and professions concerns the processes by which persons select a career. When social norms allow relative freedom to choose any occupation, it is a matter of some cogency to discern the prevailing patterns of choice, for these will illuminate questions of occupational recruitment, of social opportunity and mobility, and, more generally, of the relation of the occupational sphere to other parts of the social system (e.g., education, the family, the status order). This paper analyzes the process of choosing a career in medicine in the light of these sociological problems.

At the same time, it should not pass unnoticed that the way in which physicians come to decide on their career has long been a matter of interest to the profession itself. But to judge from the writings on this subject[1] the question doctors put to themselves and their colleagues is *why* they chose medicine. Answers to this type of question do not always prove enlightening. Even those given to introspection and having a good deal of self-awareness are often unable to fathom the reasons or the impulses that led to their choice of a career in medicine. As Brody points out:

[1] See the recent collection, *Why We Became Doctors,* edited by Noah D. Fabricant (New York: Grune and Stratton, 1954), for statements by fifty leading physicians. An excellent review of biographical and autobiographical statements is also given in Irwin Brody, "The Decision to Study Medicine," *New Eng. J. Med.,* 252:130–134, 1955.

Even many of those who claim a special calling confess that they are unable to explain why medicine so powerfully attracted them. . . . No consistent relation seems to hold between youthful predilections and future success in medicine. . . . In striking contrast to a doctor's vivid account of early lack of enthusiasm for medicine his subsequent description of his professional life may be fraught with instances of unsparing devotion to his patients and to his science. . . .[2]

It appears unproductive to look at the type and the strength of motivation leading to the decision as a direct foreshadowing of later professional competence or dedication. One alternative is to consider the manner of choosing the occupation as the earliest instance of "professional behavior" on the part of the prospective physician. Because it is the first, it is likely to be more closely linked with his non-medical status and roles than is subsequent behavior. As the novice moves closer to professional maturity, those links with the extramedical world may become so attenuated as to lose some of their usefulness in predicting the kind of doctor he will be. This points to the advisability of examining the decision process in its own terms—and only thereafter relating the various outcomes of that process to later phases of professional training and practice.

The idea of systematically analyzing occupational choice as a social and psychological *process* was first worked out by Paul F. Lazarsfeld in his *Jugend und Beruf*,[3] a review and critique of European studies on occupational choice. One of the few American studies to take up this lead is reported by Eli Ginzberg and associates in *Occupational Choice*.[4] The present analysis owes much of its form to these inquiries.

The data analyzed here were provided by six successive classes of medical students at the University of Pennsylvania. Three were questioned just prior to their entrance into the school, the others at the start of their second, third, and fourth years. All students (about 750) reported on the more objective facts about their career decision (notably, at what age the decision was made), while those in the entering classes also described their feelings

[2] Brody, *op. cit.*, p. 134.

[3] Paul F. Lazarsfeld, *Jugend und Beruf* (Jena: G. Fischer, 1931).

[4] Eli Ginzberg and associates, *Occupational Choice: An Approach to a General Theory* (New York: Columbia University Press, 1951).

about the medical profession before these attitudes were modified by their experiences in medical training. Even for the latter students, of course, much of the information is retrospective.

Because the data are restricted to medical students, they are not pertinent in inquiries concerning the differences between the process of selecting medicine and of selecting other occupations. And the analysis bears on the steps leading to a *successful* candidacy for admission to medical school, as opposed to an unsuccessful one. On these counts, and because the data are limited to one medical school, the findings cannot be prematurely generalized.

FIRST CONSIDERING A CAREER IN MEDICINE

The first thing to note about the process of deciding to study medicine is the wide variation in the time at which the process begins. Students were asked to recall how old they were when they first thought of becoming a doctor; the range of ages they reported is great, and there is no particular concentration within it. Some students were "born with a stethoscope in their ear"; others did not consider a career in medicine until they were of college age or even older (Table 1).[5]

TABLE 1. Age at Which Medical Career Was First Considered

Age	No. of students	Percentage
Younger than 10	178	24
10–13	200	27
14 or 15	134	18
16 or 17	123	17
18 or older	106	14
	741°	100

° Six students did not answer the question.

One component in this marked diversity is clearly to be found in opportunities for learning about the status and activities of

[5] Evidence from one class of students at Western Reserve School of Medicine suggests that the distribution reported here is not unique: the proportions in the same age categories at Western Reserve are 24, 22, 22, 15, and 17 per cent, respectively. Josephine Williams reports a similar distribution for 82 male students at the University of Illinois Medical School. See Josephine Williams, "The Professional Status of Women Physicians," unpublished Ph.D. dissertation, University of Chicago, 1949, p. 84.

FIGURE 2. Age at First Thinking of a Career in Medicine, According to Relationship to Physicians

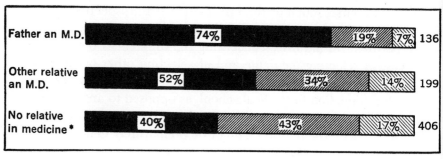

First thought of studying medicine:

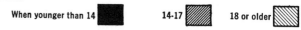

When younger than 14   14-17   18 or older

*Includes 38 students who said they had relatives in medicine, but also said they had had no contact at all with them.

Note: Numbers to right of bars indicate students.

physicians. Some students evidently enjoyed a greater degree of close and sustained contact with physicians than others. The more frequent such contacts, the easier it is to identify with physicians and to form the idea of becoming one. Having relatives (in the immediate or extended family) who are themselves doctors obviously facilitates both contacts and identification, and hence leads to earlier awakening of interest in a medical career. This of course is one of the major sources of the frequently noted trend toward inheritance of occupations from father to son.

Medical students whose fathers are doctors began thinking about a career in medicine earlier than others, and those with more distant relatives (uncles, cousins, etc.) enjoy a similar though smaller advantage over those with no relatives at all in the profession they themselves will later enter[6] (see Figure 2).

A move into the medical profession involves considerable de-

[6] Oswald Hall, discussing the awakening of interest in a medical career, states that these "ambitions were largely social in character. They had their genesis in social groups . . . one can see why doctors tend to be recruited from the families of professional workers. The latter possess the mechanisms for generating and nurturing the medical ambition." Oswald Hall, "The Stages of a Medical Career," *Am. J. Sociol.*, 53:329, 1948.

parture from the social status of their family of origin for some students, but only a small departure for others. Medical students whose fathers are *not* physicians come from families that cover a great range of occupational statuses: from well-to-do lawyers, bankers, and businessmen to wage-earning manual workers.

Where the move into the status of physician does not signify considerable social mobility, i.e., where the family of origin is of relatively high status, the presence of an uncle or cousin who is a physician seems to have little effect on arousing an early interest in medicine. But prospective physicians from lower status, *mobile* families (as indicated by the presence of at least one member who has succeeded in becoming a doctor) are more prompt than any save physicians' sons to begin thinking about the career they ultimately select. Fully 58 per cent of students from this kind of family background had begun thinking about medicine before the age of 14 (see Figure 3).

FIGURE 3. Age at First Thinking of a Career in Medicine, According to Father's Occupation and Presence or Absence of Other Relatives Who Are Physicians

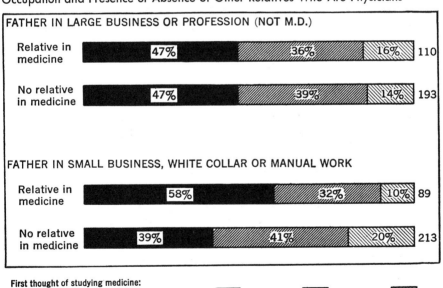

First thought of studying medicine:

When younger than 14   14-17   18 or older

Note: Numbers to right of bars indicate students.

If a mobility precedent has been set by one or more relatives, it is apparently fairly easy to come by the idea of following it. But if the precedent has not been set (lower status origins, and no relative in medicine) the delay in thinking of a career as a doctor is most marked. Another significant point develops from the similarity of the two status origin groups in the proportion having relatives in medicine. Of the sons of non-medical professionals and businessmen, 36 per cent have relatives who are doctors, compared with 29 per cent of the sons of shopkeepers, white-collar workers, and manual workers. This relatively small difference is in all likelihood not true for the total population of American families, among whom a smaller proportion of the lower occupational groups are likely to have physicians in the family. It is almost certain that the lower white-collar and manual workers' families who *do* send a son to medical school are atypical in their occupational orientation. Having seen at least one member of the family achieve professional status, they appear to be more eager and more able to see the success repeated.

THE TEMPO OF CHOICE OF A MEDICAL CAREER

Unlike the wide dispersion in the age at which medicine is first considered, the age at making the definite decision shows a marked concentration, occurring during the 16 to 20 year age period (Table 2).[7]

A more detailed distribution by single years of age is remarkably normal, with the mean, median, and mode all falling at 18 years. Fully 17.7 per cent of the students said they had decided definitely at 18. The career decision, it would appear, is most frequently experienced as final or definite when it can take the form of an overt act—typically, enrolling for a premedical course in an

[7] The Western Reserve data again parallel those for the University of Pennsylvania, although a somewhat larger proportion at the former school made up their minds after the age of 21. This may be related to the new curriculum at Western Reserve, since the older, more mature student (sometimes with an advanced degree in another field) may be regarded as particularly suited to study under this program.

On the other hand, Josephine Williams reports a somewhat younger age at final decision for students at the University of Illinois. See Williams, *op. cit.*, p. 85.

At both schools, however, the major trend being considered here is clearly noticeable: there is less dispersion in the age at final decision than in the age at first considering a career in medicine.

TABLE 2. Age at Which Definite Decision to Study Medicine Was Reached

Age	No. of students	Percentage
Younger than 10	58	8
14 or 15	73	10
16 or 17	191	26
18–20	310	41
21 or 22	77	10
23 or older	38	5
	747	100

undergraduate college. Once it is possible, through his college status, for the future doctor to identify himself as a premedical student, his hitherto private and perhaps not fully shaped intention tends to become a definite commitment.[8]

For the modal student, then, the definite career choice is keyed to the institutional requirements of the educational system. He does not prolong his choice much *beyond* the point when he must select courses appropriate to medical school prerequisites, nor does he arrive at the decision *before* the socially prescribed time. But it has also been noted that the pace of selecting an occupation is connected with the processes of social and emotional maturation. Ginzberg, for example, posits three stages in the history of an individual's career choice: a period of "fantasy choice," occurring roughly between the sixth and eleventh years; a period of "tentative choice," during adolescence; and finally a "realistic choice," made at about the age of 19 or somewhat later.[9] At first glance, personality development and institutionally induced behavior would seem to exhibit a felicitous convergence in time. But here, comparative data for the legal profession upset the reckoning. To anticipate the findings in the succeeding paper, law students make their definite career decision an average of two years later than medical students. Since there is little reason to believe

[8] In one of his stimulating papers on medical education, Dr. Alan Gregg discusses the "generic experiences that make a doctor out of a green beginner." Speaking of the years before entering medical school, he mentions occasions on which the future student comes to think of his career choice as a "responsible personal decision rather than a dream." Apparently these experiences tend to occur during the college years, and have so strong an impact that they actually date the point at which the final commitment was made. See Alan Gregg, "Our Anabasis," *The Pharos of Alpha Omega Alpha*, 18:18, February 1955.

[9] Eli Ginzberg, *op. cit.*, Chapter 7.

that the prospective physician differs from the prospective lawyer in his personality development, the discrepancy can more readily be explained by the more specialized educational prerequisites of medical schools.[10]

For some medical students, the interval between first considering and definitely deciding on their career was extremely long; for others, relatively short. As the data already presented imply, the length of this interval is greater for those who first became interested in medicine when they were children. In fact, the earlier the age at which the process of deciding was begun, the more years elapsed until the definite decision was reached. Figure 4 gives a detailed representation of the gradually increasing tempo of career choice. For example, students who first thought of becoming doctors when they were 8 years old waited, on the average, 8.2 years until they came to a final decision; students who "started" 10 years later, at age 18, waited an average of only 2 years. The initial difference of 10 years was thus reduced to 3.8. The decrease in elapsed time is so regular[11] that a good deal of the lag is made up by a more rapidly reached commitment.

But the prevailing pattern highlights the existence of a minority who made their decision years before their future classmates. About 18 per cent of medical students had already made up their minds to become doctors when they were no more than 15 years old—long before they could enroll for premedical courses in college. These youthful deciders, it can be expected, have distinctive attitudes toward the career they so early settled on. These will be examined in the last section of the analysis.

As we have seen, the sons of physicians are among the first to think of a medical career. But their deeper acquaintance with the profession does not serve to accelerate the process of coming to a final decision. Indeed, under certain conditions, the opposite seems to occur. Doctors' sons who, for whatever reasons, postponed any interest in their fathers' calling until the (for them) relatively late age of 14 or older actually took *longer* to decide than others who

[10] Wagner Thielens, "Some Comparisons of Entrants to Medical and Law School," in this volume. Other institutional sources of the discrepancy in age at deciding are also presented in that paper.

[11] For the series as a whole, the correlation between age at first considering a career in medicine and number of years until the decision was made is −.62.

FIGURE 4. Median Length of Time to Reach Career Decision, According to Age When First Considered

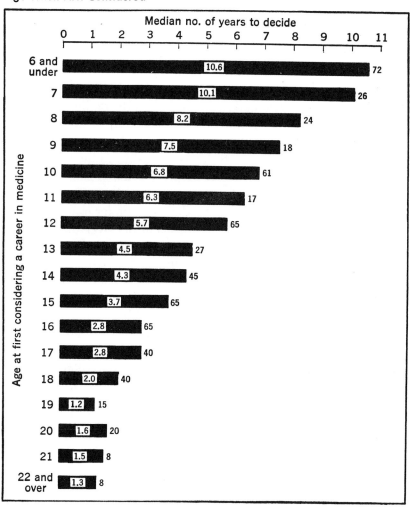

Note: Numbers to right of bars indicate students.

first considered medicine at the same time. They averaged 3.6 years until they were ready to commit themselves, as opposed to 2.7 years for students from other occupational origins.[12]

For most doctors' sons, the evidence points to family induced consideration of a medical career at an early age. But some resisted the thought until much later; if they did, it now appears that they also experienced a prolonged delay in reaching a final decision, possibly while they worked through their psychological relation to their fathers and to the family tradition.

Numerous examples of this kind of inner conflict appear in the lives of physicians, great and small. Although the definitive biography of Harvey Cushing is not rich in the details of his inner life, it contains intimations that his delay in deciding to study medicine was not unconnected with his relationship to his father. The descendant of three generations of physicians, Cushing in later life spoke of his father as "the austere, unbending, silent doctor—man we children knew."[13] During the son's undergraduate years at Yale, he had frequent run-ins with his father over the expenditure of time and money on such activities as baseball and undergraduate social clubs. Not until the summer following his graduation did young Cushing finally decide to study medicine. At that, he later acknowledged the influence, not of his family, but of a physician whom he had heard give an address at Yale during his senior year, and to whom he wrote many years later: "I well remember the informal talk you gave one night . . . on the medical career. At that time I was disposed to take up architecture, and indeed was making vague plans . . . to open an office in New York

[12] The distributions from which these medians derive are as follows: Of those first interested in medicine at 14 years of age or older:

No. of years to make decision	Percentage of doctors' sons	Percentage of all others
1 or 2	39	56
3 or 4	31	24
5 or more	30	20
	100	100
No. of students	(33)	(273)

[13] John F. Fulton, *Harvey Cushing: A Biography* (Springfield: Charles C. Thomas, 1946), p. 21.

. . . but that, like other undergraduate plans, soon went by the board."[14]

And as is well known, William H. Welch, son, grandson, nephew, and grandnephew of physicians, completed his studies at Yale with the firm intention of devoting himself to the classics as a lifework. It was only when the dim prospects of a teaching appointment in this field were wholly extinguished that "he turned at last to medicine—not a first choice but the last resort of a man thwarted in his ambition and beaten down by circumstances into conforming with the family tradition. He had held back because he had no desire at all to continue his father's work; and he only began to be happy and successful in medicine as the possibility opened out before him of a new kind of career with no precedent among the Doctors Welch and not much precedent in history."[15]

For the sons of doctors who do go into medicine, it is as though their interest in medicine, objectively facilitated by direct acquaintance with the life of a physician, is in some proportion of cases at odds with their concern to establish a separate identity of their own. To the extent that these two tendencies obtain and work at cross-purposes, they may delay the time of final commitment to medicine as a career.[16]

YOUTHFUL DECIDERS

Students who commit themselves to a medical career well before they reach college are in the minority, as we have seen. Having

---

[14] *Ibid.*, p. 51.

[15] Donald Fleming, *William H. Welch and the Rise of Modern Medicine* (Boston: Little, Brown and Company, 1954), p. 21.

[16] An interesting special case of cross-pressure may actually be involved here. In the study of political elections it has been found that voters tend to postpone their vote decision longer if they hold a combination of opinions or occupy a combination of statuses that work "against one another." One of the strongest of such cross-pressures results when an individual has leanings toward one party while other members of his immediate family prefer the opposing party. But in the case of the career decision, there may be some tendency for young persons with an interest in the *same* occupation as their fathers to experience a type of inner conflict that does not beset others. The cross-pressure may in these circumstances arise from conflicting interests and needs of the decider himself, even though he may be "in harmony" with his family. To establish this as a general trend would of course require considerably more evidence than is available here. For the effect of cross-pressures on postponement of the vote decision, see Bernard Berelson, Paul F. Lazarsfeld, and William McPhee, *Voting* (Chicago: University of Chicago Press, 1954), p. 131.

made up their minds before they could express their choice be-
haviorally (e.g., by selecting one college course rather than another), it may be assumed that these students experienced a
greater sense of a "calling" for medicine, that they found it easier
to decide that medicine was the one career to which they really
felt attracted. But it is likely that the way a youngster, as opposed
to an adolescent or young adult, comes to a decision is affected
by his age status as well. Career decisions are reached during a
period when the passage of only a year or two is accompanied by
major shifts in psychological, intellectual, and social status that
obviously exert independent influences on how an occupation is
selected. Otherwise said, differences between young persons who
decide on a career in medicine at 14 and at 18 may derive not
only from the ease with which they made up their minds, but
from the divergent statuses of 14- and 18-year-olds.

To discover whether an early decision is in fact one that was
reached with less difficulty, we consider students at three different points in time: first as they made their selection of one career
out of many, then as they waited to carry out their decision by
starting medical school, and finally as they actually "crossed the
threshold" and reflected on their choice. At all three points, those
who made an early decision appear to be more certain that studying medicine is the most appropriate choice they could make.

The more youthful the age at decision, the less frequently had
other occupations been seriously considered. Fully 83 per cent
of medical students who made up their minds about a career
before they were 14 had never given serious thought to another
occupation—in contrast to a bare 9 per cent of those, at the other
extreme, who postponed their final decision until they were 21
or older (Table 3).

There is of course nothing very surprising about this marked
divergence. After all, making a commitment to a given career
implies the exclusion of alternatives; a 21-year-old who has not
yet made up his mind[17] is unlikely to have reached that age with-

[17] Because well over 90 per cent of the medical students observed are males, the
interpretations given here may be more adequate in describing the career decisions of young men than of young women. For example, the pressure to assume an
occupational role is undoubtedly stronger on men than on women, and the latter
may postpone active deliberation about a career somewhat longer. This question is
discussed at some length in Josephine Williams, *op. cit.*

TABLE 3. Serious Consideration of Other Careers, According to Age at Decision

Age at decision	Percentage who had never seriously considered another career	No. of students*
Younger than 14	83	(29)
14 or 15	51	(39)
16 or 17	47	(106)
18–20	19	(152)
21 or older	9	(46)

* Indicates numbers on which percentages are based. In this section, the data pertain to the three classes of prospective (entering) students only. Students in the three upper classes, who were that much further removed in time from the period when they had selected their careers, were not asked the detailed questions about other behavior and attitudes before arriving at medical school.

out having given serious thought to some occupation, even if it is not the one on which he finally settles. But at the same time, the marked lack of interest in other occupations among youthful deciders indicates that a career in medicine seemed so attractive to them that it never really had any serious competitors.

Those who made an early commitment to medicine had a long time to wait until they actually began their professional training, sometimes as long as a decade. But during this prolonged interval, they were less likely than other students—for whom the "waiting time" was shorter—to have experienced doubts about their career decision. Apparently their enthusiasm for medicine not only enabled them to choose it with more alacrity, but made them less wavering, less ambivalent while waiting to put their choice into action. Again the tendency shows a direct relationship to age at decision, except for the most recent deciders, who actually had little time during which doubts might have occurred (Table 4).

TABLE 4. Doubts about Selecting Medicine as a Career, According to Age at Decision

Age at decision	Percentage who had had no doubts since deciding*	No. of students
Younger than 14	55	(29)
14 or 15	56	(39)
16 or 17	32	(106)
18–20	28	(152)
21 or older	41	(46)

* The question was worded as follows: "Once you made up your mind to become a doctor, did you ever have any doubts that this was the right decision for you?"

TABLE 5. Satisfaction with a Medical Career, According to Age at Decision

Age at decision	Percentage who feel medicine is "only career that could really satisfy" them*	No. of students
Younger than 14	86	(29)
14 or 15	87	(39)
16 or 17	62	(106)
18–20	57	(152)
21 or older	50	(46)

* Most students who did *not* endorse this statement said they felt that medicine is "one of several careers which (they) could find almost equally satisfying."

Finally, when they begin their studies, early deciders are more likely to feel that medicine is "the only career that can really satisfy them." Their initial enthusiasm, which made the decision itself easier to reach, tends to be maintained through the intervening years. Later deciders, for whom the process of choosing a career was more a matter of selecting one among several attractive alternatives, are less likely to think of medicine as uniquely gratifying (Table 5).

In certain respects, then, time of decision stands for ease in reaching the decision. But youthful deciders differ from their future classmates in other respects as well, more specifically in the relative influence on them of family and of friends. Here it will be suggested that these variations are produced by differences in the social relations typical of persons in disparate age statuses, and have relatively little to do with facilitating the decision itself.

For example, the younger the age at deciding to study medicine, the greater the importance in the decision attributed by students to their fathers (Table 6). Fathers of youthful deciders were also more prone to offer encouragement once the decision was made. On the one hand, these tendencies might signify that strong parental support actually helped to facilitate the selection of a career. But on the other, they might only indicate that father–son ties are in general closer in early adolescence than they are after the sons go off to college. As between the two processes, further evidence suggests that the latter is probably more operative. The more overt and direct part played by the families of youthful deciders appears to stem primarily from the greater intimacy between fathers and sons during the precollege years.

If paternal advice and encouragement did facilitate the choice

TABLE 6. Role of Father in Career Decision, According to Age at Decision

Age at decision	Percentage whose fathers were "very" or "fairly" important in the decision	Percentage whose fathers offered "strong" encouragement once decision was made	No. of students
Younger than 14	90	90	(29)
14 or 15	85	77	(39)
16 or 17	68	77	(106)
18–20	65	66	(152)
21 or older	35	59	(46)

of a career in medicine, they should have an effect on attitudes toward the decision irrespective of the age when it was reached. But this is not the case. Early deciders, no matter how much reinforcement was provided by their fathers, are less ambivalent than later deciders. The withholding of strong support by fathers seems to have no independent effect on students' satisfaction with their choices, or, by inference, on the ease which which they selected their future occupation (see Figure 5).

A caveat is in order before this finding can be properly evaluated. Only 2 per cent of the students said their fathers had expressed strong or even slight *opposition* to their choice of occupation; if marked encouragement was not proffered, slight encouragement, or, at the worst, indifference on the fathers' part was more typical. This suggests that outright parental opposition may be enough, in many instances, to prevent those who are interested in medicine from ever reaching medical school.[18] Our

[18] To test this idea would obviously require a study that included people who abandoned the idea of becoming doctors. One of the many justifications for this kind of inquiry comes from the fact that the proportion of medical students who said their fathers had offered strong encouragement is *smallest* (66 per cent) among physicians' sons and *largest* (84 per cent) among sons of white-collar and manual workers, with the business and professional class falling in between (76 per cent). Possibly, medical families tend to take for granted the sons' decision to carry on the profession of their fathers; overt support for such a decision may therefore be less forthcoming. Stated more generally, the less common or the less easy it is to become a doctor (on the basis of social origins) the more likely is parental support to be provided. There may in fact be a linkage between this observation and another aspect of decision processes referred to in the paper by Kendall and Selvin, "Tendencies toward Specialization in Medical Training," in this volume. There it will be shown that the prevailing decision arrived at by a particular subgroup tends to receive more social support than the atypical decision. Here, the point seems to be that the less typical decision (i.e., that of lower-class persons to enter medicine) is only infrequently carried out if social support is missing.

FIGURE 5.   Satisfaction with a Medical Career, According to Age at Decision and Encouragement Offered by Father

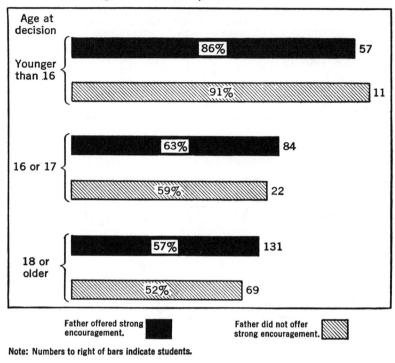

Note: Numbers to right of bars indicate students.

sample therefore consists of persons whose decision to study medicine met with, at best, a "warm" reaction and, at worst, a "tepid" one from their fathers. Only within this limited range does the father appear to have little influence on the son's own attitude toward his career.

To recall the point of this discussion, the question is whether the more prominent role which younger deciders attribute to their fathers actually eased their choice of a career, or whether it simply follows from their age status. Another type of evidence bearing on this question concerns the length of time it took to arrive at the decision.

An early decision does not always represent a "speedy" decision.

Students who finally decided at a given age, say 18, had been exposed to the possibility for varying lengths of time; depending in part on how much contact they had had with members of the profession, some had first given thought to it at a much earlier age than others. If active involvement of fathers in their sons' deliberations about a career actually makes the decision easier to reach, the effect might be to shorten the interval between the "beginning" and the "end" of the process. For example, fathers might be able to provide their sons with information, or access to information, which the latter would be slower in obtaining on their own. Yet the data do not support this inference. As the fathers' role increases in importance, there is no concomitant speeding up of the decision process.

Figure 6 distinguishes between the age at which, and the speed with which, the decision was reached. Students whose fathers played a very important role in helping them arrive at the decision to study medicine did not take less time than others to make up their minds, once the idea had occurred to them. In the case of late deciders (i.e., those who chose their career at the age of 18 or older) there appears to be a *negative* relation between importance of the father and alacrity in selecting medicine as a career. This, however, is due to the fact that, irrespective of the age at which the decision was made, the earlier medicine was *first considered,* the more important was the father. The data therefore suggest that fathers played a more important part in youthful decisions not so much because they made the decisions easier to reach, but primarily because of the close family ties between fathers and young sons.

If the fathers of younger deciders play a greater role in their offsprings' career decisions, older deciders are by the same token more subject to influence by their peers. Waiting until the college years to choose a career implies not only greater emancipation from the family, but the acquisition of friends of like age with whom information and evaluative judgments on various occupations may be exchanged. Thus, a sizeable number of later deciders attributed an important role in the decision to friends who were already in medical school, while, given the pattern of age-graded friendships, this source was, of course, almost completely inac-

FIGURE 6. Speed of Decision, According to Age at Decision and Importance of Father in the Decision

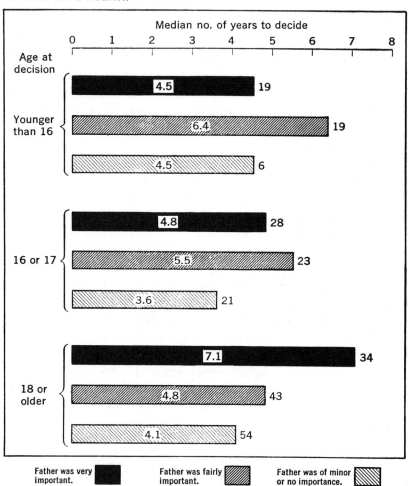

Note: This chart is based on students in only two of the three incoming classes. The exact number of years that elapsed between the time when medicine was first considered and finally selected could not be calculated for the other class. Numbers to right of bars indicate students.

TABLE 7. Importance in Decision of Friends in Medical School, According to Age at Decision

Age at decision	Percentage for whom friends in medical school were "very" or "fairly" important in the decision	No. of students*
Younger than 14	14	(22)
14 or 15	14	(28)
16 or 17	20	(65)
18–20	27	(99)
21 or older	41	(27)

* Based on two of the three classes of prospective students. The question was not asked of the remaining class.

cessible to the very youthful deciders at the time they made their commitment (Table 7).

The influence of the parental generation decreases with the age at making the career decision, while that of contemporaries increases. The difference between the relative influence of the generations may prove to have a bearing on students' perspectives on the medical profession. The possibility that youthful deciders actually form a different image of their professional training and future career is now being investigated. We start with the assumption that students' images of the profession are affected by the interests of, and information held by, those persons who influence their decision. Young adolescents and their families may be likely to look on medicine from the "outside," and see it primarily as an occupation in which one helps sick people, with emphasis on the face-to-face dealings between doctor and patient. College students, and, *a fortiori,* medical students, may be more aware of the intellectual challenge of medicine, for they are in a position to relate the content of the doctor's role to the scientific studies they are pursuing.

In support of this idea it is encouraging to observe that youthful deciders, as late as a few weeks before arriving at medical school, show a propensity for the interpersonal rather than the intellectual side of medicine (Table 8).

It is important to recall that in the interim between selecting a medical career and entering medical school, youthful deciders were exposed to the same environment as later deciders. During their years at college, they too acquired friends among those al-

TABLE 8. Patient vs. Technical Orientation, According to Age at Decision

Age at decision	Percentage who would prefer appreciative patient*	No. of students
Younger than 14	41	(29)
14 or 15	36	(39)
16 or 17	41	(106)
18–20	32	(152)
21 or older	22	(46)

* The question was posed in the form of a dilemma: "Do you think you would get more personal satisfaction from successfully solving a relatively simple medical problem for a patient who expresses great appreciation, or from successfully solving a very complicated problem for a patient who expresses no appreciation whatever?"

ready in professional training.[19] Nonetheless, they begin their studies with a greater tendency than shown by their classmates to prefer the reward of working with an appreciative patient over the reward of solving a challenging medical problem. Whether this attitude on the one hand is affected by the persons who played the greatest role in helping youthful deciders select medicine as a career, and on the other affects their actual performance in the role of medical student, will be determined by later investigation.

SUMMARY

Some medical students became interested in the profession they are to enter when they were still young children; others say the idea did not occur to them until many years later. The more contact with physicians (in the family), the earlier interest was aroused.

The final career decision was reached most often during the early college years, at which point students could carry out their decision by following a course of premedical studies. Early interest in medicine is not necessarily followed by an early commitment; in fact, the younger the age at first thinking about a medical career, the more years elapsed until the commitment was made.

[19] Fully 96 per cent of the entering students had friends at least one year ahead of them in medical school (their own school or another). In a future publication we hope to analyze the part played by these friends in giving the newcomer a set of expectations of the status he is about to assume.

A youthful decision is generally a more enthusiastic one. Other occupations are seldom considered seriously; doubts about whether a medical career is the right choice are relatively infrequent; and, on entrance into medical school, the chosen profession seems like the only one that could really be satisfying. Students who picked their career at an early age were also more likely to be influenced and encouraged by their families, and less likely to be helped by contemporaries. These seem to be matters of the difference between adolescents and young adults in their relations with family and friends, and may in turn affect the image of a medical career formed by those who decide at different ages.

Wagner Thielens, Jr.

SOME COMPARISONS OF ENTRANTS
TO MEDICAL AND LAW SCHOOL

The purpose of this paper is to compare some preliminary findings dealing with the background, attitudes, and expectations with which two groups of professional recruits—the students who entered an Eastern medical school in September 1953, and those who entered an Eastern law school at the same time—began their professional studies. The information examined here was gathered through extensive questionnaires filled in by all 124 medical entrants and by 248 of the 265 law entrants. A majority of both groups completed the questionnaires by mail before the opening of school; the remainder were reached in a relatively few days after the opening.

The findings reported here cannot, of course, be assumed to hold beyond the scope of the two schools, since without additional comparisons we do not know to what extent they must be interpreted only in terms of local situations within the two schools. But it is tentatively assumed that conditions obtaining more generally are reflected at least in part in these findings.

THE DECISION TO ENTER PROFESSIONAL SCHOOL

We begin with a difference between the medical school entrants[1] and the law school entrants which we shall later show is of con-

[1] The class of 1957 at the University of Pennsylvania School of Medicine. For greater generality, the answers of 374 upperclassmen at the University of Pennsylvania have been included in the figures throughout this section. Their decision pattern is the same as that of the more recent entrants.

131

siderable importance in a comparison of other aspects of their behavior and attitudes. The two groups were asked to indicate how long ago they had definitely decided to enter professional school.[2] As Table 9 shows, medical students were likely to make this commitment earlier than law students. About three-quarters of the medical students had decided to enter medical school at least 2 years before they actually did so, while only about one-third of the law students had made their decisions by that time.[3]

TABLE 9. Time of Final Decision to Enter Professional School

Time of decision	Medical students, per cent	Law students, per cent
Less than 2 years before entry	27	66
2–4 years before	29	19
More than 4 years before	44	15
No. of students	(496)	(248)

Evidence from another study shows that the decision pattern of our law students is typical. A nation-wide survey of some 24,000 students made in 1949 found that 50 per cent had decided to study law at age 19 or less;[4] on a later questionnaire which we administered, 50 per cent of the students likewise reported making this decision by the age of 19.

At least three factors, we believe, operate together to make for an earlier commitment to professional school by medical students than by law students: more extensive premedical course requirements, greater contact of medical entrants with their future profession, and the fact that doctors have higher standing in the community and obtain larger incomes than lawyers.

[2] Slightly different versions of the time-of-decision question were used in the two questionnaires. The medical entrants were asked, "At what age did you definitely decide to study medicine?"; the law entrants, "About how long ago did you make the final decision to enter law school?" The former answers have been converted into a form comparable to the latter.

[3] It should be noted that more law entrants than medical entrants (19 per cent compared with 4 per cent) were professional option students, entering professional school after completing three years of undergraduate study. However, this factor does not affect the time of decision: among the law entrants, 64 per cent of those on professional option had decided within the last 2 years, compared with 65 per cent of the remainder.

[4] Chief Justice Arthur T. Vanderbilt, "A Report on Prelegal Education," *New York Univ. Law Review*, April 1950.

Entrance Requirements

Because of the nature of the entrance requirements laid down by the two schools, it is often possible for a college junior or senior who has had other plans to make a belated decision to enter law school, while a similarly late decision to enter medical school is more difficult. With rare exceptions, entrants to the University of Pennsylvania School of Medicine are required as undergraduates to take at least 52 semester hours[5] of specified courses in biology, chemistry, physics, mathematics, and English. Generally, at least two years of study are needed to cover these requirements; an undergraduate making a late decision to study medicine would seldom have taken the often highly specialized courses and would need to devote the necessary time to them. The law school prerequisites, on the other hand, are neither so extensive nor so detailed. According to the school's catalog, an entrant's training "must have included satisfactory courses in English, in economics, and in English and United States history or the equivalent." Such courses might require a year's work by an undergraduate, but many upperclassmen pursuing a liberal arts program will already have taken these courses, whether planning to enter law school or not.

Of course, an undergraduate who has undertaken premedical training need not yet have made a final decision on medical school. Table 9 shows that 27 per cent of the medical students made the final decision less than 2 years before entrance; we may add that about half of this group, 13 per cent of the entrants, made their decisions less than a year before entrance. Nevertheless, the majority of those who have committed themselves to the extent of taking the specialized premedical courses have by that time also definitely decided to go to medical school.

Table 9 also indicates, however, that many students had definitely decided upon medical school more than 4 years earlier, in most cases *before* they entered college, while relatively few law students had made similarly early decisions. It seems most unlikely that this difference is more than partially due to *anticipation* by medical school hopefuls of the more demanding entrance requirements.

[5] Equivalent to 8½ or 9 full-year courses.

TABLE 10.   Students with Relatives in Each of Five Professions

| | Percentage of students with at least one relative in the profession | |
Profession	Medical students	Law students
Lawyers	34	51
Doctors	50	35
Dentists	16	14
Clergymen	21	15
Teachers	53	44
No. of students	(498)	(248)

Possible Background Differences

It is well known that sons of professional families are more likely to become professionals than are sons of families in other occupational groups, especially those of lower social standing in the community.[6] If more medical students were from medical families than law students were from law families, and if, as we might expect, the decision to enter a profession is made earlier by individuals who have relatives in the profession, this could help explain the medical students' earlier decisions. Table 10, however, indicates that nearly identical proportions of the two groups have at least one relative[7] in their own profession—51 per cent of the law students have relatives who are lawyers and 50 per cent of the medical students have relatives who are doctors. This similarity holds also within the immediate family: 15 per cent of the law entrants have fathers or mothers who are lawyers, while 17 per cent of the medical entrants have parents 'who are doctors. We note further that 35 per cent of the law students have relatives who are doctors, just as 34 per cent of the medical students have relatives who are lawyers. The figures do show that the medical students are somewhat more likely to have clergymen and teachers as relatives, but on the whole the degree to which the two

[6] For instance, Natalie Rogoff, analyzing 1938–1941 marriage applications in Indianapolis, found that 28.3 per cent of the sons of professionals were professionals, as compared with 15.8 per cent of the sons of semiprofessionals and less than 8 per cent of the sons of every other occupational group, including those of "proprietors, managers, and officials." Natalie Rogoff, "Recent Trends in Urban Occupational Mobility," in: R. Bendix and S. M. Lipset, eds., *Class, Status and Power* (Glencoe, Ill.: The Free Press, 1953), p. 445.

[7] Included as relatives: father, mother, step-parent, brother, sister, grandparent, uncle, aunt, cousin, spouse, and father-, mother-, brother-, and sister-in-law.

FIGURE 7.   Relationship between Having Professional Relatives and Time of Definite Decision

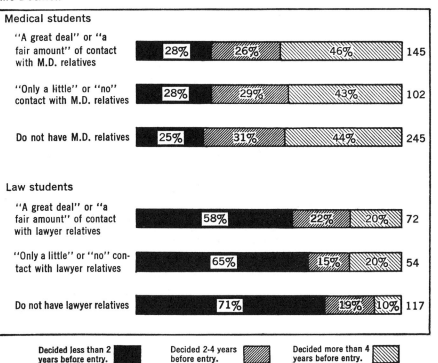

Medical students

"A great deal" or "a fair amount" of contact with M.D. relatives — 28% | 26% | 46% — 145

"Only a little" or "no" contact with M.D. relatives — 28% | 29% | 43% — 102

Do not have M.D. relatives — 25% | 31% | 44% — 245

Law students

"A great deal" or "a fair amount" of contact with lawyer relatives — 58% | 22% | 20% — 72

"Only a little" or "no" contact with lawyer relatives — 65% | 15% | 20% — 54

Do not have lawyer relatives — 71% | 19% | 10% — 117

Decided less than 2 years before entry. ▮   Decided 2-4 years before entry. ▨   Decided more than 4 years before entry. ▧

Note: Numbers to right of bars indicate students.

groups are affiliated with the professions by family relationship differs very little.

Medical students have not had more contact than law students with relatives in the respective professions, and apparently have not been more influenced by them. Both groups report about equal contact with relatives in their professions: 31 per cent of the medical students have had either "a great deal" or "a fair amount" of contact with physician relatives before entering school while 29 per cent of the law entrants report like contacts with lawyer relatives. And the data in Figure 7 suggest that having relatives in the profession, even for students who had been in close contact with them, has far less influence than we might expect. Contact with

lawyer relatives apparently may lead a few law students to somewhat earlier decisions, but contact with doctor relatives has, in
general, no effect on the timing of medical students' decisions.[8]

Other Contacts with the Professions

Though medical students have had no more contact with physician
relatives than law students with lawyer relatives, they may have
experienced greater contact with their profession in other ways.
For instance, it is evident from common observation that a larger
proportion of young Americans have at one time or another been
the patient of a physician than have been the client of a lawyer.
Virtually every child and adolescent in our society has at some
point required the services of a doctor, be it for a case of measles,
a broken bone, or swollen tonsils. Fewer, we would guess, have
been the client of a lawyer, perhaps as signer of a will, participant
in a divorce suit—or as juvenile delinquent. Replying to a question
on this matter, 87 per cent of the medical entrants can recall at
least some contact with doctors as a patient. Law entrants, presumably more likely than other young adults to be related to
lawyers, are doubtless also more familiar with lawyers' skills and
more inclined to turn to lawyers for help. Nonetheless, only 19 per
cent report a contact as a lawyer's client. Again, both groups have
very likely had considerable opportunity to observe or hear about
doctors treating relatives and friends, but have had fewer similar
contacts with lawyers; lawyers' professional services are less often
provided in the homes of clients where impressionable youngsters
may witness them. In these respects, the role of a doctor is a matter of direct experience and knowledge to a greater extent than
that of a lawyer.[9]

Social Standing and Income

Sociological studies have repeatedly shown that doctors as a group
have higher social standing in the community than lawyers. For

[8] As shown in the preceding paper, the presence of doctor relatives does affect
the age at which a career in medicine is first contemplated.

[9] In discussing the differences found between the law and medical groups, this
paper offers explanations which are in the main only indirectly supported by statistical evidence. Without further study, for instance, no data are available to provide
a table showing the extent to which greater contact of medical students with their
profession accounts for their generally earlier decision.

instance, North and Hatt[10] found that 67 per cent of the participants in a nation-wide survey gave doctors the highest of five possible ratings of an occupation's "general standing," while 44 per cent gave this rating to lawyers.[11] It would be understandable if the law students were to assign higher standing to their chosen profession. Yet when asked to assess the community's ranking of seven occupational groups, fully 50 per cent of them give first ranking to doctors; only 3 per cent put lawyers first. Even when asked, "How would *you personally* rank the standing of these groups?" more law students give first place to doctors (24 per cent) than to lawyers (19 per cent).

As with relative social standing, so with income. When asked to estimate the average yearly (after-tax) income of members of their profession, 42 per cent of the medical students pictured general practitioners as having an average yearly income of $10,000 or more, and fully 90 per cent of them pictured medical specialists as earning that sum. In contrast, only 9 per cent of the law students pictured this amount as the average income of lawyers.

Medical practice, then, is likely to be perceived by students as accompanied by both higher prestige and higher income than law practice. Insofar as these factors are inducements to students making career decisions, such perceptions may contribute to the earlier decisions of the medical entrants.

ROLE MODELS

Students, as they begin to learn and to practice the professional role, often choose a figure in the profession, a practitioner known personally or one known only by repute, as a model to imitate and an ideal with which to compare their own performance. In short, they adopt a role model.

[10] Cecil C. North and Paul K. Hatt, "Jobs and Occupations: A Popular Evaluation." Reprinted, in part, in: Logan Wilson and William L. Kolb, *Sociological Analysis* (New York: Harcourt, Brace and Company, 1949), pp. 464–473.

[11] This paper cannot attempt an explanation of *why* this difference in standing exists. We might note, however, that students have differing views of the trust accorded the two professions by the general public. While 30 per cent of the students at this medical school believe that "a large fraction of the public is suspicious of doctors," 72 per cent of the law entrants subscribe to the same statement about lawyers. It may well be true that, as Lincoln once wrote, "There is a vague popular belief that lawyers are necessarily dishonest."

FIGURE 8.   Frequency with Which Role Models Are Named, According to Time of Decision

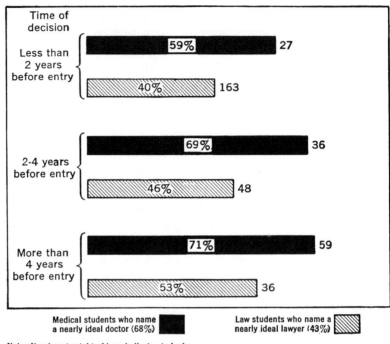

Note: Numbers to right of bars indicate students.

From the outset the two groups of entrants differ substantially in respect to having such role models. When asked, "Can you think of a doctor (lawyer) who in your opinion comes close to being an ideal doctor (lawyer)?" 68 per cent of the medical entrants[12] were able to name such a doctor, while 43 per cent of the law students could name a lawyer.

This difference is related to medical students' earlier decisions to enter professional school. Figure 8 shows that by the time students enter law or medical school, those whose decisions were made earliest are most likely to have a role model. It is possible

[12] In this section, and in the remainder of the paper, all figures apply only to the 124 medical and 248 law entrants. This paper deals with the attitudes which individuals hold before they have been influenced by direct experience at professional school. Changes in these attitudes under the impact of school attendance will be the concern of other papers.

that this relationship could develop in two ways. Great admiration for a particular doctor or lawyer might precipitate an early career decision. Or an early decision to go into a profession, made without the influence of a role model, could lead to greater interest in the profession and an increased likelihood of acquiring a model by the time of entrance into school.

However, Figure 8 shows that no matter when the decision was made, medical students name a near-ideal more frequently than law students do. This may again reflect the greater familiarity of the doctor: medical students are more likely to have role models simply because they are better acquainted with the members of their field. Or, if prominent social standing helps make a professional seem ideal to a student, again doctors might be more readily chosen than lawyers. Additional research will be needed to clarify these possibilities.

FINDING THE RIGHT CAREER

Much the same context can be utilized to interpret another finding. To estimate the proportions of students who are especially attracted to the profession they are about to enter, the two groups were asked whether or not a career as a doctor or lawyer was the "only career that could really satisfy" them. Answering this question, 64 per cent of the medical entrants felt that medicine was the only satisfactory career for them, while 30 per cent of the law entrants expressed a similar attitude toward law.

As before, this difference is related to the earlier decision of medical students to attend professional school. Figure 9 demonstrates among both law and medical students that those who decide earliest are most likely by the time of entrance to consider the profession as their only satisfactory career.

Again it is possible that the relationship could develop in two ways. Let us assume that students who regard law or medicine as the "only satisfactory career" do not consider any other career as a serious alternative. First, people who at any given time have no serious career alternatives may commit themselves definitely to professional school earlier than do those considering alternatives. Evidence from the two studies strongly supports such a conclusion. Of those medical entrants who said they did not "ever seriously consider any other occupation or profession before deciding on medicine," 77 per cent had definitely decided rather early (four years or more before entrance), compared with but 33 per cent of those who had considered alternatives. And on a similar question the comparable proportions of law students, in this case of those deciding more than two years beforehand, were 50 per cent and 16 per cent.

Second, there are undoubtedly other individuals who reach a decision to go to medical or law school while at the same time planning to keep open other career possibilities—in case, for instance, they are not accepted by a medical or a law school. But it may be that once a tentative commitment of this nature is made, such individuals subsequently experience a diminishing interest in alternatives. If so, those who made the commitment early should find that alternatives have faded most completely by the time of entrance. Here we can offer no evidence.

However, comparing the medical and law students who decided in any one of the three intervals of time, we find that medical students are still more likely than law students to regard their profession alone as satisfying. To interpret this difference we must first point out that law school training, as compared with medical school training, has a diversity of uses. Law school is widely held to be an appropriate training ground for certain fields which do not involve the practice of law. When asked what occupation they planned to enter after graduation from law school, 23 of the entrants (9 per cent) named a field outside "the practice of law."[13] And as their first choice for a permanent career, 8 per cent chose a corporation executive position and another 13 per cent a career in politics. Except perhaps for those favoring politics, these students, of course, need not think of law as their only satisfying career. On the other hand, medical school is seldom if ever taken to be a training ground for fields outside medicine.

In addition to its usefulness in specific fields, a closely related tradition holds, law training imparts to students a keen mental

[13] If these plans were known to be permanent, this group might properly be excluded from comparisons of the two schools, since our focus of attention is upon the recruits into the two professions. However, among the 23 entrants, 12 out of the 20 again answering this question at the end of their first year were then planning to practice law (and another 14 who as entrants planned to practice law had chosen some other occupation).

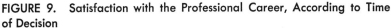

FIGURE 9.   Satisfaction with the Professional Career, According to Time of Decision

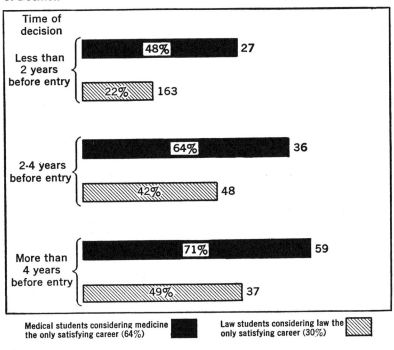

Note: Numbers to right of bars indicate students.

discipline which is useful in almost any career. Some 62 per cent of the law school student body said the thought that "a legal training will be very useful regardless of what career I go into" had been a "very important" element in their decisions to come to law school. Furthermore, with a late decision to enter law school not difficult, this tradition is useful to undergraduates whose career plans are uncertain. Some 23 per cent of the entering class report that their decision "to try law school" resulted at least in part from being "indecisive about what to do." On the other hand, with the way less smoothly paved for the unmotivated, fewer should drift into medical school; on the same question, 13 per cent had decided "to try medical school."[14]

[14] This question was asked only of three upper classes in the following form: "Below is a list of some of the reasons medical students give for their decision to

Another group of law students, presumably a small group, does not point toward a career in law. For such students it is the prestige of a higher degree, rather than the training itself, which is central. One forthright student phrased the conceptions of this group succinctly:

> The trouble these days is that there are too many lawyers and too many college graduates with A.B.'s. The idea is to go to law school, get an LL.B., and then do what you wanted to do after college.

Even when all these differences are discounted, however, entering law students still appear to be less specially drawn to law than medical students are to medicine. This can be seen when we consider *only* the 95 law students who at the same time: (1) plan at entrance to practice law after graduation, (2) have not changed this plan at the end of their first year, (3) make some form of law practice (with politics excluded) their first preference for a permanent career, and (4) did not decide "to try law school" because of uncertain career plans. Of these 95, still only 38 per cent find law the only satisfactory career, as compared with 64 per cent of the medical students.[15]

Although we are unable to identify with certainty the sources of this difference, several possible factors come to mind. Perhaps potential career alternatives are considered less satisfying by medical students in face of the unusually high prestige and income of medicine. Law students, in contrast, may find more career alternatives as attractive as the law with regard to prestige and income.

Again, medical entrants may be reluctant to change career plans once they have undertaken the specialized, expensive, and time-consuming premedical training. Since this training might go largely wasted in other careers, they may already feel constrained to seek satisfaction only in medicine. Law entrants, by contrast,

---

study medicine. For each, is it a very important factor to you, a somewhat important factor, or not a factor at all: I was indecisive about what to do and decided to try medicine."

[15] We may add that this group of 95 shows very little difference from the total group of 248 entrants in both the time of their decision to enter law school and the frequency with which they name a "nearly ideal" lawyer: 60 per cent decided two years or less before entrance (compared with 66 per cent of the total group) and 47 per cent named an ideal lawyer (compared with 43 per cent).

with little or no investment in special training, may feel more free to continue consideration of other careers.

Finally, observation suggests that the recruits of the medical profession are expected by our society to be more dedicated to their work than law recruits, to feel an exclusive devotion to their task which is quite apart from such practical considerations as income, social prestige, or previous investment. Perhaps medical students include, as a part of their own self-images and self-expectations, an appropriate reflection of the expectations that others have of them.

THE PERCEPTION OF COMPETITION

Entrance into an occupation typically involves a number of sorting devices by which candidates are screened for their qualifications to take up the occupation. Physical, mental, and temperamental characteristics are often carefully examined, both before the candidate is permitted to begin work or training, and on through his indoctrination into the occupation. This is especially true of the professions; widely sought after as careers, they generally have stringent sorting procedures.

As seen from the point of view of candidates, the selective sorting devices inherently require some sort of "competition," a striving to emerge from the sorting process in a favored position. But little is known about competition among candidates for professions—about the circumstances under which it becomes acute, the strains it imposes on the competitors, or the mechanisms by which it is regulated.

To provide baselines for study of these processes, the two sets of students were asked to assess the academic competition they had experienced as college undergraduates.[16] Among medical students almost three times as many—49 per cent compared with 18 per cent of the law entrants—reported a "great deal" of competition in college.

At least two considerations are evidently involved here: the undergraduate situations in which the two sets of ultimate professional school entrants find themselves, and the circumstances of entrance to the two kinds of professional schools.

[16] "How much competition did you find among your classmates in college?"

The Undergraduate Situation

Quite apart fi·m the actual amount of undergraduate competition, prospective students of law and of medicine may be expected to perceive it differently. Presumably most students with definite plans to apply to professional school will tend to regard any existing academic competition as having serious and direct significance, since a good undergraduate scholastic record is required for entrance both to medical school and to law school. But students with less definite plans, though they may of course wish to compile a good record, might well attach less significance to competition. If this is the case, the eventual medical entrants, more often already committed to professional school than the eventual law entrants, should more often perceive competition as being "real" competition aimed toward admission to professional school.

Differences in the composition of classmates may also affect the sense of competition of the two groups. In satisfying their relatively small number of prerequisites, prospective law students may choose from courses which are suited as well to students with a variety of other career plans; premedical students, whose prerequisites are larger in number and sometimes highly specialized, have by comparison a relatively unchanging group of classmates composed mainly of other premedical students. Such circumstances may well contribute to a sense of *direct* competition among premedical students which is less often found among prelaw students.

Entrance to Professional School

The greater competition experienced by medical school aspirants undoubtedly also reflects a widespread belief that there are, in general, more candidates for each of the openings available at the medical schools of the nation than there are for those at the law schools. The available evidence, though not conclusive, supports this belief.[17] At the University of Pennsylvania Medical School the ratio of applications to entrants for each new class is typically a

---

[17] The national *applicants*-acceptances ratio is available for medical schools, but not for law schools. National *applications*-acceptances ratios, while available for both, do not eliminate multiple applications by single applicants. However, inferences drawn from these ratios and from data for our two schools suggest that while individual medical aspirants make more applications than law aspirants, there

great deal higher than is true for the law school we studied; in 1953, for instance, the ratios were 16 to 1 and 3.2 to 1, respectively. A comparison of undergraduate records also supports the depiction of the medical entrants as a somewhat more highly selected group; some 30 per cent of them compiled an undergraduate grade average of A or A–, compared with 10 per cent of the law entrants.

Expectations of Competition in Professional School

It seems apparent that the over-all sorting processes governing entrance into a profession should be found to undergo a shift in character as candidates make the transition to professional school. As one clue to such a shift, both sets of students were asked to estimate how much competition they anticipated in their first year at professional school. A reversal of position and an even greater contrast than that found for undergraduate competition is revealed here: fully 83 per cent of the law entrants, compared with 35 per cent of the medical entrants, expected to find "a great deal" of competition.

Subsequent reports from these students, we may say at once, show that these expectations were in the main borne out. At the end of their first year, 74 per cent of the law students, and 19 per cent of the medical students, found that there had been a great deal of competition among classmates during the year.[18]

These widely differing perceptions of first-year competition can perhaps best be accounted for by two sets of factors, involving differences between the two professional schools and differences between the professions for which they train.

Differences between Professional Schools

The first year of law school has a significance today quite different from that of the first year of medical school. At one time there

are still considerably more applicants for each medical school opening than for each law school opening.

For national medical applicants-acceptances ratios, see for example, John M. Stalnaker, "The Study of Applicants, 1954–1955," *J. Med. Educ.*, 30:625–636, November 1955. For applications-acceptances ratios at both types of schools, see William S. Guthrie, "Applications to the Professional Schools and Colleges," College of Arts and Sciences of Ohio State University, Columbus, Ohio, 1953.

[18] These figures are based on answers given by 212 of the original 248 law entrants, and 123 of the 124 medical entrants.

existed in the majority of both medical and law schools a policy
of winnowing; this, so tradition has it, found pungent expression
in a stern admonition to entering freshmen:

> Look to the gentleman on your left, sir, and look to the one on your
> right. One of the three of you will not be here next year!

At the law school studied (and many others) an element of this
tradition remains, for the first year of school is still likely to be
regarded by both students and faculty as a trial year. During this
year an appreciable number of students, many with low grades,
leave school,[19] and at the end of the year another group flunks out.
By the start of its second year, a typical law class will decrease in
size by from 15 to 20 per cent. In contrast, many medical schools,
including the one studied, attempt today by careful screening to
select at entrance the entire group of students who will graduate.
Once he has been accepted for admission to the school, a student
has an extremely good chance of remaining there, since the decrease in size of recent entering classes over their entire four years
of school has seldom been greater than 5 per cent. Clearly there
is less of the "try it for a year" approach to medical school.[20]

The first year of law school is also a trial year in another sense
not paralleled in medical school. At the end of the year the top-
ranking students, making up about 8 per cent of the class, are
invited to join the staff of the school's Law Review. No further
members are chosen in later years.[21] Yet fully 49 per cent of the
entering class had received advice from various quarters to "make
every attempt to get on the Law Review." Law Review membership is widely considered to be of great consequence, in providing

[19] The self-selection which occurs among first year law school students is undoubtedly paralleled to some extent by a similar self-selection among *premedical*
students. It may be that many parallels for significant aspects of the first year of
law school can be traced in the phase of training preceding medical school.

[20] These differences may also contribute to the differing levels of career commitment among the two groups, as noted above. Knowing that they may leave school,
law students may want to keep open in their minds the possibility of finding satisfaction in another career. At the medical school, where flunking out is rare, students
can more safely commit themselves exclusively to medicine.

[21] Technically, students may be invited to become Law Review candidates at
the end of their second year; in practice this occurrence is rare. It should be added
that certain other awards, such as research assistantships to school professors, are
made at this time, and these too are likely to depend at least in part on students'
marks.

special legal training and experience not otherwise available in law school, and also, later on, in helping graduates get jobs. As one student expressed it, "If you make Law Review, you're in; if you don't, you're out in the cold." Without minimizing the importance of competition in medical school, no such highly regarded and permanently valued reward is given there to first-year students of topmost rank.

For both successful and unsuccessful first year students in law school, then, the stakes are higher—the prize for outstanding performance greater, the penalty for less successful performance more severe. Such circumstances should indeed add impetus to competition.

One further difference between these schools, possibly more idiosyncratic, may be reflected in entrants' differing expectations of competition. At the law school, there is a general expectation that entering students should strive, within the bounds of fair play, to outdo their classmates; they are strongly encouraged to "work just as hard as you can." But the medical school does not expect quite such an all-out effort; entrants are advised, for instance, to "work hard, but relax on weekends."

Differences between the Professions

Not only differences in professional training, but also differences between the practicing professions may be reflected in students' differing expectations of competition. In the eyes of many lawyers, the field of law is overly crowded and competitive. For instance, Reginald Heber Smith, director of the recent Survey of the Legal Profession, writes in a study for the Survey:

> Of all professions, the legal is the most competitive. A client who is dissatisfied with his lawyer can easily find another. Competition is so keen that many Bar Associations have committees on "The Economic Condition of the Bar," and a perennial topic among lawyers is whether their profession is not badly overcrowded.[22]

Similar sentiments are less common, it would appear, among doctors, although no systematic evidence is available to establish the difference. In any case, the entrants consider the two professions to be different. Asked about disliked features of their profession,

[22] Reginald Heber Smith, "Complaints against Lawyers," 1949, mimeographed.

TABLE 11. Student Views on Faculty Assessments of Importance of Several Factors in Making a Good Doctor or a Good Lawyer

Factor in making a good professional	Percentage of students saying faculty would consider the factor "very important"	
	Medical students	Law students
High intelligence	73	73
Pleasing personality	40	44
Good appearance	23	23
Good social background	6	4
Medical (legal) tradition in family	1	2
Extensive experience as a patient (client)	0	0
High grades in professional school	36	55
No. of students	(124)	(248)

some 15 per cent of the law entrants wrote of "cut-throat competition," "overcrowding," and "scarcity of jobs"; only 2 per cent of the medical entrants voiced similar sentiments.[23] This competition, of course, becomes an especial concern for most law students; it is seen as reducing their chances either of getting jobs in established law firms or of successfully setting up new practices. A few law entrants (11 per cent) are already assured of jobs in the firms of relatives or friends. But for the rest, students, professors, and the firms which will hire the students alike agree that acceptable jobs may be hard to find.

In consequence, compiling a good scholastic record takes on added importance for law students. Notices of employment opportunities on law school bulletin boards frequently announce that openings are limited to students in the top quarter or fifth of their class. Good grades are of course also desired by many medical students, who see them as opening up opportunities for internships in top-ranking hospitals. But, as Table 11 shows, they are not as likely to be considered of singular importance. The medical and law entrants, when asked how their teachers would rate a number of factors in "making a good doctor" or "a good lawyer," agree

[23] This difference, too, may help explain why fewer law students find law their only satisfying career: if they see the field as a highly competitive one in which they may not be able to succeed, they may of course desire to keep open other career possibilities. In addition, many of these students anticipate that success in law may require distasteful ethical compromises: fully 37 per cent agree that "competition among lawyers is so intense that even among those who would like to be scrupulously ethical many have to compromise to earn a living."

closely on every factor with the exception of grades. To these the law entrants attribute substantially more importance.

A more nearly inherent characteristic of the legal profession may also underlie law entrants' anticipation of greater competition in the school. It has often been said that dispute and conflict are, in a double sense, an intrinsic part of American law. As Professor Llewellyn has written, the basic "business of law" is to deal with these elements:

> Our society is honeycombed with disputes. Disputes actual and potential; disputes to be settled and disputes to be prevented. . . . Disputes call for somebody to do something about them. . . . This doing of something about disputes, this doing of it reasonably, is the business of law.[24]

And the disputes are settled by disputation; our courts make use of an adversary system in which justice and truth are considered to be best served by "the open fires of controversy" between opposing counsel. In two senses, then, lawyers must deal in forms of competition. In medicine, on the other hand, the only *inherent* conflict, in terms of professional principles, is with disease. In their relations with each other, doctors are *expected* to cooperate, not to compete. Thus, as a reflection of the nature of the two professions, law entrants may well expect to find an appropriately contentious atmosphere in law school, and medical students a more cooperative one in medical school.

THE SHIFT FROM COLLEGE TO PROFESSIONAL SCHOOL

It is apparent from the foregoing that the move from college to professional school has quite different meaning, at least in anticipation, for medical students than for law students. From their reports on competition, brought together in Table 12, we note that medical students, taken as a whole, anticipate a decrease in the level of competition after their entrance to medical school. Perhaps this reflects a feeling on the part of students that, though competition will of course continue into professional school, they are "over the hump": they have already won out in the competition to enter medicine. Although their success in obtaining pres-

---

[24] K. N. Llewellyn, *The Bramble Bush: Some Lectures on Law and Its Study* (New York: Columbia University Press, 1930), pp. 2–3.

TABLE 12. Amount of Competition Experienced in College and Expected in Professional School

	Percentage of students answering "a great deal" of competition	
	Medical students	Law students
Reported from college	49	18
Expected in professional school	35	83
No. of students	(124)	(248)

tigeful internships may depend in part on their standing in school, their future as members of the profession should not, since neither flunking out of school nor subsequent struggle for a livelihood is likely. Law entrants, by contrast, now anticipate a very sharp increase in competition, having encountered little in college. They believe, it appears, that only marked success in law school can insure them a place in the legal profession, and that most of their classmates will also be striving for top ranking; with the first year of school expected to prove decisive, competition during that year receives a strong impetus.

Since competition is seldom a matter of indifference to the competitors, it is natural that students, perceiving the competitive situations in which they are engaged, might well react to them with feelings of concern. In this connection, the two groups were asked how much they had been "concerned, as an undergraduate in college, about how well you were doing in comparison with the other students in your courses," and also, in like vein, about the coming year in professional school. As Table 13 demonstrates, the medical students on the whole expected to make the transition from college to professional school without increased concern. The law students, however, anticipated considerably increased pre-

TABLE 13. Concern with School Standing Experienced in College and Expected in First Year of Professional School

	Percentage of students answering "deeply concerned"	
	Medical students	Law students
Reported from college	13	14
Expected in professional school	13	40
No. of students	(124)	(248)

occupation with their performance. This result, if hardly surprising, can perhaps be further clarified. Concern for something may have two aspects: it may involve a deep and serious interest, and it may also involve worry. Our previous analysis suggests that law entrants might have special reason for increased concern in both these regards. Insofar as they expect their standing in the first year to have exceptionally important consequences, they may plan an even more serious devotion to their studies than do medical students. And if they anticipate greater competition from fellow students, they have reason, perhaps, to be more worried.

Thus, entrance to law school is viewed by students, in some ways at least, as a sharper break with the past than is entrance to medical school. In consequence, more of the law students are preparing for accommodation to a significant change. Asked whether they thought they were "going to have to make definite adjustments during your first year" of professional school, 32 per cent of the law entrants anticipated a great deal of adjustment, as compared with 15 per cent of the medical entrants. And 41 per cent of the law entrants expected to find these adjustments difficult, against 14 per cent of the medical group. As this paper is written, continuing analysis indicates that law students' expectation of increased competition is, as we might expect, the predominant source of their anticipation of greater over-all adjustment. A comparison of students' expected adjustment to other unfamiliar features of law and medical school, once the effect of differing levels of competition has been discounted, is also in progress.

SUMMARY

Typically, the decision to enter medical school is made much earlier than the decision to enter law school. Three factors appear to contribute to this difference: course requirements for admission to medical school are more extensive than those for admission to law school, medical entrants have had more contact with representatives of their future profession, and physicians have higher standing in the community and larger incomes than lawyers.

As they enter professional school, far more medical students than law students have picked out a role model in their profession to emulate. They are also more likely to feel that the profession they have chosen is the "only career that could really satisfy" them. Though the medical entrants' earlier decisions enter into these differences, other factors, similar in fact to those which affect the time of decision, also appear to be involved.

Medical entrants report a more competitive atmosphere surrounding their undergraduate studies than law entrants, but the law entrants are considerably more likely to anticipate sharp competition in the first year of professional school. These differences are tentatively traced to variations in the undergraduate situations of the two groups, contrasting admissions policies in the two types of professional schools, differing emphasis on the importance of grades, and dissimilar features of the two practicing professions.

Patricia L. Kendall and Hanan C. Selvin

TENDENCIES TOWARD SPECIALIZATION IN MEDICAL TRAINING

Within the last decade, the number of medical specialists in this country has greatly increased. According to Deitrick and Berson, the number of physicians certified by various specialty boards more than tripled between 1940 and 1951, and, during the same period, the number of residencies designed to provide specialized training more than doubled.[1]

To what extent has this trend reached down to medical students? One may speculate on at least two answers to this question. Because the trend has apparently had such far-reaching consequences for the medical profession as a whole, one might expect that even entering medical students, the extreme novices of their field, would have felt its influence. Such is likely to be the case in most professional fields where an older tradition of practice has been replaced by a newer one. For example, it is difficult to conceive that present-day students of architecture develop an interest in functional design only after giving up an earlier interest in ornate styles of the Victorian period. If the trend toward specialization has had this kind of uniform influence on all levels of professional candidates, then we should expect to find that intentions to specialize, to add oneself to the trend, so to speak, will be ex-

---

[1] John E. Deitrick and Robert C. Berson, *Medical Schools in the United States at Mid-Century* (New York: McGraw-Hill Book Company, 1953), pp. 276–277 and *passim*.

pressed as frequently by entering as by graduating medical students.

But quite the opposite is also possible. The trend toward specialization has had important influences on the medical profession; but it also has had a relatively short history. For this reason, it may have had little impact on the students who are entering medical school today. Their desires to become physicians may have been influenced by older conceptions of medical practice; and the practitioners whom they took as their models are likely to have come from the older tradition. In this case, we should expect entering medical students to show relatively little interest in specialization, and to modify their attitudes only gradually as they learn more about the profession for which they are training themselves.

Because both of these possibilities seem plausible, we cannot tell, in advance of studying the intentions of medical students, which fits the actual situation better.

THE TREND TOWARD SPECIALIZATION

There are a number of ways in which we might go about the task of deciding between these alternative possibilities. One way is to consider the plans which medical students have for their later careers, to see whether, as they advance through medical school, they are more and more likely to say that they plan to enter specialty practice. In the not too distant future, every medical student must reach some decision about his later career; and, if he plans to become a practitioner (as the very large majority do), general practice and specialty practice are the major alternatives open to him.[2]

Or we may consider a more concrete indicator of the student's

[2] It is important here to indicate that there seem to be two parallel trends in modern medical training and practice which, at first glance, might appear to be contradictory. On the one hand, there is a trend toward *increasing* specialization, in the sense that, at the present time, more young physicians receive intensive training in a particular field of medicine. At the same time, however, there seems to be a beginning trend toward *decreasing* specialization, in the sense that physicians are urged to assume greater responsibility for their patients, and to serve them as family physicians.

Specialization, in the context of the present paper, refers to the kind of training which is sought and received, and not to the kinds of functions which the physician serves or to the sorts of responsibility which he may assume.

long-range plans—the kind of internship experience he wants to obtain. Nearly every medical student is required to take an internship when he has completed medical school, regardless of his plans for his later career. Usually, however, he has a certain degree of latitude in deciding what kind of internship to apply for.[3] He may seek a rotating internship in which, typically, he divides his time between four different fields (such as medicine, pediatrics, surgery, and obstetrics and gynecology). Or he may apply for a more specialized internship in one of the fields of medicine. The obvious advantage of a rotating internship is that it provides varied training and experience; the correlative disadvantage is that the training obtained in any particular field, while usually adequate, is necessarily limited. Because of this, some major teaching hospitals do not offer rotating internships, and some will not award residencies to students who have served such internships. As a result, the expressed desire to obtain a rotating internship may be taken as an approximate index of the intention *not* to specialize, or of the postponement of that decision.[4]

Actually, as it turns out, it makes little difference which of these career orientations one chooses to examine. For, at least at Cornell University Medical College, from which the data reported here were collected, the same general result is found whether one looks at the kind of training the student hopes to obtain following his graduation from medical school or at the kind of practice he expects to establish in the future. Stated most simply it is this: most students enter Cornell Medical College with intentions *not* to specialize, and only modify these intentions gradually during the course of their training.

With regard to their plans for their later careers, each of the students was asked the following question: "When you have finished your formal medical training (including work beyond your M.D.) to what type of professional activity do you expect to give most of your working time?"[5] Table 14 compares the answers given by different classes of medical students.

[3] A major exception is the state of Pennsylvania which requires students intending to practice in that state to serve rotating internships.

[4] Deitrick and Berson say of rotating internships that they are "designed to train (the student) for general practice." (*Op. cit.*, p. 266.)

[5] This question was asked in May 1952. Answers to a second part of the question,

TABLE 14.   Plans for Later Careers, According to Class in Medical School

Expect to devote most of working time to:	Percentage in each class			
	First year	Second year	Third year	Fourth year
General practice	60	56	39	16
Specialty practice	35	41	56	74
Other (teaching, research, etc.)	5	3	5	10
No. of students*	(75)	(73)	(82)	(76)

* A few students in each of the classes failed to answer this question correctly or at all, and were therefore excluded from consideration here.

The differences are indeed quite striking. Well over half the first year students, but less than a fifth of those about to graduate, said that they expected to go into general practice. At the other extreme, only slightly more than a third of the beginning students, as contrasted with fully three-quarters of the graduating class, told us that they expect to practice some specialty.[6]

The same general pattern shows in comparing internship preferences of the first three classes of medical students (Table 15).[7] Although no other type of internship is sought nearly as frequently, there is a marked decrease, from the earlier to the later stages of medical school, in the number of students expressing a preference for rotating internships. (These, as we recall, usually suggest an intention not to specialize.) And there is a correlative increase in

---

dealing with the kinds of professional activities to which the students would *prefer* to give most of their working time, reveal the same general pattern, although in somewhat less dramatic fashion.

[6] This question was also asked of students at the University of Pennsylvania School of Medicine and at Western Reserve School of Medicine, with virtually the same results. For example, in May 1955, 59 per cent of the first-year students at the University of Pennsylvania, 52 per cent of the second-year students, 35 per cent of those in their third year, and 29 per cent of those about to graduate said that they expected to give most of their professional time to general practice. The comparable figures from Western Reserve, in May 1955, are 51 per cent, 51 per cent, 35 per cent, and 26 per cent for the first to fourth years, respectively.

[7] These data also come from the first administration of our questionnaire, in May 1952. The question on internship choices was not asked of the graduating students, for they had already received their internship assignments. For reasons which are beyond the scope of this paper, the internship preferences of students at the University of Pennsylvania School of Medicine and at Western Reserve School of Medicine cannot be directly compared with those expressed by students at Cornell Medical College.

TABLE 15. Internship Choices, According to Class in Medical School

	Percentage in each class		
Type of internship	First year	Second year	Third year
Rotating	72	59	49
Straight medical	10	17	18
Straight surgical	5	1	10
Straight pathology	—	3	1
Mixed medical and surgical	11	11	13
Obstetrics and gynecology	—	1	2
Straight pediatrics	1	3	5
Other	1	5	2
No. of students	(79)	(76)	(83)

the number choosing internships in medicine, surgery, pediatrics, and other specialized fields.[8]

Cross-sectional analyses of the kind reported in Tables 14 and 15 sometimes involve a difficulty which can never be completely settled without the assistance of additional data. This is the problem that observed differences between the classes, which are attributed to various levels of training, may in fact be due solely to differences in the composition of the several groups. As noted earlier, panel techniques have been developed to cope with this kind of difficulty. These involve the successive observation of the same group of individuals at different points in time. In the present instance, instead of comparing the preferences which different classes have expressed at the same time, we compare the preferences which the same students have expressed at different times.[9] If the same trend is noted when such panel analysis is carried out, then greater confidence will attach to the finding.

Exactly one year after expressing the preferences recorded in Table 15, some of the same students were again asked what kind of internship they would like to obtain. Table 16 summarizes the

[8] As a matter of fact, of the factors which we have investigated, stage of training stands almost alone as an important determinant of internship plans. As we shall see later, for example, the students' cumulative grades have no discernible influence on the preferences which they express: good students are no more likely than less capable ones to say that they hope to obtain specialized internships.

[9] This kind of analysis also makes it possible to identify the individuals who have changed their preferences. Later on in this paper we shall exploit this possibility, and begin to analyze what kinds of students are most likely to shift in one direction or another.

TABLE 16. Changes in Internship Choices (May 1952—May 1953)

Type of change	Percentage
Consistent preference for *rotating* internship	39
Shift from *rotating* to *specialized* internship	25
Shift from *specialized* to *rotating* internship	9
Consistent preference for *specialized* internship	27
No. of students	(150)

changes—and consistencies—in their choices.[10] First of all, it is quite apparent that most of the medical students in these two classes maintained a consistent preference during the one-year interval between their two interviews. Some 39 per cent said on both occasions that they hoped to obtain rotating internships; an additional 27 per cent expressed a consistent preference for a more specialized internship.[11]

But a second, and perhaps more important, point concerns the *direction* of change among those who did not make the same sorts of choices in the two interviews. Table 16 indicates clearly that changes in internship plans usually involve a shift from a general toward a more specialized kind of training. Among the students in these two classes who did change, some three-quarters shifted from rotating to more specialized internships; only one-quarter made the opposite kind of change. Adding the first two figures, we see that at the time of the first interview, 64 per cent of these students expressed preferences for a rotating internship; adding the first and third figures shows us that at the time of the second

[10] Table 16 is based on only two classes of medical students—those who were first- and second-year students at the time of the first interview, in May 1952, and who had advanced to the second- and third-year classes by May 1953. The exclusion of the other classes is easily explained: the class of 1952, who were fourth-year students at the time of the first interview, left the medical school shortly after that time. The class of 1953, who were third-year students in the first panel wave, had received their internship assignments by the time of the second interview and therefore were no longer in a position to express their preferences. The class of 1956, who were first-year students at the time of the second interview in May 1953, had entered the medical school the previous fall, and therefore were not available for interviewing in May 1952.

[11] By combining all of the specialized choices into one category, the actual amount of observed change is somewhat underrated. If only *identical* choices are classified as consistent preferences (and not shifts from one specialized field to another), then it develops that 51 per cent of the students remained constant.

interview, about one year later, only 48 per cent hoped to obtain such general training. This is a restatement of the panel result in a form comparable with Table 15.

This series of findings points to a trend among the students of this medical school at least. As they advance through the school, they become increasingly interested in specialized training and in specialty practice. It is almost as if each of these students were experiencing, on an individual level, the kind of change which has been taking place in the medical profession as a whole. And because this trend is not at all an obvious or self-evident one, it requires considerable exploration.

Two kinds of explanations are needed. On the one hand, we must make an effort to understand why it is that beginning students in this medical college seem to have much less interest in specialization than do more advanced students, or than they themselves have at later stages of their training. On the other hand, we must try to find out what happens to these students during the course of their studies so that, by the time they are ready to leave medical school, most are interested in receiving specialized training. Attempts to answer these questions will occupy the remainder of this paper.

Before turning to that task, however, we must make a decision. The two questions—the one on later career plans and the other on internship choices—can be used interchangeably, first, because both yield the same general results, and second, because they are substantially correlated with each other.[12] Therefore, to make

[12] The extent of this correlation is shown in the following table:

| Later career plan | Percentage distribution internship choice | | |
	Rotating	Specialized	Total*
General practice	40	13	53
Specialty practice	20	27	47
Total	60	40	100

* This table is based on 219 students. Seven students, with miscellaneous plans for their later careers, have been excluded from consideration. Two-thirds of these students—the 40 per cent who said that they wanted to take a rotating internship and then go into general practice and the 27 per cent who said that they wanted to take a specialized internship and then enter specialty practice—gave consistent answers to the two questions. To this extent, then, the answer to one of the questions indicates the answer to the other as well.

our analysis as economical as possible, and to avoid unnecessary repetition, one should be chosen to stand for both. Now, each question has distinct points in its favor. On the one hand, the question regarding later career plans is a relatively direct measure of the kind of attitude with which we are concerned—interest in specialization. But it has the disadvantage of referring to the more or less distant future; and we know from other studies that the more remote a decision, the less likely it is to have received serious thought.[13] As a result, the answers which medical students give to such a question on later career plans may, in some cases, be almost perfunctory.

The alternative question, that on internship choices, has the disadvantage that it is only an indirect measure of the attitude with which we are concerned here; we can only infer that preferences for a rotating rather than a specialized internship are more indicative of an intention not to specialize. At the same time, however, the question possesses a unique advantage. Two of the classes in the medical school, a total of approximately 160 students, were followed from the end of the third to the end of the fourth year. (Actually, one of these classes was observed periodically from the end of the second year through graduation.) In addition to knowing the kinds of internship preferences which they expressed at the end of their third year, therefore, we also know what assignments they actually received. And, as we shall see later, this collateral information adds an entirely new dimension to our analysis. We can begin to study how many, and what kinds, of students obtained assignments which were different from their earlier preferences; and we can also begin to explore the processes by which such changes came about. These possibilities are so promising that they seem to outweigh whatever disadvantages the question has. For the balance of this paper then, we shall concentrate our attention on internship preferences.

We turn first to the question of why beginning medical students are so much less interested in specialization than are their colleagues in the more advanced classes.

[13] A relevant study, from a very different field, dealt with decisions to purchase automobiles. A report on this study, carried out by Elmo Roper and associates, will be published in a volume on panel analysis, now in preparation at the Bureau of Applied Social Research.

BROAD INTERESTS AND THE AVOIDANCE OF
PREMATURE COMMITMENTS

One important reason why so many beginning medical students
express a preference for the most general, all-encompassing kind
of internship is that they do not want to commit themselves yet
to any particular field of medicine. They have not yet had sufficient experience to judge whether they are more interested in internal medicine than in pediatrics, or more skilled in surgery than
in psychiatry. They avoid a premature decision by making plans
to obtain an internship which can give them experience in virtually
all of these fields. The comments of a first-year student, made
shortly after his entrance into medical school, are relevant in this
connection. He was asked which special fields in medicine attracted him, and he replied:

> Fields in which there's great personal contact—general practice,
> maybe, or pediatrics, because I like kids a lot, or psychiatry, because
> I don't have to use my hands, for one thing. [Have many of your
> classmates crystallized their ideas about the medical sub-fields which
> interest them?] *Don't get me wrong—I haven't either.* I used to be
> asked that question a lot of times before I came here—what field I
> was interested in—and I'd usually flare up at that. *I'm certainly not
> in a position to know yet.* Maybe I'm making judgments on a false
> basis. *I won't really be qualified to judge until we get into the spe-
> cialties in the third and fourth years.*

Had this first-year student been asked what kind of internship he
hoped to obtain four years hence, he might very easily have answered that, at that point, a rotating internship seemed most ap-
pealing to him.[14] This illustrates what is meant by the tentative

[14] There is some suggestion (though little more than an intimation) in the opening phrases of this comment—that he is most interested in those fields of medicine
which involve "great personal contact"—that beginning students enter medical
school with the conviction that they want to have sustained and intimate contact
with their patients, a conviction which may become less strong in time. Some support for this is found in the answers to an item in the questionnaire. Members of
all classes in the medical school were asked, "Would you prefer a patient who
wants to know you only on a doctor–patient basis, [or] one who wants to know
you also on a friend-to-friend basis?" The answers given by the different classes
indicate that it is the less advanced students, those in their first or second year of
medical school, who feel that it is possible and appropriate to have their patients
as friends: 47 per cent of the first-year students, 46 per cent of those in their second
year, 29 per cent of the third-year, and only 19 per cent of the fourth-year students
said that they would like to know their patients on a friend-to-friend basis as well
as professionally.

assumption that, in the early years of medical school at least, selection of a rotating internship may indicate "suspended judgment" regarding fields of specialization which may later prove attractive, rather than a complete lack of interest in specialization.[15]

Furthermore, it is fairly likely that first-year students do not have a very clear idea of what one actually does during his fifth year of training, let alone of what the alternative types of internships consist. In other words, he may as yet know little about his own interests and talents and equally little about the specialized training available to meet such interests.

This first hypothesis pertains to beginning students and the reasons why they start out in medical school saying that they want to obtain broad and general experience in their internship assignment. We now turn our attention to advanced students, to consider why it is that they become progressively more oriented toward specialized training and specialty practice.

INTEREST IN SPECIALIZATION AND RECOGNITION
OF MEDICAL COMPLEXITIES

What leads so many of these medical students to abandon their early interest in general, comprehensive training, and to turn instead to specialized fields? A full answer to this would, of course, be premature. But part of the answer seems to be their growing appreciation of the complexity of modern medicine, and increased awareness of their inability to master all of these complexities personally.

Medical students may genuinely want to receive as broad and general training as possible, and they may preserve this desire throughout their stay in medical school. But as they are introduced successively to internal medicine, to surgery, to psychiatry, and to other specialized fields, they may develop awareness of the virtual impossibility of achieving equal competence in all fields, and may therefore feel compelled to select one branch of medicine

---

[15] This points to an interesting methodological problem, namely, that the choice of a rotating internship appears to have different implications in different social contexts. It is our assumption that, in the later phases of medical training, the selection of this kind of internship represents a positive decision, while in the earlier phases it represents, in many cases, a way of avoiding any decision.

in which to concentrate. A first-year student shows the beginnings of such awareness in his reactions to an exhibit of clinical projects which he visited. He reported in his diary:

> Well, the rest of this day was almost lost to other subjects than medicine. I did take advantage of an opportunity to view some of the project exhibits at the Alumni meeting—but most of the projects were over my head and the head of the first-year student. They were primarily clinical exhibits. *Yet they did point out in a striking fashion how completely variegated the field of medicine is, and how absolutely impossible it would be for one person to be a specialist in everything.* That old axiom of "the more you know, the more you know you don't know" holds quite true here.

Although this student did not understand much of what he saw, he did come away from the exhibit with a greater appreciation of the complexity of medicine, and perhaps with a greater sense that he would need specialized training.

A more advanced student, in the early months of his third year of medical school, was quite explicit in stating how his own study experiences led him to better understanding of why, as he put it, "specialization is the rage today." His diary entry for one Sunday in October reads as follows:

> I slept late until noon and then got up to eat lunch. At 1:00 I returned and debated what I should review. Since tomorrow is the last day on Pediatrics, I decided that I would review everything that I had learned during my 5½ weeks there. This took the whole afternoon and part of the evening until 9:30. I decided that I had learned quite a bit during the 5½ weeks, but nothing even resembling what I should know as a bona fide pediatrician. This seems to be one of the faults of the third year—we're learning so much very quickly; yet we wish we knew even more than is possible during such a short time, *since we feel very inadequate in Pediatrics even at the termination of the course. I can see why specialization is the rage today. Medicine is so large now that a doctor doesn't feel confident unless he knows at least one field extremely well, rather than just a little about all subjects.*

What is significant in this student's comment is that his sense of inadequacy and personal limitation, developing as a result of his own learning experiences, led him to appreciate increasingly the value of and need for specialized training.

And finally a fourth-year student made it quite plain that, in his view, it would be difficult for anyone aware of his own limitations to feel comfortable as a general practitioner. As he put it in an interview:

> In general I'd say [students going into general practice] are a more easy-going group. They're not sloppy. But, by Jove, they have to be easy-going! That's why there are some people going into general practice whom I can't visualize in it—like A. S. for example. If he does finally decide on general practice, I think he's going to be pretty uncomfortable in it. *Because an extremely conscientious man who is aware of his limitations is bound to be uncomfortable in general practice.* ["When does such 'awareness of limitations' begin in medical school?"] I would say when graduation becomes imminent—early in the fourth year—when I left Obstetrics, for instance, and realized that this would not only be all the obstetrics I'd be taking here, but that my limitations in obstetrics were thereby defined. . . . In the second year, for instance, you don't think much about limitations . . . *you realize that there are a lot of things you don't know now, but you have the feeling that this will come in time.*

Of particular interest is the last part of this comment. This student suggests that he and his classmates become progressively aware of the limitations of their knowledge and training during the course of medical school.[16] And the underlying implication is that, as such awareness developed, so did a parallel uneasiness about going into general practice.

So far we have described the trend toward specialization, using internship choices as our approximate indicator, and have considered how this trend might be explained. We put forth the notion that beginning students know too little about their interests and capacities to commit themselves regarding specialization, while more advanced students know too much about their limitations *not* to develop specialized interests.

Internship preferences pertain only to the first three classes in medical school. During their fourth year students apply for and receive the internship assignments which they will actually have in the year following their graduation. This fact provides us with an entirely new kind of data, and raises new questions. First, we

[16] For a fuller discussion of this point, see Renée C. Fox, "Training for Uncertainty," in this volume.

shall want to see whether the trend toward specialization, found in the internship *preferences* of first-, second-, and third-year students, is accelerated or arrested when actual internship *assignments* are made. Secondly, we shall want to explore the kinds of influences which have bearing on these internship assignments. Up to this point, our provisional hypotheses have been stated largely in terms of the individual student's maturation and development. As we shall see, the internship assignments which graduating students receive seem to be determined, to a degree not true of earlier internship preferences, by influences from faculty members in the medical school.

SPECIALIZED INTERNSHIPS AND FACULTY INFLUENCE

If the trend discernible in internship choices were continued through the period in which actual assignments are made, one would expect a considerable majority of the graduating students at Cornell to seek and to receive specialized internships. But this is not the case. Although a majority of the fourth-year students do end up with specialized internships of one kind or another, it is actually a somewhat smaller number than had expressed preferences for such internships at the end of their third year in school. In line with the trend noted earlier, we find here that 20 of the 71 students who had expressed a preference for rotating internships at the end of their third year ended up the following March with specialized assignments. But what we had not observed before (compare with Table 16) is that the trend in this direction is counterbalanced—even slightly outweighed—by a trend in the opposite direction. Of the 91 students who had originally said that they hoped to obtain specialized internships, 27 ended up with rotating assignments.

TABLE 17. Internship Assignments Compared with Third-Year Preferences of Same Students

Actual assignments in fourth year	Third-year preferences		
	Rotating	Specialized	Total
Rotating	51	27	78
Specialized	20	64	84
Total	71	91	162

The reason for this is that the trend toward specialized interests is not, as the evidence up to this point would suggest, a simple one. When the final commitments must be made, when the students must make calculations about where their best chances lie and the faculty must decide which students to recommend for what kinds of internships, then a selective process is set in motion. Under these conditions, some students who have already developed an interest in specialized internships reverse the trend and end up with an assignment to a rotating internship. The starting point in our efforts to demonstrate how this selectivity operates is a fact mentioned earlier, namely that, by and large, there is no relationship between performance in medical school, as graded by the faculty, and the internship preferences which are expressed. This fact can be documented in a number of ways. For the present purposes, it is most convenient to show that, at the end of their third year, high-ranking students were almost as likely as low-ranking students to say that they hoped to obtain rotating internships.[17]

As Table 18 shows, at the end of the third year in medical school, there is little linear relationship between class standing and internship preferences. Although the bottom students, those in the fourth quartile, were most likely to say that they would like to take a rotating internship, the top-ranking students, those in the first quartile, were almost as much attracted to the same general kind of training. And quartile differences in the two major kinds of specialized internships—in medicine and surgery—are neither large nor consistent. This finding is consonant with the notion that the trend toward specialized interests affects all students equally up until the fourth year.

Quite a different picture emerges when we examine the situation a year later, when we consider the relationship between class standing and the *actual* internship assignments which these students received. As Table 19 indicates, a consistent and marked relationship is then observed.

Here, then, is a definite relationship. Approximately one-third of the top-ranking students received rotating internships, while,

[17] The same result is found when we examine the first- and second-year classes. Among those students too there is no consistent relationship between the internship preferences which they express and the grades which they have received in medical school.

TABLE 18. Third-Year Internship Preferences, According to Cumulative Grades

Internship choices	Percentage in each quartile			
	Top quartile	Second quartile	Third quartile	Bottom quartile
Rotating	49	35	36	56
Straight medicine	22	26	18	15
Straight surgery	7	9	10	8
Other specialized (pathology, pediatrics, obstetrics and gynecology, etc.)	22	30	36	21
No. of students	(41)	(43)	(39)	(39)

TABLE 19. Actual Internship Assignments, According to Cumulative Grades

Internship assignments	Percentage in each quartile			
	Top quartile	Second quartile	Third quartile	Bottom quartile
Rotating	32	43	51	71
Straight medicine	41	33	18	7
Straight surgery	12	14	18	12
Other specialized (pathology, pediatrics, obstetrics and gynecology, etc.)	15	10	13	10
No. of students*	(41)	(42)	(39)	(42)

* Minor discrepancies in the sizes of the quartile groups from one table to another are due to the fact that the composition of the classes changes somewhat from year to year, and also that, in any one year, a few students will fail to answer questions asked on our questionnaire.

in contrast, more than twice as many of the lowest-ranking students were assigned to this general kind of training. And the picture with regard to medical internships is just the opposite. Less than one in ten of the fourth-quartile students, but nearly six times as many of those in the first quartile, had received internships in internal medicine. Furthermore, the relationship is consistent. From the top to the bottom quartiles, there is a steady increase in the proportion of students assigned to rotating internships, and a steady decline in the percentage who were going to serve their internships in internal medicine. The result of Table 18 was consistent with the conclusion that, through the first three years of medical school, the trend toward specialization is a simple one, affecting students on all academic levels equally; in contrast,

FIGURE 10. Coincidence of Actual and Preferred Internship, According to Third-Year Choices and Cumulative Grades

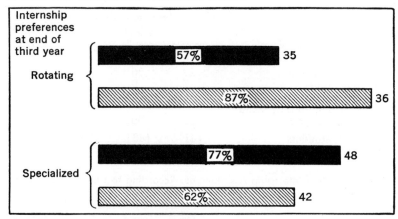

Students who received kind of internship preferred at end of third year:

In upper half of class ■   In lower half of class ▨

Note: Numbers to right of bars indicate students.

the finding of Table 19 is consistent with the notion that, after that point, actual internship assignments are highly selective.

The full picture is obtained when these three variables—third-year internship preferences, actual internship assignments, and cumulative grades—are considered simultaneously. This results in a panel finding, and reveals the changes which took place in *individuals* rather than in whole quartile groups.

What does Figure 10 show? Stated most simply, it is this: good students, those in the upper half of the class, were most likely to end up with the kind of internship they wanted when, at the end of their third year, they had expressed a preference for specialized internships. Among these good students, over 75 per cent of those who had chosen specialized internships, but less than 60 per cent of those who had selected rotating internships, received the kind of assignment they had wanted. Exactly the reverse was true of the lower-ranking students. Those in the bottom half of their class were most likely to end up with the kind of assignment they wanted when they had expressed a preference, at the end of their third year, for rotating internships. Within that group, 87 per cent of those who had chosen rotating internships, but only 62 per cent of those who had expressed a preference for specialized training, received actual assignments which coincided with these earlier preferences.[18]

We must be somewhat speculative about the mechanisms through which this selectivity operates, because the materials at hand do not offer more than slight clues. One thing which seems clear, however, is that, by and large, the selection takes place between the end of the third year of medical school and the *middle* of the fourth, *before* formal internship applications have been submitted.[19] It does not often happen at Cornell that a high-ranking student who has applied for a rotating internship is denied this request and assigned, instead, to a specialized internship. Nor, which is perhaps more surprising, does it often happen that a low-ranking student who has applied for a specialized internship is turned down in his request, and instead given a rotating assignment. Evidence for this is the fact that, with few exceptions,

---

[18] The findings of Figure 10 have broader implications than is immediately apparent. If we try to state the finding in a more general form we might say that the preferences (or intentions) of individuals are more likely to be predictive of final behavior when these preferences (or intentions) are consistent with the modal pattern of the groups to which the individuals belong. We know from Table 19 that it is typical for good students to end up with specialized internships, while it is typical for lower-ranking students to end up with rotating internships. Figure 10 reveals that third-year internship preferences were most likely to be realized in actual internship assignments when these preferences coincided with the most probable outcome for the quartile group to which the individual belonged. Among the good students who, as a group, were most likely to end up with specialized internships, preferences for such specialized training stood a better chance of being realized in actual assignments than did preferences for the general training of a rotating internship. Among students in the lower half of their class who, as a group, were most likely to receive rotating internships, the selection of such general internships was more apt to be fulfilled than the selection of specialized internships.

Exactly the same sort of finding appears in quite different contexts, especially in voting studies. An empirical generalization with some stability is that Catholics are more likely than Protestants to vote for Democratic candidates. If one conducts a panel study, one finds that Catholics are most likely to carry out their early voting intentions if these intentions were to vote for Democratic candidates, while Protestants are most likely to carry out their early intentions if these intentions were to vote for Republican candidates. See Bernard Berelson, Paul F. Lazarsfeld, and William McPhee, *Voting* (Chicago: University of Chicago Press, 1954), p. 283.

[19] The deadline for filing internship applications comes in January of the final year of medical school. Actual assignments are made known in March.

medical students receive the *kind* of internship they finally ask for, even though they may not always be selected to intern in the *hospital* of their first choice. In one of the classes being considered here, 64 of the 82 graduating students received their first choice internships. Only 8 of the remaining 18 (most of whom received their second choices) were not assigned to the kind of internship which they had asked for. In other words, approximately 80 per cent of this class were chosen to intern in the field and in the hospital which they had designated as their first choice; over 90 per cent were chosen to intern in the field which they had applied for. To be sure, some students did not receive the kind of internship they asked for. But this seems to happen in only a few cases which have not been effectively filtered through prior screening processes.

There are two kinds of selective processes to be sought. One of these must explain how it happens that low-ranking students finally decide not to apply for specialized internships in as large numbers as do high-ranking students; the other must explain how it happens that high-ranking students decide not to apply for rotating internships in as large numbers as do the lower-ranking members of their class.

To explain why it is that the low-ranking students are less likely than the high-ranking students to end up with specialized internships, we must remind ourselves that there is considerable competition for the best internships—particularly for the specialized internships in large, prestigeful hospitals. Now, although the students in Cornell Medical College do not know their exact standing in their class, they do know in which quartile they rank. They can therefore estimate their chances of obtaining a desirable internship. Those in the upper half of the class can generally count on getting good recommendations from the dean and faculty of the medical college, and favorable comparison with graduates of other medical schools. Those in the bottom half of the class cannot be so sure of either of these advantages.

But the students need not rely only on their own estimates of their chances. It is customary at Cornell that fourth-year students, before submitting their formal internship application, discuss their plans with a member of the faculty or with an administrative officer. During the course of these discussions, students may be discouraged from some of the plans which they have developed, and encouraged in others. For example, a low-ranking student may be advised not to apply to a hospital which normally receives so many applications that it can select only top-ranking students.

As a result of these self-estimates, corrected or reinforced by discussions with faculty members, when the day of crucial decision approaches, low-ranking students seem to scale down their intentions to meet the probable reality; and, as we saw in Table 19, the reality for most of the students in the bottom half of the class is a rotating internship.

Our materials do not contain any systematic evidence on this adjustment of aspirations, as it might be called, at least so far as it involves the selection of a rotating, instead of a specialized, internship. However, a conversation between two students during the fall of their fourth year suggests that decisions to enter one specialty rather than another are sometimes based on the same kind of anticipatory scaling-down of preferences which, we provisionally assume, explains in large measure why so many of the students in the bottom half of their class decide to apply for rotating internships. This conversation took place after a session in which the students, along with an instructor, had discussed the examination in third-year medicine which they had taken the previous spring:

A: You know, it's very strange . . . when I took that exam last spring, I was the first one finished and out of the room. That never happened to me before. I read it very fast—half-read it, in fact—and got done very early. At first I thought I'd done well. But as the week wore on, I began to realize some of the terrible things I'd done. By the end of the week, I repressed the exam completely, and I hadn't thought of it since—until today. *This exam probably ruined my chances with Dr. G.*

B: I went through it quickly too, thinking it was the kind of exam where, if you don't know the right answer immediately, it wouldn't do you much good to think too hard about it. But the exam wasn't written that way. *I did well, but I don't think that improved my chances with Dr. G. any.*

A: Are you interested in medicine?

B: No, pediatrics.

A: Then it's not too important.

B: *Well, I would have been interested in medicine if I'd thought I had a chance.* I was ambivalent about it actually. But I talked to the people on pediatrics and on medicine both; *I felt them out. And I got the impression that I was better liked on pediatrics than on medicine.*

This conversation illustrates the process by which a number of low-ranking students feel impelled to apply for rotating internships. Student B would have liked to go into internal medicine; but through a subtle probing of judgments of significant faculty members, he decided, rightly or wrongly, that he was more likely to get good recommendations and support from physicians in the Department of Pediatrics. He therefore decided to shift his interests to the field in which, he felt, he had better chances of success.

Actually, this student modified his preferences still further when it came to choosing an internship—he was assigned a rotating internship at a hospital not closely connected with a university.

High-ranking students presumably engage in the same process of appraising their chances. But, if they are realistic, they know that there is a good probability that they will end up with the kind of internship which they want. Why, then, do so few receive rotating internships, even among those who several months previously had said that they wanted this type of internship? The answer seems to be that they are given strong encouragement by the faculty to apply for specialized internships.

Even though the Cornell student is not necessarily taught explicitly to develop specialized interests, there are diverse tendencies which propel him in that direction.[20] Indeed, the student's development of a specialized orientation may be as much a part of his indoctrination in medical school as is his acquisition of certain technical skills and knowledge. He may start out with a strong desire to serve a rotating internship; but he may subsequently learn that New York Hospital, the teaching hospital associated with his medical college, considers such internships relatively poor preparation for a residency, and therefore does not offer them;

[20] One important question is the extent to which the findings reported in this paper would be duplicated in another kind of medical school, one for example, which considers its primary objective to be to turn out well-trained general practitioners.

as a result, he may gradually lose his original interest and develop new preferences.[21] He may have come to medical school with the firm conviction that he will work as a general practitioner; in medical school, however, he probably has little opportunity to see, at first hand, what general practice is like; his clinical instructors, and the other physicians with whom he comes in contact, have all received highly specialized training; taking them as his models, he may gradually revise his original plans and intentions. In the larger profession as a whole he sees that the physicians who receive acclaim are again those who are either highly specialized in some limited area, or who have made some contribution in a specialized field.

It appears that high-ranking students are particularly sensitized to this general atmosphere in the medical school, for they, particularly, are encouraged to recognize the positive value of specialization in modern medicine. In some cases, members of the staff express their values in the judgment that a rotating internship is less desirable than a specialized one, and they may respond in terms of these values when they learn of the plans of a high-ranking student to apply for a rotating internship. In contrast, the high-ranking student who expresses a preference for a specialized internship will, on occasion, receive support and encouragement from the faculty. Consider, for example, the experience of one top-ranking student who planned to take his internship in internal medicine; he reported the following conversation with a faculty member whose opinion he greatly respected:

> After we had seen the patient and decided on his disposition, Dr. F. lowered his voice and said to me, "What do you intend to do after medical school?" I told him internal medicine, and he said "Good!" *So far as I am concerned, this is a big fat pat on the back,* and I don't know whom I'd rather have it come from. . . . *It is nice to know that Dr. F. approves of me.*

In other words, the high-ranking student at Cornell who maintains an interest in a rotating internship must to some extent go counter

[21] The staffs of Cornell Medical College and of New York Hospital distinguish between specialized training and the practice of narrow subspecialties. They believe that medical candidates should proceed through an internship in a specialized field and through the several levels of residency training, but should then devote themselves to broad and general practice within the field of their specialty. This is related to the trend noted earlier (see footnote 2 above) calling on physicians to assume greater and more comprehensive responsibility for their patients.

to the expectations and advice of the faculty and administration, while the good student who has already developed specialized interests receives support and encouragement.

SUMMARY

We have found that, as they proceed through Cornell Medical College, students are increasingly likely to express an interest in specialized training. Several hypotheses were offered to account for this trend. It was suggested, first of all, that one of the reasons why so many beginning students say that they would prefer to receive general training is that, as yet, they know so little about their own capacities or the requirements of various specialties; their preference for a rotating internship is thus a way of avoiding a premature commitment on their part.

To explain why it is that more advanced students express a preference for specialized training, we set forth a second hypothesis. We suggested that, as these students learn more in medical school, they come to recognize both the vast complexities of modern medicine and their own limitations in being able to cope with all of these complexities effectively. As a result of this new-found awareness, they feel compelled to select a particular field in which to develop their competence.

When we came to examine the actual internship assignments received by fourth-year students at Cornell, then the trend observed in the first three years was no longer so apparent. In fact, the number of graduating students who received specialized assignments was actually somewhat smaller than the number who had said, at the end of their third year, that they hoped to obtain such specialized training. To explain this we offered a third hypothesis. We set forth the notion that, to some unknown degree, the staff of Cornell Medical College, both directly and indirectly, influences the decisions which these fourth-year students make before actually submitting their internship applications. We suggested that low-ranking students who indicated a preference for a specialized internship might be discouraged from actually applying for one, while, correlatively, high-ranking students who expressed interest in such specialized training might receive encouragement and support from the staff.

Part III

Processes of
Attitudinal Learning

INTRODUCTION

Medical educators are paying increasing attention to the processes whereby students acquire attitudes and values in keeping with the role of physician. It is now widely recognized that students learn more than medical facts, techniques, and concepts: they come to have particular ways of thinking about themselves, their patients, and their profession. Physicians and educators have often commented insightfully on their own experiences and those of students whom they have observed, but little in the way of systematic knowledge of how attitudes are learned in medical school is now available. The following papers, still provisional and representing only the first phases of ongoing research, all bear on this question.

By the time they leave medical school, most students can hear themselves addressed as "Doctor" without feeling any qualms about their right to the title. Not so, of course, four years earlier. The first paper, by Mary Jean Huntington, deals with these self-images and analyzes some of the processes by which students, in some cases even as early as their first year, come to feel that they are acting out the doctor's role and hence to define themselves as doctors. In part, of course, the development of a professional self-image as a doctor is a function of the actual distance from the M.D. degree. But it is also a response to particular experiences in medical school. It is the identification of some of these experiences which Huntington takes as the central problem of her paper.

In addition to modifying their attitudes about themselves, medical students also acquire particular attitudes toward patients over

177

the course of their training. From instructors they may learn that some patient-oriented attitudes are considered more appropriate than others; from their own experience they may learn that their attitudes affect their ability to work effectively with patients. The second paper, by William Martin, is concerned with one of these patient-oriented attitudes—the affective neutrality of students toward the type of patient with whom they are called upon to deal. It is assumed, to start with, that advanced clinical students will fulfill their role most ably, and will derive most gratification from it, when they have no strong preferences about different kinds of patients. The central problem here, as in Huntington's paper, is to isolate some of the factors and experiences that lead to such neutrality.

Just as students develop new self-images and attitudes toward patients as they pursue their medical studies, so they also acquire attitudes toward the field of medicine as a whole. The final paper in this section, by Renée C. Fox, deals with an important orientation among these—a developing awareness and acceptance of uncertainties in medicine. To the layman it may seem that the primary purpose of medical training is to replace the uncertainties of the acknowledged novice with the certainties of a mature physician. But this is not the case. As Fox points out, there are various kinds of uncertainty that every practicing physician encounters. The process of becoming aware of these and learning to accept them is gradual, extending over the four years of medical school. In this paper once more, the central concern is to identify some of the experiences that contribute to this learning process and enable medical students to cope with the uncertainties of which they are made aware.

The three papers in this section make use of different sorts of data. Those by Huntington and Martin are based almost entirely on the questionnaires, with Huntington focusing on first-year students and Martin on fourth-year students. In contrast, Fox's paper is a qualitative analysis. It is based entirely on her observations of medical students at different stages in their training, on the journals which a number of medical students kept for the purposes of our study, and on intensive interviews focused on the experiences that students had in institutionally patterned situations.

Mary Jean Huntington

THE DEVELOPMENT OF A
PROFESSIONAL SELF-IMAGE

Interest in some of the processes through which medical students come to regard themselves as doctors stems in part from consideration of the importance of a fully developed professional self-image in later medical practice. Presumably, the physicians who consistently feel and think like doctors are able to carry out the doctor's role more effectively than those who have not fully incorporated such a self-image. Thinking of themselves as doctors may help practitioners maintain confidence in their capacity to deal with difficult medical tasks. This, in turn, probably reduces the amount of personal strain they might otherwise experience in conforming to the exacting obligations of their professional role.

If defining themselves as physicians enables practitioners to perform their work more easily, it is useful to investigate how a professional self-image first develops. This paper will discuss some of the first phases in the gradual transformation of young neophytes, who define themselves as students, into physicians able to identify themselves fully with their professional role.

CHANGES IN SELF-IMAGES

It is of course evident to all that students typically think of themselves primarily as students at the beginning of their medical training and come progressively to think of themselves as doctors as they advance through medical school. Students at three medical schools[1] were asked: "In the most recent dealings you have had with patients, how have you tended to think of yourself, primarily as a doctor rather than as a student, or primarily as a student rather than as a doctor?" A substantial minority of students in the first two years of training, approximately 30 per cent, reported that they felt primarily like doctors; by the end of the third year, 59 per cent indicated that they felt more like doctors, and just prior to graduation, this proportion had increased to 83 per cent. These figures are shown in Table 20.

TABLE 20. Self-Images in Dealing with Patients, According to Class in Medical School

Class in medical school	Percentage of students who thought of themselves "primarily as doctors"	No. of students*
End of 1st year	31	(162)
End of 2nd year	30	(159)
End of 3rd year	59	(752)
End of 4th year	83	(759)

* Percentages are based on the aggregation of two classes of first-year students, and two classes of second-year students at Western Reserve University School of Medicine, and on eight combined classes of third-year and of fourth-year students at Western Reserve, University of Pennsylvania School of Medicine, and Cornell University Medical College—all of whom were asked the question stated above.

The central fact of this progression of self-images scarcely requires explanation. But these figures also exhibit a collateral pattern which is not self evident: an appreciable number of students report that they felt more like physicians than students while still in their early years of training. What, then, accounts for this fact that some students and not others see themselves primarily as doctors as early as the end of their first year of medical school?

SELF-IMAGES AND ROLE SET

In the course of their first-year studies, medical students have sustained contact with persons holding other statuses within the medical school and, occasionally, in the teaching hospital: other students, faculty members, nurses, and patients.[2] The relationships students have with persons in each of these statuses are by no

[1] See footnote, Table 20 for details.
[2] Many of the current innovations in medical school curricula are changing the relationship of students to those in some or all of these statuses.

means identical. Patients, for example, obviously differ from faculty members in their images and expectations of medical students. And, in turn, these expectations diverge from those of classmates or of nurses. Such a complex of role relationships which persons have by virtue of occupying a particular status has been described as their *role set*.[3]

Because they find themselves in situations calling for widely disparate attitudes and behavior, students *at any one stage in their training* tend to think of themselves now as students, now as physicians, as they work in diverse social contexts.

The first-year student who thought of himself as a doctor while in contact with his instructors or classmates is clearly the rare exception. The tendency is somewhat more common in relation to nurses, and most marked in connection with patients. The second column in Table 21 suggests one explanation of the "unstable" self-image held by students at a single point in their medical training, for there is a consonance between the status that students believe others in their role set assign them and the status to which students assign themselves.[4] This tendency for individuals to live up to the role expectations of those with whom they are interacting and to come to perceive themselves in accordance with these expectations has long been recognized but little investigated.[5] The evidence in Table 21 and other material to be presented below lend support to this proposition.

Fully aware that they are just beginning their medical training, first-year students when interacting with classmates think of each other primarily as students. This is reflected in their self-definitions. When students interact with instructors, furthermore, the disparity between their own competence, experience, and status, and those of faculty members is apparent to both.

The data concerning nurses and patients require a word of

[3] The concept of role set has been formulated by Robert K. Merton, *Social Theory and Social Structure* (Glencoe, Ill.: The Free Press, 1957, rev. ed.), pp. 368–384.

[4] Of course, it would be of even greater value to obtain independent reports from individuals in the other statuses. Interviews with patients before and after being examined and treated by student–physicians are now being analyzed by Lois Pratt of the Cornell Comprehensive Care and Teaching Program. Research is also being conducted on faculty members' images of students.

[5] See Charles H. Cooley, *Human Nature and the Social Order*, rev. ed. (New York: Charles Scribner's Sons, 1922), pp. 183–185; and George Herbert Mead, *Mind, Self, and Society* (Chicago: University of Chicago Press, 1934), pp. 138–139.

TABLE 21. Self-Images and Attributed Images of First-Year Students in Diverse Role Relationships

In their dealings with:	Percentage who thought of themselves as doctors*	Percentage who thought others defined them as doctors*
Faculty	2	2
Classmates	3	0
Nurses	12	8
Patients	31	75
No. of students	(162)	(162)

* Percentages are based on the aggregation of two classes of first-year students at Western Reserve University School of Medicine. The percentages in column 2 are based on answers to the following question: "In your recent dealings with (patients, classmates, instructors, nurses), how have they thought of you, by and large, primarily as a doctor rather than as a student, or primarily as a student rather than as a doctor?"

explanation about the special circumstances of the first-year student at Western Reserve School of Medicine. Every student is provided with the opportunity of having patient contacts early in his first year. Each is assigned a family to follow during his first year and preferably through all four years of medical school. This serves to introduce students to the patient–physician relationship, and allows them to act in a role approximating that of physician, although it of course involves only limited responsibility in helping a family cope with health problems that might arise. In the assigned families, the wife is pregnant, but there is no serious or long-standing history of medical, emotional, or social pathology.[6] Students are expected to *observe* their patients during the course of pregnancy, the delivery, and the early growth and development of the child. These continued observations in the hospital and in the home of the family provide students with early clinical experience which is correlated with didactic instruction by clinical preceptors.

When students see their assigned patients in the hospital, they are acting out some limited aspects of the role of physician while nurses are acting in their professional role as a member of the medical team. Nurses tend, in such a situation, to expect of students the behavior appropriate to physicians. In conforming to

[6] For some indications of the problems that may arise when this criterion is not in effect, see Mary E. W. Goss, "Change in the Cornell Comprehensive Care and Teaching Program," in this volume, pp. 251–254.

these expectations, so far as their medical student status allows, first-year students—about 12 per cent of them—begin to think of themselves more as doctors than as students.

PROFESSIONAL SELF-IMAGE VIS-A-VIS PATIENTS

It is vis-à-vis patients, more than with any other status in their role set, that medical students even as early as the end of their first year of training tend to see themselves as physicians. Some 31 per cent of the students reported this self-image. However limited the medical knowledge of first-year students, and they are usually aware that it is severely limited, it is, in general, considerably greater than that of the patients with whom they have contact. Moreover, the fact that students partly serve in the capacity of physician leads some patients to assign them the status of doctor. To the extent that patients define students as doctors and expect them to conform to the behavior appropriate to that role, students are likely to act as if they were doctors.

Thirty-nine per cent of the 117 first-year students who thought that their patients regarded them primarily as doctors also thought of themselves primarily as doctors, whereas only 6 per cent of the 35 first-year students who thought that their patients regarded them primarily as students thought of themselves as doctors.

Self-images appear, then, to be in part "reflections" of the expectations of others. As students are defined by their patients, so do they tend to define themselves. But we are on less than firm footing with this inference, because it is not based on reports from patients. The data might be interpreted in quite another way: as students define themselves so do *they think* patients define them. Other data in hand permit a rough test of this second interpretation. The same students had been asked a year earlier, before they had actually entered medical school, whether they *expected* to think of themselves primarily as students or as doctors when they came to work with patients. This information provides a clue to the initial "definition of the situation"[7] with which students began their dealings with patients.

[7] The term, "definition of the situation," first introduced by William I. Thomas and Florian Znaniecki in *The Polish Peasant in Europe and America* (Boston: Richard G. Badger, 1918), Vol. 1, pp. 68–69, refers to the individual's prior conception of and attitudes toward a given situation that influence his behavior when he meets that situation.

These initial states of mind do not appear to have colored students' impressions of the image which patients have of them. Of those who expected to play the role of doctor, 78 per cent felt, a year later, that they had been so defined by patients; of those who expected to play the role of student, almost exactly the same proportion, 77 per cent, felt that they had been defined, contrary to their own expectations, as doctors.

At the same time, self-confirming tendencies do appear when anticipated and actual *self*-images are compared. The majority —51 per cent—of the 41 students who had expected that they would feel more like doctors reported at the end of the year that they so defined themselves, compared with only 24 per cent of the 111 students who had anticipated that they would feel more like students than doctors.

First-year medical students tend to maintain their expected self-conceptions; however, as we saw earlier, they are not immune to the cues furnished by the limited contacts they have with patients. When these two factors are considered simultaneously, it appears that the majority of students maintain their expected self-image throughout the first year. This was somewhat more marked if they felt that patients also perceived them in this role rather than in another role. Specifically, 78 per cent of the 58 students whose expected self-image corresponded to the image they felt patients had of them maintained the same self-image from the beginning to the end of the first year, whereas only 64 per cent of the 94 students whose expected self-image differed from the image they felt patients had of them maintained the same self-image throughout the year.

There is the further question of elements in the student's relationships with patients which promote the formation of one or another self-image. As was indicated earlier, at Western Reserve occasions arise even as early as the first year of medical school, where students put into effect some peripheral skills of the medical role. It is these types of occasions that will be considered.

In addition to observing patients during the course of pregnancy and the delivery and subsequent development of the child, students are expected to develop a sense of responsibility for the continuing care of their patients; if the mother or other family member needs medical attention at any time, the student is reached directly by the family and is expected to make the necessary arrangements for the patient to get appropriate medical care. The students do not of course practice medicine. They have only limited medical responsibility when dealing with patients, and their performance is closely supervised.[8]

Since each student has only one family to follow, this allows for fairly wide variation in the objective experiences students meet. By tracing the developing self-images of those who report different types of experiences with their families, we can begin to detect what it is in their first contacts with patients that facilitates a sense of growing doctorhood among some students.

Merely having a family assigned to them is hardly likely to help students feel like doctors—unless occasions arise in which they are called upon to exercise the obligations of their new role as quasi-physician. Aside from providing students with the opportunity to observe the medically interesting processes of pregnancy and birth and development of a child, certain families will not present distinct problems that require the further services of students. When this is the case, students may have little chance to establish ongoing relationships with their patients, and consequently, to perform their assigned role.

From all this we can understand why students who reported that no medical problems arose in their families were not as likely to think of themselves primarily as doctors as those whose families presented medical problems during the course of the year. This should be seen in perspective. After all, these are first- and second-year students and this overarching fact keeps the great majority of them from adopting an image of themselves as physi-

---

[8] At the beginning of their first year, students are given a set of instructions indicating what is expected of them in their contacts with the assigned family. The following statements are extracted from "Family Clinic Procedures, Syllabus, Phase I," Western Reserve University School of Medicine, pp. 1–2 and *passim*.

". . . the student must obtain a complete history, which is elicited through interviewing techniques. Since talking to a patient in the hospital setting usually gives one only a single facet of the patient, it is helpful to make observations in the home. . . . You will be expected, therefore, to make regular visits each month to see your patient in her home. . . .

"The patient usually turns first to the physician-in-training when any difficulty arises in the home. Here he can be of real assistance by getting help for the patient or for a member of her family."

cians. Nevertheless, differences in the run of experience with patients do appear to affect the formation of such self-images. Thirty per cent of the 129 first- and second-year students whose families had definite medical problems came to see themselves primarily as doctors, in comparison with a bare 5 per cent of the 22 students whose families did not present medical problems.

The opportunity to establish a quasi-physician–patient relationship and to test out one's ability in this role is not enough to lead most students to think of themselves primarily as doctors rather than students. The amount of difficulty they experience in handling patients further affects the formation of the self-image. For some students, the requirements of the assigned task may outrun their still very limited capacities in both the technical and the interpersonal spheres. Such experiences will probably impede their developing a sense of doctorhood. But where the task and their abilities seem to the students to be matched, they are likely to feel they have handled the situation well—not very differently from the way a doctor would. Even in the first year, fully 45 per cent of the 29 students who reported having had no difficulty in handling patients indicated that they felt more like doctors than students; this compares with 29 per cent of the 91 who had little difficulty and 25 per cent of the 32 who had a fair or considerable amount of difficulty in handling patients. (The question read: "From your own experience, how much difficulty would you say you have in handling patients?")

SUMMARY

As students move through medical school, they of course tend to develop an image of themselves as doctors rather than as merely students, especially in their clinical years when they have substantial contact with patients. We find that at each phase of their training, students' self-images tend to vary as they interact with faculty members, classmates, nurses, and patients, i.e., with persons in their role set who have varying expectations of them.

The relationships of students with patients were chosen for more detailed analysis of some of the factors facilitating the formation of a professional self-image in this social context. The professional relations of preclinical students at Western Reserve with families assigned to them provide a suitable set of materials, allowing us to isolate processes operating in student–patient relationships which are not readily distinguishable when students come to have wider experience with numerous patients. In accord with the hypothesis that individuals tend to develop a self-image which reflects the images others have of them, it was found that students who noted that their patients assigned them to the role of physician were more likely than other students to begin to think of themselves as doctors.

It was further found that, within this context, the requirements of the patient also affected the development of a professional self-image by the student. The opportunity to act in the role of quasi-physician facilitated the sense of growing doctorhood; specifically, those students whose families presented medical problems were more likely than others to think of themselves primarily as doctors rather than students. Furthermore, students who felt they handled the problems of their assigned families without difficulty showed a greater tendency to develop this professional self-image, even as early as the end of their first year.

Further inquiry is being directed to additional factors entering into the early development of the professional self-image. It will then be in order to find out how these self-images, developed early in the training period, affect the pace and character of students' subsequent learning in medical school.

William Martin

PREFERENCES FOR TYPES OF PATIENTS

This paper deals with the question of how medical students come to acquire attitudes which make it possible for them, with greater or less ease, to live up to one of the norms governing the physician's role.

The norm under study is the physician's obligation to provide appropriate care for *all* patients, whether young or old, of high or low social status, or with one or another kind of illness. Whatever his social or personal attributes, the patient should be given the medical attention he requires. *The Principles of Medical Ethics,* for example, incorporates the statement of Sir Thomas Watson, who expressed a well-established norm when he wrote in 1843 that medicine "dispenses its peculiar benefits, without stint or scruple, to men of every country, and party and rank, and religion, and to men of no religion at all."[1] Whatever the physician's likes and dislikes, he should accord interest and care to all his patients.

It would, of course, be easier for the physician to live up to this obligation if he liked every patient about as well as any other. If there are certain kinds of patients to whom he feels less favorably disposed, however, the physician may give them the proper amount of attention but will presumably experience some strain

[1] *Principles of Medical Ethics of the American Medical Association* (Chicago: American Medical Association, 1953), Ch. I, Sec. 2.

in having to work with them. He might eliminate this source of strain by neglecting the patient or discharging him, but the norm enjoins him not to do so. It would be easier to adhere to the norm if, in the first place, he did not have strong preferences for some kinds of patients over against others.

But a physician, like anyone else, can be expected to form likes and dislikes for those with whom he interacts. A physician might come to prefer those with whom he can most easily work, and the temptation might arise to avoid patients who make his task more difficult. He would thus feel more strain in living up to the obligation not to discriminate against any who seek help from him.

Serving in the capacity of junior physicians in their clinical years, medical students have substantial professional contact with patients. They too, presumably, find it easier to deal with all kinds of patients if they do not regard some as being preferable to others. They will probably be better prepared for the role of practitioner if they adopt, while in medical school, the attitude that it makes no difference what the attributes of the patient are—all patients should be taken in stride.

ATTITUDES TOWARD PATIENTS: PREFERENTIAL OR NEUTRAL

The following study deals with two successive fourth-year classes in the University of Pennsylvania School of Medicine and two in Cornell University Medical College, as well as one fourth-year class in the Western Reserve University School of Medicine. These consist of a total of approximately 500 students completing their fourth year of undergraduate medical training. These students were asked about their preferences concerning various characteristics of patients. As shown below, some of the questions pertain to the patient's type of illness; others, to his relationship with the doctor:

> Would you prefer a patient who is a close personal friend, a casual acquaintance, a complete stranger, [or does it make] no difference?

> Would you prefer a patient who asks for detailed explanations, accepts the explanations you give him without further question, [or does it make] no difference?

Would you prefer a patient who wants to know you only on a doctor-patient basis, wants to know you also on a friend-to-friend basis, [or does it make] no difference?

Would you prefer a patient whose illness is entirely physical, whose illness is chiefly emotional, [or does it make] no difference?

Would you rather be assigned a patient with positive physical findings who is beyond medical help, negative physical findings who can be helped, [or does it make] no difference?

Although it would also be of interest to compare those who prefer one type of patient with those who prefer another, our purpose is somewhat different—we shall compare students who *prefer any type of patients* with those who do not make such distinctions. On each set of alternatives, some students expressed a preference one way or the other, while others said they had no preference between the two. Moreover, it seems that students vary in the extent to which they *generally* tend to single out attributes of patients which they prefer. Some students, as Table 22 shows, expressed no preferences whatever, while others made a definite choice on all five.

This approximates a so-called normal distribution, which suggests that the questions differentiate students according to their preferential attitudes toward patients. Those at the upper end of the distribution appear to commit themselves to a preference for some patients over others, while those at the lower end tend to feel that any one type of patient is as desirable as any other.

We provisionally assume that students are expressing varied attitudes toward working with particular types of patients. Those with few preferences are apparently saying that, no matter what

TABLE 22. Extent of Student Preferences for Patients

No. of preferences expressed	No. of students	Percentage
0	54	11
1	81	16
2	98	19
3	120	24
4	87	17
5	69	13
No. of students	(509)	100

the varying courses of action involved in working with diverse kinds of patients, these make no difference in their evaluations.

Some of these differing courses of action can be seen by briefly examining the case of patients with primarily emotional rather than primarily physical illnesses. (This is the fourth item in the list; see page 191.) Compared with the patient with discernible physical illness, the emotionally ill patient requires the doctor to explore a wide array of possible organic disturbances, for he must guard against the failure to uncover a serious organic illness in the course of practicing an immature psychiatry. Further, the physician frequently must rehear the same account of diffuse symptoms, often from the lips of a distressed, anxious patient. And finally, it may not be clear what, if anything, can be done for the patient. As one fourth-year student puts it:

> It's very discouraging to try to work with such patients. They come in with aches and pains just about everywhere. So you have to do a long series of lab tests on them when you know that they've had at least six urines and six EKG's and six blood counts done already. You're obliged to do these tests for safety's sake. Not for the patient's safety so much, but for the doctor's. Because God help the doctor who misses out on an organic condition. . . . Well, after the lab tests come back, then you have the patient to put up with. He wants to come back time after time. And what he tells you gets boring after a while—the same complaints over and over. You know you're not accomplishing anything, except support maybe, and that gives you small satisfaction.

Interpersonal relations with such a patient take on a crucial character more often than would be the case with a patient having definite organic problems. A fourth-year student remarks:

> When you have an elderly lady with . . . an average of 3 bodily complaints per every square inch of bodily surface, that's very discouraging. In cases like that you have to gauge yourself not by measurements like the level of blood pressure or blood sugar, but by how the patient feels.

That is, the student finds himself compelled to rely primarily on the patient's reactions to decide whether or not he is accomplishing anything.

It comes as an instructive if not surprising fact that the choice between patients with physical or with emotional illnesses is so heavily weighted that almost no student *prefers* the latter; there are some, however, who maintain that they are equally willing to deal with either kind. Unlike the problems involved in working with emotional versus physical illnesses, the other clinical situations about which students were asked present more evenly balanced sets of alternatives, so that some students prefer one or the other type of patient—for example, the patient who asks for detailed explanations or the patient who accepts without question the physician's formulation. However, as we have seen, some students maintained an attitude of neutrality, no matter what the alternatives. It is this attitude, the tendency to be neutral rather than preferential, which is at the focus of this study.

Of course, "neutrality" may result in part from unawareness of what it means for the effective performance of the medical role to have one type of patient rather than another. But it is probable that, owing to their experience with patients, relatively few fourth-year students would be unable to perceive that such differential demands exist; that there are, for example, different types of problems in the performance of their role when dealing with a patient who has an emotional, rather than a physical, illness.[2]

It is therefore advisable to focus this inquiry upon the preferences of fourth-year students for various types of patients. For them, the response "it makes no difference" is not likely to mean "I can't see how the differences are relevant," as it well might for first-year students. Rather it seems to indicate the attitude, "there are differences, but I can accept one kind of patient as well as another." A further reason for studying fourth-year students particularly is that their preferences represent a cogent summing up of their clinical experience as undergraduates, consisting of actual contact with patients, formal presentation of clinical cases, and informal discussion of patients with other students, faculty, and staff.

---

[2] On a questionnaire administered at only one medical school, students were given the option of saying that they were unable to form an opinion on the kinds of patients they prefer. This response indicates inability to perceive differences among patients as relevant to the performance of the physician's role. In the preclinical years, when students have relatively little contact with patients, the average percentages reporting that they have no opinion on preferences among patients are 11 and 8 for the first- and second-year students, respectively. In the clinical years, these percentages are 4 and 6 for the third- and fourth-year students, respectively.

It can be assumed that by the end of the fourth year all students have seen about the same range of patients in the inpatient and outpatient services of a teaching hospital. Nevertheless, students react differently to this "reality situation," which is approximately the same for all.[3] Our major objective is to account for these differences in response to the same situation. More generally, our purpose is to shed light on the processes by which students acquire attitudes that facilitate or hinder meeting one of the norms governing medical practice; for if the students feel that no patient is distinctly preferable to any other, they can more easily fulfill the obligation to treat all patients with equal consideration. But to the extent that they have marked preferences and dislikes, having to deal with patients they dislike may exact a psychic toll.

PREFERENCES AND ROLE PERFORMANCE

When fourth-year students single out types of patients they would like or dislike treating, they are probably indicating that they can more successfully act out the role of physician with some rather than other patients. Students who express few preferences can be thought of as attesting that they can fulfill their role-obligations in good fashion with almost *any* type of patient. Before investigating the general import of this hypothesis, we shall consider an example of the way in which students' assessments of their ability to carry out a specific task influence their preferences for particular types of patients.

To return to the example cited before, the patient who has chiefly an emotional illness presents particularly difficult problems for the student–physician. Many of these problems are in the realm of the interpersonal relations between physician and patient. Sometimes, patients may not accept the physician's statement that there is nothing organically wrong with them. In the words of one student:

> If their bodily complaints are symptoms of neurosis, they will be dissatisfied. They question you—is this or that possible. They won't accept a diagnosis of being well. They are dissatisfied with your findings and are sure they are physically sick and need medicine.

[3] For a description of the "reality situation" of the fourth year at one medical school, see Renée C. Fox, "Training for Uncertainty," in this volume.

If the student–physician is to carry out his obligation to care for the patient, he must be able to retain his composure in the face of what he might regard as intransigence on the part of the patient.

Furthermore, with an emotionally ill patient, there is greater likelihood that the student will have to handle acute psychic distress, overt aggression, or other trying behavior of the patient. It is at this point that students' self-confidence becomes an important consideration.[4] This situation might present a problem to *any* student, but more so, presumably, to the student who does not feel sure that he can, in the normal course of events, cope with a situation of this kind. To the extent this is so, it can be hypothesized that students who *feel confident that they can perform the tasks of control and reassurance* will be more inclined toward "neutrality" between a patient with an emotional illness and one with a physical illness. Correlatively, students who are less confident of their ability in this respect will prefer to work with the kind of patient who creates less stress for them, that is, the patient with a distinctly physical illness. The more the student is confident of his skill in dealing with emotional problems, the less it is likely that he will prefer the physical to the emotional illness.

The evidence supports this conception. Students with a great deal of confidence in their ability to deal with a patient who has an emotional outburst[5] are in fact less concerned than others about whether their patients have physical or emotional illnesses. Among the completely confident students, 62 per cent have no preference between a primarily physical or primarily emotional illness, in comparison with only 32 per cent of those with little confidence (Table 23). The latter more often prefer patients with entirely physical illnesses with whom this problem is less likely to occur.

---

[4] Self-confidence refers to a judgment based on the matching of a self-perception and a standard. Standards represent "benchmarks" with which students compare their ability and performance. These benchmarks may be provided by the faculty, by classmates, or by students' own conceptions of the level of achievement appropriate to their stage of training. The student who judges his ability and performance in the light of the standard he has adopted and arrives at a favorable verdict has a high degree of self-confidence.

[5] The specific wording of this question is given on p. 197, below.

TABLE 23.   Attitude toward Patients with Physical or Emotional Illnesses, According to Confidence in Ability to Deal with Patients Who Have Emotional Outbursts

Type of patient preferred	Percentage according to degree of confidence		
	Complete	Moderate	Little or none
Entirely physical illness	32	50	68
Chiefly emotional illness	6	2	—
It makes no difference	62	48	32
No. of students*	(79)	(356)	(68)

* In this and all following tables, the few students who did not answer are omitted.

This example illustrates two points. (1) Students seem to experience, or learn from the experience of others, the fact that certain types of patients make it difficult to carry out particular requirements of the physician's role, such as the control of the doctor–patient relationship. (2) Some students are not fully confident of their ability to perform such a task as controlling patients' behavior, and therefore prefer to avoid the kinds of patients who put the greatest strain on this capacity.

This finding may be provisionally extended to this hypothesis: the wider the range of tasks students feel competent to perform, the less marked should be their tendency to prefer *certain types of patients to others*. There are, in fact, differences among fourth-year students in the range and extent of situations with which they feel able to cope. This was ascertained not by asking students about their degree of self-confidence in the abstract, but by summarizing their self-evaluations of ability to handle the following specific situations.

Being able to do a venipuncture without difficulty.

Deciding on appropriate medication and dosage.

Having a doctor as a patient.

Deciding what to tell a patient who has a serious and irremediable illness.

Knowing what to do in an emergency.

Having to tell a patient that the tests performed on him do not reveal the cause of his problems.

Making a diagnosis in a difficult case.

Preventing a patient from becoming embarrassed during a pelvic examination.

Dealing with a patient who has an emotional outburst of some kind.

For each of these problems, students indicated whether they felt "completely confident," "fairly confident," "not really confident," or "completely lacking in confidence." As Table 24 shows, a majority of students felt at least fairly confident of their ability to handle most of the problems.

Since the listed problems are not very difficult for fourth-year students, the distribution is markedly skewed. In contrast with the 48 per cent of *fourth-year students* who are relatively sure of their ability to manage at least 8 of the situations, only 26 per cent of one class of *third-year students* feel confident of handling as many problems. Nevertheless, even at the end of the fourth year, there is considerable variation among students in the number of problems they feel well equipped to handle. This variation, we have suggested, may account in large measure for differences among students in the tendency to be preferential toward patients.

Figure 11 shows that students who feel confident in most or all respects are less given to partiality in their attitudes toward patients than their classmates. In general, the higher the degree of confidence, the smaller the average number of preferences. (Some students, it will be recalled, expressed as many as five preferences; others, none at all.)

TABLE 24. Confidence in Ability to Handle Medical Problems

No. of problems which student is at least fairly confident he can handle	No. of students	Percentage
Only 1	1	—
Any 2	1	—
" 3	3	1
" 4	23	5
" 5	50	10
" 6	79	16
" 7	104	20
" 8	97	19
All 9	148	29
No. of students	(506)	100

FIGURE 11.   Mean Number of Preferences, According to Number of Problems Students Feel Confident of Handling

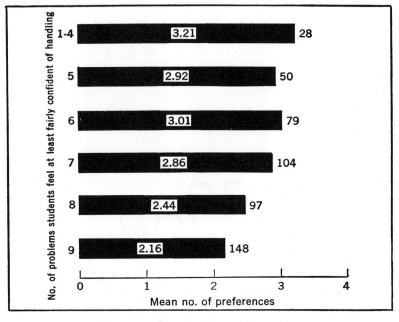

Note: Numbers to right of bars indicate students.

SELF-CONFIDENCE, AFFECT, AND PREFERENCES FOR PATIENTS

Preference for particular types of patients, we have suggested, in part reflects motivated avoidance of patients who make the performance of role-tasks difficult and stressful. However, fourth-year students are assigned to patients, and therefore have no opportunity to choose those who actually conform to their preferences. Under these circumstances, the level of gratification from patient contacts attained by students with preferences should be less than that attained by those who are equally willing to work with all types of patients, as Table 25 shows to be the case.

Although students may find it satisfying to work with patients who accord with their preferences, this seems to be outweighed by the necessity of dealing with others who do not. Furthermore, the expression of preferences for certain kinds of patients is evidently not a matter of casually held opinions, but derives from experiences that have had a marked impact. In dealing with cer-

TABLE 25. Amount of Satisfaction Derived from Patient Contacts, According to Number of Preferences

No. of preferences expressed	Percentage reporting great satisfaction*	No. of students
None or 1	64	(122)
2 or 3	55	(203)
4 or 5	44	(151)

* The question was: "How much satisfaction have you derived from the physician–patient relationships you have had during the current semester—a great deal, a fair amount, only a little, or none at all?"

tain patients assigned to them, students have on occasion become profoundly irritated, even though they well know Osler's precept of equanimity. It is of direct interest, then, to consider the types of students who are most vulnerable to this loss of detachment and the types of patients, "uncooperative" ones, most likely to evoke this response.

The concept of the "uncooperative patient" is deeply embedded in medical practice. In a study recently conducted in the outpatient clinic of a teaching hospital, for example, it was found that students, faculty, and other medical personnel could readily describe the uncooperative patient. As they formulated it, a patient is uncooperative "when he is stubborn," "when he won't recognize that help is being given to him," "when he refuses to accept his condition," or when he fails to appreciate the effort that has been expended on his behalf.[6]

Excerpts from the diary of a fourth-year student, describing a sequence of clinic visits by a patient whom he came to define as uncooperative, exemplify the process of losing a sense of professional detachment. (The italics are supplied.)

Monday, Dec. 7. [My patient] is a woman who has been followed for several months with globus hystericus. She is still bothered by this, but has noted some improvement in the frequency of attacks and feels that she is improving. This was only a brief interview most of which was devoted to learning her problem, and a little of her home and family life. *She is a very pleasant person*, tending toward hyper-

[6] Doris Schwartz, "The Use of Nursing Care Plans with a Group of Fifty Non-Conformist Clinic Patients," Cornell University Medical College, Comprehensive Care and Teaching Program Research Memorandum No. 2, Series B, December 1955. The definitions of uncooperative behavior given above are responses by medical personnel to the questions, "If the term 'uncooperative patient' is used in this clinic, of whom do you think? Why do you consider them uncooperative?"

activity. . . . *I have hopes that I may be able to continue her progress,* give her a little more insight into her problem and make her adjust to this entire situation.

Monday, Dec. 14. My usual patient visit for the morning with a 38-year old woman with globus hystericus. This woman is very unhappy about husband's lack of interest in her, etc. and wonders if she loves him. . . . I think that if I can relieve this doubt of her love for her husband, much of her anxiety may be relieved and in turn, her globus should improve.

Monday, Jan. 4. My other patient, the woman with the unhappy home situation and difficulty in swallowing returned. We talked about her home situation, nothing new! *I don't know how successful this therapy is going to be with this girl.* By that I mean I'm not too certain whether we will ever get this woman over some of her anxious moments. I mean I don't think she'll be cured completely.

Monday, Jan. 18. At 11:00 A.M. I had my weekly appointment with Mrs. B. and her problems. *This woman is beginning to get on my nerves.* She is a chronic complainer and in some instances shows very poor judgment in her relationships with her husband. I have tried to point out how she may show more interest in him, etc., but she's always not feeling well, or has some difficulty which prevents her doing as she knows she should. However, I realize that by letting her come weekly and ventilate, she seems to have achieved some measure of improvement.

Monday, Jan. 25. The other patient was my weekly revisit, who came in with a new raft of symptoms, worrying about what's going to happen next, etc. *I really have difficulty at times restraining myself* from telling this woman that she's far too concerned with herself, and in no uncertain terms. I shouldn't react like this and I would like very much to think that I have helped this woman but as soon as she is assured that one symptom has no organic basis she immediately digs up some new ones.

Monday, Feb. 15. Also saw my weekly revisit. . . . She still is over-reactive to any form of symptom and I think she'll continue to be. . . . *I look forward to the end of this period of treatment.*[7]

[7] As is evident from the above excerpts, this particular outpatient clinic provides opportunities for fourth-year students to follow the same patient for an extended length of time. We see, then, the development of strain in the student in considerable detail. Some of the problems peculiar to an extended relationship between fourth-year student and patient are discussed in Renée C. Fox, "Training for Uncertainty," in this volume.

By the time ten weeks had elapsed, this student was motivated to end the relationship with his patient. In the interim, he had become increasingly pessimistic about the prospect of bringing about marked improvement in the patient, he had been confronted by what seemed to him a never-ending stream of bodily complaints, and he had found himself faced with the serious problem of controlling his own affect. The student's detachment and confidence seem to have been closely interrelated in the gradual unfolding of this case; as the patient failed to conform to the normative expectations of the student–physician, both detachment and confidence diminished.

There is some statistical evidence to suggest that detachment and confidence in handling some kinds of uncooperative patients are related. Students who feel relatively unable to control the emotional outbursts of patients more often report irritation with some of the patients they have seen (Table 26).[8]

TABLE 26. Irritation with Uncooperative Patients, According to Confidence in Ability to Deal with Patients Who Have Emotional Outbursts

Degree of confidence	Percentage reporting irritation	No. of students
Complete	56	(48)
Moderate	62	(213)
Little	69	(39)

As we have seen, lack of confidence and lack of detachment seem to develop when students work with patients whom they define as uncooperative, that is, patients who do not conform to their expectations. Students may, on the one hand, come to doubt the adequacy of their ability to handle such patients. At the same time, they may feel some annoyance at patients whose behavior they consider deviant. Each of these reactions in turn, we have also seen, motivates students to avoid working with particular types of patients. Now it appears that when both reactions are present, they reinforce each other. Students who lack self-confidence with patients *and* have difficulty maintaining detachment

[8] Students were asked whether they agreed or disagreed with the following statement: "I sometimes became very irritated with patients who were uncooperative."

FIGURE 12.   Mean Number of Preferences, According to Confidence and
Irritation with Uncooperative Patients

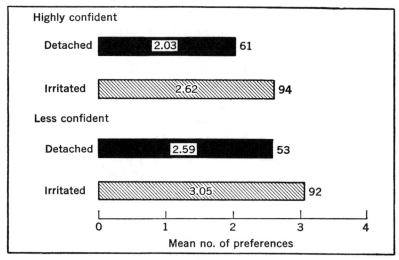

Highly confident:	Less confident:
Students who expressed confidence on any 8 or 9 problems	Students who expressed confidence on 7 or fewer problems

Note: Numbers to right of bars indicate students.

are most likely to prefer certain kinds of patients to others (Figure
12).

Students who were able to carry out their work with the least
strain, both confidently and without undue affective involvement,
also have the fewest preferences. Those who lacked both confidence and the ability to remain detached have the largest number of preferences. They are, it would appear, the least able to
work easily with all types of patients.[9]

[9] The doctor–patient relationship is, of course, a two-way affair. Our data tell
us only of the student–physician's perceptions of patients and reactions to them.
But the course of the interaction is also influenced by the patient's views of the
physician. This gives rise to further questions: what kinds of doctors do various
types of patients prefer? What behavior in physicians causes patients to become
affectively disturbed? Do patients feel differentially equipped to play the role of
patient, and does this influence their reactions to particular kinds of doctors? Investigation of how the patient views his visits with the doctor is currently under
way. See footnote 4, page 181.

SELF-CONFIDENCE AND FACULTY JUDGMENTS OF
COMPETENCE

Self-confidence refers to the way in which an individual judges himself. Since the clinical performance of students is rated by the faculty and expressed in the grades they give, the question naturally arises: to what extent do faculty judgments and self-judgments of students' performance agree?

The data show no relationship between degree of self-confidence of students and the fourth-year grades they received. As can be seen from Table 27, students who have relatively low average grades are about as confident of their abilities as classmates with high academic averages.

Among students in the top quartile, 28 per cent have high estimations of their ability to perform as a doctor should (Table 27). But as many (29 per cent) of those in the bottom quartile also feel quite confident. It is therefore not the case that self-evaluations correspond closely to the faculty's judgments as embodied in grades.

The reasons for this disparity are far from evident; they require further inquiry. At this time, two immediate possibilities suggest themselves. (1) The two measures, self-confidence and grades, may not be tapping the same dimension of performance, either because of differences in the skills taken into account or differences in the criteria used in measuring these skills. (2) Standards of excellence may differ among students and these may influence the manner in which they evaluate their performance. The standards

TABLE 27. Degree of Self-Confidence, According to Fourth-Year Quartile Standing

| | Percentage in each quartile | | | |
Degree of confidence	Top quartile	Second quartile	Third quartile	Bottom quartile
High (confident of ability to handle all 9 situations)	28	37	23	29
Moderate (confident of ability to handle any 7 or 8 situations)	39	36	47	38
Low (confident of ability to handle 6 or fewer situations)	33	27	30	33
No. of students	(130)	(126)	(124)	(124)

may be closely related to the individuals that students employ as standards in evaluating themselves. (It may make a difference whether the student takes members of the house staff of the teaching hospital as bases for comparison or personal friends in his own class.) Whatever the reason for the absence of a close relationship between faculty evaluations and students' self-perceptions of adequacy in dealing with patients, the fact that the disparity exists is an interesting and challenging one.

Moreover, fourth-year grades seem to have no bearing on the tendency of students to categorize patients as more or less desirable. As Table 28 suggests, students with high grades have as many preferences as students with lower academic *averages*.[10]

TABLE 28.   Mean Number of Preferences, According to Fourth-Year Quartile Standing

Quartile standing	Mean no. of preferences	No. of students
Top	2.65	(130)
Second	2.67	(126)
Third	2.50	(125)
Bottom	2.62	(126)

We have noted that students whose self-judgments of performance are quite favorable—who believe that they can manage many of the problems faced by the practicing physician—are more willing than the rest to work with all kinds of patients. It is now evident that those students who receive the most favorable judgments *from the faculty* are *not* more likely than others to hold this neutral attitude toward patients. It becomes clearer that it is not academic superiority as such that disposes a student to think of all patients as equally preferable, but the psychological *perception of himself* as a capable physician—a perception which apparently is not merely a reflection of judgments made by the faculty in the form of grades.

SUMMARY

We started with the assumption that students will be under less strain in providing uniformly good care for all patients if they feel

[10] Part of the explanation for this may be provided by the institutional fact that students are not ordinarily told their *precise* grades, but only their quartile standing. This allows some variability in students' perceptions of their places *within* the designated quartile; cf. page 210 of this volume.

equally willing to work with all. Their neutrality toward patients is fostered by confidence in their ability to perform many of the duties of the physician. Contributing further to this attitude of impartiality is the ability of students to remain detached even when patients behave in a way that is defined as uncooperative. Thus it appears that neutrality of fourth-year students toward several attributes of patients derives in large measure from their sense of having mastered certain core tasks of the physician's role.

Medical educators have long known that the physician must develop the attitudes and values appropriate to his calling if he is to provide optimum care of the patient. Sociologists have long known that a social role is best performed by those who satisfy the attitudinal as well as the technical requirements of the role. From the preliminary findings reported in this paper this concept seems to hold for the student–physician in his relation to the patient: students who feel best equipped to meet the technical demands of the role are also those who find it least difficult to meet its attitudinal requirements.

Renée C. Fox

TRAINING FOR UNCERTAINTY

"There are areas of experience where we know that uncertainty is the certainty."

—James B. Conant

Voluminous texts, crammed notebooks, and tightly-packed memories of students at Cornell University Medical College attest to the "enormous amount"[1] of established medical knowledge they are expected to learn. It is less commonly recognized that they also learn much about the uncertainties of medicine and how to cope with them. Because training for uncertainty in the preparation of a doctor has been largely overlooked, the following discussion will be focused exclusively on this aspect of medical education, but with full realization that it is counterbalanced by "all the material [students] learn that is as solid and real as a hospital building."

There is of course marked variation among students in the degree to which uncertainty is recognized or acknowledged. Some students, more inclined than others to equate knowing with pages covered and facts memorized, may think they have "really accomplished a lot . . . gained valuable knowledge," and that what they have learned is "firmly embedded and clear in their minds." Other

[1] Unless otherwise indicated, all the quoted phrases and passages in this paper are drawn from the diaries that eleven Cornell students at various points along the medical school continuum have kept for us over the course of the past three years; from interviews with these student diarists and some of their classmates; and from close-to-verbatim student dialogue recorded by the sociologist who carried out day-by-day observations in some of the medical school situations cited in this paper.

students are more sensitive to the "vastness of medicine," and more conscious of ignorance and superficiality in the face of all they "should know," and of all the "puzzling questions" they glimpse but cannot answer. Many students fall somewhere between these two extremes, half-aware in the course of diligent learning, that there is much they do not understand, yet not disposed "at this point to stop and lament." Discussion will be limited to the training for uncertainty that seems to apply to the largest number of students, admitting at the outset that inferences from the data must be provisional.

THE KINDS OF UNCERTAINTY THAT THE DOCTOR FACES

In Western society, where disease is presumed to yield to application of scientific method, the doctor is regarded as an expert, a man professionally trained in matters pertaining to sickness and health and able by his medical competence to cure our ills and keep us well. It would be good to think that he has only to make a diagnosis and to apply appropriate treatment for alleviation of ills to follow. But such a Utopian view of the physician is at variance with facts. His knowledge and skill are not always adequate, and there are many times when his most vigorous efforts to understand illness and to rectify its consequences may be of no avail. Despite unprecedented scientific advances, the life of the modern physician is still full of uncertainty.[2]

Two basic types of uncertainty may be recognized. The first results from incomplete or imperfect mastery of available knowledge. No one can have at his command all skills and all knowledge of the lore of medicine. The second depends upon limitations in current medical knowledge. There are innumerable questions to which no physician, however well trained, can as yet provide answers. A third source of uncertainty derives from the first two. This consists of difficulty in distinguishing between personal ignorance or ineptitude and the limitations of present medical knowl-

---

[2] It is not only the doctor, of course, who must deal with the problem of uncertainty. To some extent this problem presents itself in all forms of responsible human action. The business executive or the parent, for example, has no assurance that his decisions will have the desired results. But the doctor is particularly subject to this problem for his decisions are likely to have profound and directly observable consequences for his patients.

edge. It is inevitable that every doctor must constantly cope with these forms of uncertainty and that grave consequences may result if he is not able to do so. It is for this reason that training for uncertainty in a medical curriculum and in early professional experiences is an important part of becoming a physician.

An effort will be made to identify some experiences as well as some agencies and mechanisms in medical school that prepare students for uncertainty and to designate patterns by which students may gradually come to terms with uncertainty. In the initial inquiry we shall content ourselves with a general view of the sequence through which most students pass, but in a concluding section we shall suggest some variations that might be considered in further investigation of training for uncertainty.

THE PRECLINICAL YEARS

Learning to Acknowledge Uncertainty

The first kind of uncertainty which the student encounters has its source in his role as a student. It derives from the avoidance of "spoon-feeding," a philosophy of the preclinical years at Cornell Medical College (as at many other medical schools).

> You will from the start be given the major responsibility for learning [students are told on the first day that they enter medical school]. Most of your undergraduate courses to date have had fixed and circumscribed limits; your textbooks have been of ponderable dimensions. . . . Not so with your medical college courses. . . . We do not use the comfortable method of spoon-feeding. . . .[3] Limits are not fixed. Each field will be opened up somewhat sketchily. . . . You will begin to paint a picture on a vast canvas but only the center of the picture will be worked in any detail. The periphery will gradually blur into the hazy background. And the more you work out the peripheral pattern, the more you will realize the vastness of that which stretches an unknown distance beyond. . . . Another common collegiate goal is to excel in competition with others. . . . [But] because an overly-competitive environment can hinder learning, student ratings are never divulged [in this medical school], except to

---

[3] This particular sentence was taken from the "Address of Welcome to the Class of 1957" delivered by Dr. Lawrence W. Hanlon. Everything else in the paragraph quoted above is extracted from "Some Steps in the Maturation of the Medical Student," a speech delivered by Dr. Robert F. Pitts at Opening Day Exercises, September 1952.

the extent that once a year each student is privately informed as to which quarter of the class he is in.

From the first, the medical school rookie is thus confronted with the challenge of a situation only hazily defined for him. Information is not presented "in neat packets";[4] precise boundaries are not set on the amount of work expected. Under these conditions the uncertainty which the beginning student faces lies in determining how much he ought to know, exactly what he should learn, and how he ought to go about his studies.

This uncertainty, great as it is, is further accentuated for the beginner by the fact that he does not receive grades, and therefore does not have the usual concrete evidence by which to discover whether he is in fact doing well:

> In college, if you decide to work very hard in a course, the usual result is that you do very well in it, and you have the feeling that studying hard leads to good grades. You may tell yourself that you don't give a damn about grades, but nevertheless, they do give you some reassurance when you ask yourself if the work was worth it. . . . In medical school, there is no such relationship. Studying does not always lead to doing well—it is quite easy to study hard, but to study the wrong things and do poorly. And if you should do well, you never know it. . . . In my own case, I honestly think the thing that bothers me most is not the lack of grades, but rather the feeling that even after studying some in a given course, I always end up knowing so little of what I should know about it. . . . Medicine is such an enormous proposition that one cannot help but fall short of what he feels he should get done. . . .

Thus, it would seem that avoidance of spoon-feeding by the preclinical faculty encourages the student to take responsibility in a relatively unstructured situation, perhaps providing him with a foretaste of the ambiguities he may encounter when he assumes responsibility for a patient.

From the latter parts of the comment under review it would appear that the same teaching philosophy also leads to the beginning awareness of a second type of uncertainty: by making the student conscious of how vast medicine is, the absence of spoon-feeding readies him for the fact that even as a mature physician he will not always experience the certainty that comes with knowing "all

[4] Pitts, *ibid.*

there is to know" about the medical problems with which he is faced. He begins to realize that no matter how skilled and well-informed he may gradually become, his mastery of all that is known in medicine will never be complete.

It is perhaps during the course of studying Gross Anatomy that the student experiences this type of uncertainty most intensely. Over the centuries this science has gradually traced out what one medical student describes as the "blueprint of the body." As a result of his struggle to master a "huge body of facts," he comes to see more clearly that medicine is such an "enormous proposition" he can never hope to command it in a way both encompassing and sure:

> ... Men have been able to study the body for thousands of years ... to dissect the cadaver ... and to work on it with the naked eye. They may not know everything about the biochemistry of the body, or understand it all microscopically ... but when it comes to the gross anatomy, they know just about all there is to know. ... This vast sea of information that we have to keep from going out the other ear is overwhelming. ... There's a sense in which even before I came to medical school I knew that I didn't know anything. But I never *realized* it before, if you know what I mean—not to the extent that it was actually a gripping part of me. Basically, I guess what I thought before was, sure, I was ignorant *now*—but I'd be pretty smart after a while. Well, at this point it's evident to me that even after four years, I'll still be ignorant. ... I'm now in the process of learning how much there is to learn. ...[5]

As in this case, the student's own sense of personal inadequacy may be further reinforced by the contrast he draws between his knowledge and that which he attributes to his instructors. Believing as he does that "when it comes to the gross anatomy, they know just about all there is to know," he is made increasingly aware of how imperfect his own mastery really is.

There are other courses and situations in preclinical years which acquaint the Cornell student with uncertainties that result, not

[5] Such a felt sense that there will always be more to learn in medicine than he can possibly make his own, is the beginning of the medical student's acceptance of limitation. It might also be said that this same realization is often one of the attitudinal first signs of a later decision on the part of a student to enter a specialized medical field. This is of some relevance to the discussion of specialization by Patricia L. Kendall and Hanan C. Selvin, "Tendencies toward Specialization in Medical Training," in this volume.

from his own inadequacies, but from the limitations in the current state of medical knowledge. For example, standing in distinction to the amassed knowledge of a discipline such as Gross Anatomy is a science like Pharmacology, which only in recent years has begun to emerge from a trial-and-error state of experimentation:

> Throughout the history of pharmacology, it would appear that the ultimate goal was to expedite the search for agents with actions on living systems and to provide explanations for these actions, to the practical end of providing drugs which might be used in the treatment of the disease of man. As a result of many searches there now exist such great numbers of drugs that the task of organizing them is a formidable one. The need for the development of generalizations and simplifying assumptions is great. It is to be hoped that laws and theories of drug action will be forthcoming, but the student should at this point appreciate that few of them, as yet, exist.[6]

The tentativeness of Pharmacology as a science, then, advances the student's recognition that not all the gaps in his knowledge indicate deficiencies on his part. In effect, Pharmacology helps teach medical students that because "there are so many voids" in medical knowledge, the practice of medicine is sometimes largely "a matter of conjuring . . . possibilities and probabilities."

> When Charles was over for dinner last week, I remarked at the time that I was coming to the conclusion that medicine was certainly no precise science, but rather, it is simply a matter of probabilities. Even these drugs today, for example, were noted as to their wide range of action. One dose will be too small to elicit a response in one individual; the same dose will be sufficient to get just the right response in another; and in yet another individual, the same dose will produce hyper-sensitive toxic results. So, there is nothing exact in this, I guess. It's a matter of conjuring the possibilities and probabilities and then drawing conclusions as to the most likely response and the proper thing to do. And Charles last week agreed that a doctor is just an artist who has learned to derive these probabilities and then prescribe a treatment.

In Pharmacology (and in the other basic medical sciences as well) it is assumed that "laws and theories will be forthcoming" so that the uncertainties which result from limited knowledge

[6] Joseph A. Wells, "Historical Background and General Principles of Drug Action" in: Victor A. Drill, ed., *Pharmacology in Medicine* (New York: McGraw-Hill Book Company, 1945), p. 6.

in the field will gradually yield to greater certainty. However, the "experimental point of view" pervading much of early teaching at the Cornell Medical College promotes the idea that an irreducible minimum of uncertainty is inherent in medicine, in spite of the promise of further scientific advance. The preclinical instructors presenting this point of view have as a basic premise the idea that medical knowledge thus far attained must be regarded as no more than tentative, and must be constantly subjected to further inquiry. It is their assumption that few absolutes exist:

> If you were having a great deal of trouble finding some simple sort of cell in histology and you asked him about it, Dr. A. always made a point to give you information from the experimental point of view. He would (a) point out that this cell has five different names; (b) point out that this cell might actually be a ——— cell or a ——— cell that has undergone a transformation and that indeed, this cell might be able to change into almost anything; (c) also mention that even though the cell has five names, it may not, in fact, exist in the first place—perhaps it's just an artifact.

> Or, take the way the Bacteriology Department pushes the theme of "individual differences"—how one person will contract a disease he's been exposed to, while another one won't. The person may have a chill, or not; the agent may be virulent or not; and that determines whether pneumonia will occur or not. . . . "The occurrence, progression and outcome of a disease is a function of the offense of the microorganism and the defense of the host." That's the formula they keep pounding home. . . .

> . . . In the course of the demonstration of drugs affecting respiration, Dr. S. quoted Goodman and Gilman [a pharmacology textbook universally recommended and respected] as to the dramatic effect of one certain drug in respiratory failure. And then, they proceeded to show the falsity of that statement. So pharmacologists are now debunking pharmacologists! Heretofore they simply showed the drugs commonly used by many physicians had no effect. If this keeps up, we will all be first-class skeptics!

This is not to say, a student cautions, that we don't learn "a lot of established facts . . . tried and true things about which there is little or no argument." But in course after course during the preclinical years at Cornell, emphasis is also placed on the provisional nature of much that is assumed to be medically known. The experimental point of view set forth by his teachers makes it more apparent than it might otherwise be that medicine is something less than a powerful, exact science, based on nicely invariant principles. In this way, the student is encouraged to acknowledge uncertainty, and, more than this, to tolerate it. He is made aware, not only that it is possible to act in spite of uncertainties, but that some of his teachers make such uncertainties the basis of their own experimental work.

Up to this point we have reviewed some of the courses and situations in the preclinical years at Cornell which make the beginning student aware of his own inadequacies and others which lead him to recognize limitations in current medical knowledge. The student has other experiences during the early years of medical school which present him with the problem of distinguishing between these two types of uncertainty—that is, there are times when he is unsure where his limitations leave off and the limitations of medical science begin. The difficulty is particularly evident in situations where he is called upon to make observations.

Whether he is trying to visualize an anatomical entity, studying gross or microscopic specimens in pathology, utilizing the method of percussion in physical diagnosis, or taking a personal history in psychiatry, the preclinical student is being asked to glean whatever information he can from the processes of looking, feeling, and listening.[7] In all these situations, students are often expected to see before they know how to look or what to look for. For, the ability to "see what you ought to see," "feel what you ought to feel," and "hear what you ought to hear," students assure us, is premised upon "a knowledge of what you're supposed to observe," an ordered method for making these observations, and a great deal of practice in medical ways of perceiving. ("We see only what we look for. We look for only what we know," the famous Goethe axiom goes.)

Nowhere does this kind of uncertainty become more salient for medical students during their preclinical years than in Physical Diagnosis:

> Physical Diagnosis is the one course I don't feel quite right about. I still have a great deal of difficulty making observations, and I usually

---

[7] The physician is called upon to use his sense of smell and of taste on occasion, too, but not as frequently as those of sight, touch, and hearing.

don't feel certain about them. . . . Dick and I had a forty-year-old woman as our patient this morning. Though I thought we were doing better than usual at the time, we nevertheless missed several important things—a murmur and an enlarged spleen. . . .

"This sort of thing happens often in a course like Physical Diagnosis," the same student continues, and "it raises a question that gives me quite a bit of concern—*Why* do I have . . . difficulty making observations?"

There are at least two reasons for which a student may "miss" an important clinical sign, or feel uncertain about its presence or absence. On the one hand, his oversight or doubt may be largely attributable to lack of knowledge or skill on his part:

One of the problems now is that we don't know the primary clinical signs of various disease processes. . . . For example, today we suspected subacute bacterial endocarditis, but we didn't know that the spleen is usually enlarged, and as a result, we didn't feel as hard as we should have. . . .

On the other hand, missing a spleen, for example, or "not being sure you hear a murmur" is sometimes more the "fault of the field" (as one student puts it) than "your own fault." That is, given the limitations in current medical knowledge and technique, the enlargement of a spleen may be too slight, the sound of a murmur too subtle, for "even the experts to agree upon it."

The uncertainty for a student, then, lies in trying to determine how much of his own "trouble . . . hearing, feeling or seeing is personal," and how much of it "has to do with factors outside of himself." (Or, as another student phrases the problem: "How do you make the distinction between yourself and objectivity?")

Generically, the student's uncertainty in this respect is no different from that to which every responsible, self-critical doctor is often subject. But because he has not yet developed the discrimination and judgment of a skilled diagnostician, a student is usually less sure than a mature physician about where to draw the line between his own limitations and those of medical science. When in doubt, a student seems more likely than an experienced practitioner to question and "blame" himself.

His course in Gross Anatomy, it has been suggested, gives a Cornell student some awareness of his own inadequacies; Pharmacology emphasizes the limitations of current medical knowledge; and his training in observation, particularly in Physical Diagnosis, confronts him with the problem of distinguishing between his own limitations and those in the field of medicine. But in his second year his participation in autopsies simultaneously exposes the student to all these uncertainties. The autopsy both epitomizes and summarizes various other experiences which together make up the preclinical student's training for uncertainty.

Before witnessing their first autopsy, second-year students may, on occasion, sound rather complacent about the questions which death poses. For example, speculating on the causes of death, one group of Sophomores decided to their satisfaction that the cessation of life could be explained in simple physiological terms and that, armed with this knowledge, the doctor stands a good chance of "winning the fight" against death:

> We found that one very important matter could be traced back to one of two basic actions. The important matter—death. The two basic actions—the heart and respiration. For death is caused, finally, by the stopping of one of these two actions. As long as they both continue, there is life. . . . It's all a fight to keep the heart beating, the lungs breathing, and, in man, a third factor—the brain unharmed. . . . With all the multitude of actions and reactions which are found in this medical business, it seems strange and satisfying to find something that can really be narrowed down. . . .

But the conviction that death "can really be narrowed down" is not long-lasting. Only a short time later, commenting on an autopsy he had just witnessed, one of these same students referred to death with "disquietude" as something you "can't pinpoint" or easily prevent.

One of the chief consequences of the student's participation in an autopsy is that it heightens his awareness of the uncertainties that result from limited medical knowledge and of the implications these uncertainties have for the practicing doctor. This is effected in a number of ways. To begin with, the experience of being "on call" for an autopsy ("waiting around for someone to die") makes a student more conscious of the fact that, even when death is expected, it is seldom wholly predictable:

> In groups of threes, we all watch at least one autopsy—and my group is the third one in line. The first group went in for theirs this morning;

this means that ours may come any time now. You can't be sure when, though, so you have to stay pretty close to home where you can be reached. . . .

In other words, although ultimate death is certain, medical science is still not far enough advanced so that the physicians can state with assurance exactly when an individual will die.

Of even greater importance, perhaps, in impressing the student with the limitations of current medical knowledge is the fact that, although the pathologist may be able to provide a satisfactory explanation of the patient's death, the student usually finds these "causes of death" less "dramatic" and specific than he expected them to be:

> While our case was unusual, it was a bit of a letdown to me, for there was nothing dramatic to be pointed to as the cause of death. The clinician reported that the patient had lost 1,000 cc. of blood from internal bleeding in the G.I. tract. . . . Well, we saw no gaping hole there. There was no one place you could pinpoint and say: "This is where the hemorrhage took place." . . . Rather, it was a culmination of a condition relating to various factors. I suppose most causes of death are this way. But still . . . (though I'm not really sure why it should be) . . . it was somewhat disquieting to me.

A third limitation of the field is implied in lack of control over death. For example, the student observes that "the various doctors connected with the case being autopsied . . . wander in while the procedure is going on." This serves to remind him that the "body on the autopsy table" belongs to a patient whose death no physician was able to prevent.

It is not only the limits of the field which are impressed upon the student during his participation in an autopsy. This experience also serves to make him aware of the personal limitations of even the most skilled practitioners. For instance, an autopsy gives a student an opportunity to observe that "the doctors aren't always sure what caused the patient's death"; rather, as one student puts it, "they come . . . to find out what was really wrong." Furthermore, the student may be present at an autopsy in which the pathologist's findings make it apparent that the physician was mistaken in his diagnosis (when, for example, the pathologist "doesn't find any of the things in the doctors' diagnoses"). From experiences such as these the student learns that, not only he, but also his instructors have only an imperfect mastery of all there is to know in medicine.

These varied aspects of the autopsy, in other words, give it central significance in the student's training for uncertainty.

Learning to Cope with Uncertainty

In describing the various kinds of uncertainty to which a student is exposed during his preclinical years at Cornell, we do not mean to portray him as groping helplessly around in the midst of them. On the contrary, as time goes on, a student begins to develop effective ways of dealing with these forms of uncertainty, so that, gradually, he becomes more capable of meeting them with the competence and equipoise of a mature physician.

To begin with, as a student acquires medical knowledge and skill, some of his uncertainty gives way. "A more complete and satisfying picture of the organism takes shape" in his mind. Gradually, "the missing jig-saw puzzle pieces seem to fall into place, and [he] sees interconnections and interrelationships between all subjects." The student also feels more at home looking in a microscope; he finds it easier to draw slides; he begins to have more confidence in what he sees and hears in Physical Diagnosis; and he becomes more adept at talking to patients. In all these respects, cognitive learning and a greater sense of certainty go hand in hand.

Growing competence and more experience decrease the student's uncertainty about his personal knowledge and skills; this, in turn, modifies his attitude toward the uncertainties which arise from limitations in the current state of medical knowledge. It will be remembered that, at first, the preclinical student goes through a period in which he is inclined to regard his uncertainty as reflecting his personal inadequacy. During his early days in Physical Diagnosis, for example, a student is likely to dismiss the uncertainty he may feel about "how much percussion tells [him]" in a particular instance, by saying that he thinks he is "probably wrong" to have doubts in the first place and that giving vent to these doubts might make him "look like a fool":

> For example, I can see that percussion *does* tell you a lot, and that in most cases, the borders of the heart *can* be percussed. What it

amounts to really is not that I doubt it, but that I can't do it. . . . It's all very well and good [to express your doubt], but if it turns out that you're the only one who seems to be having so much trouble, you begin to look like a fool after a while if you do. . . . We don't really know enough yet so that we can afford not to take a positive stand. . . .

With the growth of his knowledge and skill, however, and the widening and deepening of his experience, a student's perspective on his own uncertainty changes. Now that he "knows a little more" and is a "little more sure of himself," a student says, he realizes that although some of his uncertainty is attributable to his "ignorance," some of it is "really well-justified." By this he means that he is better able to distinguish between those aspects of his uncertainty that derive from his own lack of knowledge and those that are inherent in medicine. He is therefore less apt to think of his uncertainty as largely personal and now considers it more appropriate to give voice to the doubts he feels.

This more "affirmative attitude" toward doubting (as one student calls it) is not only a product of book knowledge and skill in the techniques of physical diagnosis. It also results from what a student learns about the uncertainties of medicine through his daily contact with members of the faculty. From time to time in the classroom, for example, a student will ask what he considers a "well-chosen question" only to discover that his teacher "does not have immediate command of the known medical facts on that point" or to be told that the problem into which he is inquiring "represents one of the big gaps in medical knowledge at present." In the autopsy room, as we have seen, a student is struck by the fact that the pathologist cannot always explain the causes of death and that, although the "doctors' diagnoses are often right, they can also be wrong." Examining patients under the supervision of clinical faculty, a student discovers that when "different instructors listen to (or feel or see) the exact same thing, they frequently come up with different impressions . . . and have to consult one another before they reach a final conclusion."

In short, observing his teachers in various classroom and clinical situations makes a student more aware of the fact that they are subject to the same kinds of uncertainty that he himself is experiencing. Furthermore, the student notes that when his instructors experience these uncertainties, they usually deal with them in a forthright manner, acknowledging them with the consistency of what one student has termed a "philosophy of doubting." Thus, a student's relationship to the faculty, like his advances in knowledge and skill, encourages him to accept some of his uncertainty as "inevitable" and thoroughly "legitimate" and to handle that uncertainty by openly conceding that he is unsure.

Another process by which the student learns to face up to uncertainty in an unequivocal manner is connected with his membership in the "little society" of medical students, for a medical school class is a closely-knit, self-regulating community, with its own method of "tackling a big problem" like that of uncertainty.

Through a process of "feeling each other out," the group first establishes the fact that uncertainty is experienced by "everyone," thereby reassuring a student that his own difficulties in this regard are not unique:

> As always, the biggest lift comes from talking to other students and finding that they have felt the same way. You may do this by a few casual jokes, but you know there is more to it than that. . . .

Secondly, out of the more than "casual joking, asking around and talking to others" that constantly go on among students, a set of standards for dealing with uncertainty gradually emerges—standards that tend to coincide with those of the faculty:

> Suppose I should talk real enthusiastically about the job of dissection I did [a Freshman explains]. Well, Earl will say, "Gee, I'm a great guy, too, you know," or something to that effect. From that remark, I can tell I'm bragging too much. That cues me in, so I make a mental note not to brag so much the next time. . . . Because you don't talk about your successes to the group as a whole. It's sort of understood that you don't try to impress each other. . . . A lot of the fellows belittle themselves. . . . I mean, a fellow will say, for example, that he thought a certain structure was a lymph node and that it turned out to be something entirely different. Then he and everyone else will laugh a lot over that. . . .

If he acts presumptuous about his knowledge, a student will be reproached by his classmates whereas an admission of ignorance on his part may evoke their approval. From their positive and negative reactions, a student learns that his classmates, like his teachers, expect him to be uncertain about what he knows and candid about his uncertainty. (As one student puts it, "It really isn't fashionable to believe much or to be overly sure.")

"Summing up is pretty tough," a Sophomore writes, taking stock as his second year draws to a close:

> The uncertainty of first year is missing. You feel now as though you have a very shaky hold on a great deal of knowledge. You rather expect that the next two years will be spent getting a better hold on the things you are already familiar with. . . . We are half way through. To some people this is quite a milestone. . . . The realization that one day we will be doctors—finished with medical school—is now in the back of our minds. But few people have a definite idea of what they want to do. . . . For the most part, I think our class is looking forward to the third year, although there is a certain uneasiness about the idea of presenting yourself to the patient as a doctor. . . .

In some respects confident and knowing, in others uneasy and not sure, a student feels variously certain and uncertain as he makes the transition from the preclinical to the clinical years of medical school.

THE CLINICAL YEARS

The Kinds of Uncertainty Facing the Third-Year Student

The kinds of uncertainty experienced by a third-year student are qualitatively the same as those he encountered in his preclinical years. First, there is the uncertainty that comes with realizing that, despite all the medicine a student has mastered and all he will learn, he can never hope to "shovel out more than a corner of what there is to know":

> Studying medicine is a lot like digging a hole in the sand. You get down there and start digging, but it seems as though for every shovelful you toss out, some more slides in. And of course, when you dig *any* hole, you never get to the bottom. . . . If you were to ask me how I felt about medicine now, and you happened to catch me in a moment of honesty, I'd tell you that I'm completely overwhelmed by a feeling of lack of knowledge. . . .

Secondly, when he meets clinical problems that "even stump the experts," a third-year student is confronted with uncertainty that derives from the limitations of medical science:

> Ted and I got to talking about some of the revelations of third year, and one of the things that has struck him is that there isn't a diagnosis for everything. He has more or less assumed that there was always a diagnosis that could be made, and especially that a resident or attending should have no trouble making one. But this year, he has discovered that even a sharp attending like Dr. ——— can be stumped. . . .

Uncertainty over how to distinguish his own inadequacies from those which are general to the field continues to pose a problem for the student. If he has trouble with a venipuncture, for example, or does what he considers a "hack-job" in "working up" a patient, a student wonders if "it's mostly due to the fact that [his] talents just don't run toward being a doctor" or if his difficulty is largely attributable to the poor condition of the patient's veins and to the objective intricacy of her case.

But if the uncertainties of third year are like those with which a student is already acquainted and to which he has become partly inured, there is a sense in which the third year at Cornell seems to intensify the *degree* of uncertainty. As one student puts it:

> Starting third year is a little like starting medical school all over. Everything is new, and you don't know what to expect or to plan for. . . .[8]

[8] Within the limited confines of this paper, we have chosen to treat the third year as a unit—for the most part ignoring the fact that it is actually made up of a series of microcosms. The third year at Cornell is divided into three terms: (1) Medicine; (2) Surgery; (3) Obstetrics-Gynecology; Pediatrics; Public Health; Psychiatry. And the class itself is divided into three groups that rotate through these various terms—some taking Medicine first, some Surgery, some Obstetrics-Gynecology, etc. Further, these three groups are, in turn, subdivided—half taking their medical clerkships at New York Hospital first, half at Bellevue first (and then interchanging); half taking Pediatrics first, half Obstetrics-Gynecology first (and interchanging, too). Again, within each of these terms, even more subdivisions take place. For example, the students go two-by-two to the palpation clinic while on Obstetrics-Gynecology; on Medicine, they are broken up into tutorial groups containing five students apiece, and so on. In the section that follows, we will only allude to the differences between the trimesters of the year and the wide dispersion of the student group. Though our discussion of it here is cursory, the effect that the "geometry" of third year has on students merits future study.

Because the third year represents a major transition point in a student's training—it is the beginning of his total immersion in clinical medicine—the uncertainties he encounters at first seem greater to him than those he encountered as a Sophomore.

In spite of his enthusiasm over working on the wards and in the clinics of the hospital, a third-year student looks back somewhat wistfully on what he regards as the relative "organization and continuity of the academic classroom." How do you "approach learning," he wonders, "now that things are no longer grouped by courses—and the choice of what to study is so completely your own?"

> For example, suppose you want to read up on headache. . . . You can read a two-page section in the Merck Manual, a five-page section in Cecil,[9] a thirty-page section in a book called *Signs and Symptoms*, or recent articles in the journals. . . .

"Which is best is very hard to decide." Part of the student's difficulty in evolving a plan of study lies in the fact that what he is really seeking is nothing less than an organized way of learning to think like a doctor. During the third year at Cornell the student reaches out to make the process of differential diagnosis and the logic of rational treatment more conclusively his own.

As a student quickly discovers, however, the way of thought of the doctor is something other than a sum total of the ideas he has already mastered. Neither the principles he has learned in the basic medical sciences nor his book knowledge of disease processes automatically equip him to think like a doctor:

> The basic principles of medicine are very difficult things to catch hold of [a third-year student writes]. In engineering, once you really understand a principle, it stays with you, and you feel confident you will be able to use it in attacking a wide range of new problems. If you really understand mechanics, you can do anything with it, and you don't have to worry so much about whether certain things are true in one case and not in another. . . . The problems may be new tomorrow, but the basic principles don't change (much). . . . With medicine, it's different. . . . There are as many exceptions as there are rules . . . and the important things in one case don't count in another. . . . You can't read the chapter and "figure out the problem"

[9] Russell L. Cecil, Robert F. Loeb, and associates, *Textbook of Medicine* (Philadelphia: W. B. Saunders Company, 1955).

in medicine. And it is the greatest folly to argue with an instructor (a good one) with only the chapter behind you. You can say, "Cecil says . . . " but if he's seen patients with such-and-such for twenty years, then he probably has you. In other words, years of experience don't modify the principles of the engineering book, but in medicine they do. . . .

Along with the change in organization and the different way of thought, the divided nature of the third year augments the uncertainty to which a student is subject:

> The class is pretty split up these days. . . . Lunch is the only time you see friends you are otherwise completely out of contact with. You are all doing different things, and it is really very nice to get a chance to eat together and talk about them. . . .

Separated from some of the people on whom he depended for confirmation and support and now asked to see patients alone, a third-year student is called upon to meet uncertainty in a more solitary fashion:

> Last year, if you thought you felt a liver, for instance, but you weren't quite sure, there were always two or three other fellows there, and you could ask them if they felt it too. But this year, we see patients alone. So we're more on our own now. . . .

Perhaps most important of all in quickening a student's sense of uncertainty is his conviction that "third year is the year when the whole jump is made, and you learn to be a doctor." What is called for now, he says, is "knowing enough to do justice to your patients."

> . . . You get to the point where you say I should know these things. . . . Otherwise I'll be cheating my patients. . . . In that respect, I feel like a doctor already. . . .

In general, then, the uncertainty of third year is compounded for a student by his "developing sense of responsibility." As he becomes aware of the imminence of his doctorhood, "gaps in [his] knowledge" or unsureness on his part seem more serious to a beginning third-year student than they formerly did.

The Certitude of the Third-Year Student

Although a student may tell you at the outset of the third year that he feels "a little bit like a pea on a griddle" (dwarfed by medicine and alone in some ways), he does not continue to sound so unsure of himself. As the year unfolds, a student's initial uncertainty gradually gives way to a manner of certitude. One gains the impression that students are more uncertain during the first part of the third year than they were before, but that they become less uncertain than before during the later part of the third year. There seem to be several reasons for this.

In the atmosphere of the "clinical situation," a student can feel his medical knowledge take root. The "chance to see many of the things [he] has read about" reinforces what he has previously learned; and the fact that "there is a patient lying there in bed proves" to him that what he is currently learning is "really important."

However, the growing assurance of a third-year student does not result only from his greater knowledge and his conviction that what he is doing is important. It results also from the fact that in the third year he is relatively insulated from some of the diagnostic and therapeutic uncertainties he will encounter later. For one thing, the acute illnesses he sees on the wards and the explicit problems he handles in the clinics are often "classic" or so manifest that he says they seem almost "obvious" to him. For another, the responsibilities a third-year student is asked to assume are carefully circumscribed. Although he now has more responsibility than he did when he was a preclinical student, he has considerably less than he will have later, as a fourth-year student or practicing physician. His duties on the wards do not go beyond taking a history, doing a physical examination, and carrying out indicated laboratory tests. When it comes to the problems of treating a patient, the student is largely an onlooker. He does not have to decide upon medicaments and other therapeutic procedures—weighing the potential risks involved against the possible benefits that may accrue to his patients. A student's responsibilities in the clinic are equally limited and specific. In the Surgery specialty clinics, for example, his diagnoses are restricted to those facets of a patient's problems that are encompassed by the particular specialty he is representing at the time. The only therapy for which he is responsible is "fairly simple and concrete": treating infections, removing sutures, and dressing wounds, for example, such as he does on Minor Surgery.

In effect, the delimited nature of his responsibilities frees a student from the necessity of coping with diagnostic and therapeutic uncertainties that fall outside a narrow orbit.[10] Even in the General Surgery clinic where he deals with a wider range of medical problems in a more comprehensive way, the student is protected from many clinical uncertainties. In General Surgery (and in his other clinics as well) a student rarely sees a patient more than once. It is usually only in retrospect that he catches a glimpse of the uncertainties he might have encountered had his relationship with patients been continuous. For example, reviewing the charts of patients he examined in General Surgery as a Junior, a fourth-year student was "amazed to discover" that some of the cases he saw were never resolved:

> . . . One poor woman had a negative GB series (I thought she had gall bladder disease); was seen by someone else and had a negative GI series (he thought she had an ulcer); was seen by someone else and had a negative proctoscopy and Ba. enema (he thought she had Ca. of the colon). She then went to another clinic and had two more negative GI series because someone there thought she had a Meckel's diverticulum. On her last visit, someone wrote down "irritable colon" and treated her with "reassurance." . . .

His close relationship to the clinical faculty is another source of a third-year student's increasing assurance:

> During the first two years it was possible to remain completely removed from the faculty and yet still do O.K. by reading and going to lectures. While some departments made an effort to develop a close student–faculty relationship, you never had to depend on this to get the things you were supposed to. But now only 50% of what we need can come from books. The other 50% has to come from the teachers we work with. And so, there is a 180-degree shift in the class' relation to the faculty. . . .

[10] One of the factors that may persuade a student to enter a specialized field within medicine is that narrowing the scope of practice also narrows the range of potential uncertainty with which he will have to deal as a doctor. For further discussion of this point, see Patricia L. Kendall and Hanan C. Selvin, "Tendencies toward Specialization in Medical Training," in this volume.

Because he finds that listening to experienced doctors reason out loud is the only way he can get "a sense of how to approach clinical problems," the third-year student welcomes the opportunity to learn through direct contact with his instructors. Meeting with members of the faculty or house staff in small intimate groups and discussing patients with them is "the heart of clinical medical education," so far as a student is concerned. Sessions like these, he says, "give [him] insight into how a doctor organizes and uses his information," and a "real sense of colleagueship." ("You catch the feeling you must have in a craft: the father passing the secrets of the craft on to the son.") The closeness of his relationship to the faculty in the third year helps a student to think and feel more like a doctor, and consequently fosters his sense of certainty.

In these respects, the student acquires greater assurance during the course of his third year at Cornell. He also adopts a *manner* of certitude, for he has come to realize that it may be important for him to "act like a savant" even when he does not actually feel sure. From his instructors and patients alike a student learns this lesson: that if he is to meet his clinical responsibilities, he cannot allow himself to doubt as openly or to the same extent that he did during his preclinical years. Instead, he must commit himself to some of the tentative judgments he makes, and move decisively on behalf of his patients:

> Dr. T's philosophy goes something like this. . . . "You boys are to handle the case as you see best. I put no restrictions on you from this point of view. You do the work-up, decide what's to be done, and whatever you decide is all right. But I insist on this much—you must stand up for your decisions, never apologize for what you are doing, and never start getting humble and say you don't know. . . ."

The third-year student learns from his instructors that too great a display of unsureness on his part may elicit criticism; from his patients he learns that it may evoke alarm:

> To say that the patient "searches your face" for clues is no overstatement. An example—while on OB, when trying to palpate a baby once, I got a little confused and frowned in puzzlement. Sensed at once that the mother saw the frown and was alarmed. So, I reassured her that everything was all right. I have always tried to remember not to do it again. . . .

Yielding to the point of view of his instructors who enjoin him to be "firm and take a position," to the desire of his patients to be assured, and to his own "need for definiteness" as well, a third-year student generally makes it his policy to "believe."

> I'm sure that on the higher levels of medicine you *do* admit your ignorance and avoid stereotyped thinking. But we are at the point now where you have to believe in the rule rather than the exception. . . . Perhaps this is a phase you must pass through on the way up, just as you must learn that the heart *does* have a pacemaker before you learn that it *doesn't*. . . .

In sum, the assurance of a third-year student results from his progress in learning and his unawareness of many clinical uncertainties. He assumes a sure manner also because of his belief that "it is a mistake for a medical student at [his] stage of the game to doubt too much."

Training for Uncertainty in the Comprehensive Care and Teaching Program

The sense of sureness expressed by students about to complete their third year at Cornell is, in some respects, premature. At any rate, the fourth-year student's perspective on the uncertainties of medicine is usually different from that of a Junior:

> Experience makes you less sure of yourself, [a Senior explains]. What you realize is that even when you've been out of medical school twenty years, there'll be many times when you won't be able to make a diagnosis or cure a patient. . . . Instead of looking for the day, then, when all the knowledge you need will be in your possession, you learn that such a day will never come. . . .

A fourth-year student who faces up to uncertainty in this way has departed considerably from his third-year self. Part of this change seems attributable to experiences in the Comprehensive Care and Teaching Program.[11] A central feature of the Program is the extensive responsibility for patients which it allows students. Each student is assigned a number of patients who are defined as *his* patients, and he is expected to deal with all the problems that each

[11] Though the fourth year at Cornell is made up of three terms, we will discuss only the Medicine semester (Comprehensive Care) in this paper. The qualitative data (diaries, interviews, and observations) are not sufficient to do justice to the Surgery and Obstetrics-Gynecology terms that also form part of the fourth year.

case presents.[12] Stemming from this degree of responsibility are varied situations and experiences which make the fourth-year student more aware of the uncertainties of medicine.[13]

One important way in which students exercise the broad responsibility offered them is by following their patients over a period of months. This gives them more insight into the prevalence of uncertainties in the practice of medicine. What began as the "classical case" of Mrs. B., for example, illustrates this fact:

> My new patient arrived first . . . Mrs. B., a thirty-two year old housewife and mother of two children, who had a sudden onset of typical thyroid symptoms complete with the physical findings to go with them. . . . I ordered several diagnostic tests for her and advised her to return in a week. . . .

In this initial contact, the student–physician considered Mrs. B.'s case "typical," and the tests which he ordered were presumably intended merely to confirm his diagnosis. There is no indication that he anticipated special difficulty in handling Mrs. B.'s problems.

On the second visit the student and the attending physician who was supervising him agreed that Mrs. B.'s case was clear-cut, and that surgery would be appropriate. But they did not reckon with the response of the patient to that proposal:

> By the time I got to my second re-visit, Mrs. B., my toxic thyroid case, she had been waiting some time. . . . She gave me the story of continuation of her previous symptoms with shaking even more apparent at present. Of the tests ordered, only the BMR came back, but this was conclusive, being 59% above normal. I informed her that all her problems were related to these findings, and after discussing her with Dr. D. told her that hospitalization and surgery were her best

[12] For a more detailed description of the Comprehensive Care and Teaching Program and the kinds of experiences which students have in it, see the following papers in this volume: George G. Reader, "The Cornell Comprehensive Care and Teaching Program," and Margaret Olencki, "Range of Patient Contacts in the Comprehensive Care and Teaching Program."

[13] The types of uncertainties a student encounters in the Comprehensive Care and Teaching Program seem to be like those he has dealt with recurrently since his days as a Freshman. However, it is no longer so easily possible to distinguish which fourth-year experiences are salient for which types of uncertainty. Rather, in the situations in which the fourth-year student finds himself all types of uncertainty seem to converge and to be intertwined. For this reason we have found it necessary here to modify the pattern set in earlier sections of this paper, and we talk now largely in terms of undifferentiated uncertainties.

chance for a permanent cure. At this she broke down in tears, and after composing herself, made many arguments against surgery. . . . Dr. D. and I quickly agreed that I should treat her with propylthiouracil on an ambulatory basis until she has quieted down. This is an unnatural response to hospitalization and surgery, and I'll be interested in seeing if she becomes more logical with the quiescence of her toxic symptoms. . . .

The patient's fear of an operation forced the student and the attending physician to adopt a plan of therapy which they believed was less effective than the one they originally set forth.

On a later visit the full complexity of Mrs. B.'s case became more apparent:

I went in to see Mrs. B. and found that the threat of her husband's quitting his job was related to hysterical crying most of the day. She admitted that her reaction wasn't wholly because of her disease state, but that she had been easily unnerved prior to this. I assured her that although this might be so, her thyroid was making it much worse, and that we would shortly be rid of part of it. . . . She mentioned that a lump on her daughter's wrist was bothering her, and I suggested that she bring her in on the next visit. . . . We discussed surgery at her initiation, and arrived at the same conclusion as before: my insisting that surgery was the best solution to her problem, and her insisting that she, her husband and friends all agree that if a cure is possible without surgery, that it is to be embarked on. . . .

Mrs. B.'s emotional response to the diagnosis and recommendations made by the student–physician, her eagerness to accept the antisurgical opinions of her family and friends, her anxiety over her husband's job and her daughter's health all proved relevant to the appraisal and management of her case. With each visit it became more apparent to the student–physician that Mrs. B.'s problems were psychological as well as physical, and this realization evoked new questions. Was Mrs. B.'s long-standing nervousness wholly attributable to her disease state? Would it be possible to "ever get this woman over some of her anxious moments," and thus ready her for a needed operation? "I'm not too certain about any of these things," Mrs. B.'s student–physician reported at the end of his third visit with her. But had he seen her only once, this student would not have had any reason to alter his original impression that the case of Mrs. B. was diagnostically and therapeutically "clear-cut."

The continuous nature of his contact with patients in the Program, then, alerts a student to some of the clinical uncertainties that lie beyond first medical judgments and the appearance of things. Furthermore, it confronts him with the problem of managing a long-term doctor–patient relationship in the face of these uncertainties. For example:

> I saw Mr. T. again and gave him the sad news—no ulcer demonstrated. What could this be if it wasn't an ulcer? I tried my best to put him off so that I wouldn't be obligated to further diagnostic procedures which would be useless and expensive. I did my best to convince him that it sounded like nothing but ulcer, and that we planned to treat it as such because not all ulcers are demonstrated by x-ray. This wasn't good enough. . . .

> Mrs. J. puts up a pretty good front, but I think she worries a good deal about her problem. And today she asked me what she had. I was kind of up a tree. . . . I told her that what she had was somewhat different in that it didn't respond to the usual therapy—but that we had many other weapons and she shouldn't be concerned. . . .

With every revisit, the need for a solution may grow more intense in both the patient and the student–physician. Mr. T., for example, becomes harder to convince or reassure. Mrs. J. shows evidence of worrying a great deal and begins to press her doctor for an explanation of her problem. And the student, feeling responsible for the welfare of this man and woman (defined by the Program as *his* patients), is likely to feel frustrated and disappointed by his inability to resolve their cases.

These frustrations may be all the more provoking because the student has not been completely prepared for them by his earlier experiences. His relatively brief and circumscribed contact with patients in the third year had led him to assume that a good doctor ought to be able to arrive at a "definitive diagnosis" and to evolve a successful plan of treatment for most of the cases with which he deals. But the broad and continuous experience provided by the Program teaches a student that cases like those of Mr. T. and Mrs. J. are more widespread than he had supposed them to be.

Not only do his continuing relationship with patients and the growing magnitude of his responsibility for them increase a student's awareness of the uncertain aspects of the cases with which he deals; they often lead to his being deeply affected by these uncertainties. Because he is working with patients in a sustained way, a student is more susceptible to positive and negative countertransference than he was before entering the Program. As time goes on, he may become attached to some patients and alienated from others. Furthermore, the relatively large degree of responsibility assigned to him by the Program makes a student feel more accountable for what happens to patients than he formerly did. As a result, the uncertainties that a student experiences in the Program "make an emotional impact on [him]," so that he is sometimes inclined to react subjectively to the uncertain features of cases he cannot bring to a satisfactory conclusion. Usually these reactions involve the placing of "blame," either on himself or on his patient:

> I blame myself, not Mrs. H. [her student–physician declares]. I can't get her to reduce, and I don't know what I'm doing wrong. I have remained pleasant and sympathetic, but have applied strong urging and have registered disappointment (not wrath) at her failure to cooperate. . . . The reason I find her so difficult is that I feel if someone else were handling her, he could get the pounds off her. . . .

> Mrs. C. has caused me quite a bit of consternation [another student asserts]. Though we have taken adequate physical measures to ascertain that her difficulty is on an emotional basis, she's still showing bodily overconcern. . . . She complains of pains in her legs; that her arms are too weak; that she's tired; that she feels pressure in her abdomen. . . . And then, these gripes about her husband. I can understand them in a way—because he's the type of man who comes home from work, picks up his paper, looks at TV for a while, and then goes to bed without saying a word. . . . But she makes no effort to do anything about the situation. . . . She just sits there and tells me, "That's the way he is. . . ." Another thing about this woman is, in all instances she will discontinue whatever treatment you prescribe and proceed on her own conception. . . .

The "failure" is his, the first student claims; it's the "fault" of the patient and her environment, says the second.

As the cases of Mrs. H. and Mrs. C. suggest, a student is particularly apt to respond in one or the other of these affectual ways when the uncertainty he faces concerns either the social and psychological aspects of a patient's illness, or his own management of the doctor–patient relationship. Partly because psychiatry and the social sciences are in a more embryonic stage of development than the disciplines from which medicine derives its understanding of the human body, the student encounters uncertainty more frequently in trying to handle the emotional and environmental components of his patient's disorder than in trying to cope with problems that are largely physical in nature. The classification of psychological disturbances thus far evolved, for example, is not precise enough to permit a high degree of diagnostic exactitude. The relationship between social factors and illness is only beginning to be systematically explored. And most of the available methods for treating sociopsychological difficulties are still grossly empirical, their relative merits and demerits a focus of present day medical controversy, interest, and concern.

Intellectually, a student is aware of these things before he enters the Comprehensive Care Program; but he has not yet fully learned to acknowledge the uncertainties and limitations in this realm, or to proceed comfortably within the framework of such a realization. This is partly because, prior to his semester in the Program, a student has had little opportunity to take active responsibility for the "personal problems" of his patients. In the third year, for example, as we have seen, a student's work centers primarily on physical diagnosis. The only personal therapy he has occasion to administer to his patients is a simple and limited form of reassurance, which, on the whole, he judges to be effective. His success in this respect he deems "understandable" for he is inclined to feel that the so-called art-of-medicine skills are based not so much on trained experience as they are on personal qualities. Such an attitude is reflected, for example, in the way that a number of third-year students look upon their psychiatry instructors:

> There is a general feeling of great respect for most of the psychiatry people we have come in contact with [one student tells us]. We are impressed to note that the psychiatrist almost always suggests the honest, straightforward, direct approach to things . . . and most of us feel these people make sense. . . .

Yet "the regard we have for psychiatrists is not the same as the respect we have for surgeons," this student goes on to say. In the case of surgery, "it's a matter of respecting skill," in the case of psychiatry, "respecting common sense."

This distinction is one that students carry with them into the Program. It helps explain the observed tendency of many students in Comprehensive Care to reproach themselves when they are unable to formulate the "human aspects of a patient's case" or to decide upon an effective way of dealing with those aspects. ("I can't get Mrs. H. to reduce . . . and I don't know what I'm doing wrong.") For a student who tends to regard problems like "getting the patient to lose weight" as more contingent on personal attributes than on learned skill, the case of Mrs. H. may seem to represent a personal failure on his part.

The more common tendency of a student to blame the patient under such circumstances is a different manifestation of the same emotional involvement. In the face of medical uncertainties that may impede his attempts to be decisive about the sociopsychological dimensions of the cases he handles, a student often projects his own sense of inadequacy upon the patient. In Comprehensive Care, for example, students frequently apply the epithet "crock" to "patients who do not have an organic lesion" or whose behavior appears to be "psychoneurotic." "The central feature in all these patients we call 'crocks' is that they threaten our ability as doctors," one student points out. This is both because such patients do not respond to the diagnostic and therapeutic efforts of the student–physician in the way he would like ("You don't get a foothold anywhere and do something to give them a better adjustment. . . ."), and because the student is emotionally "more vulnerable when thinking about the human aspects of a case, rather than just the strict medical problems involved."

> Whether you're conscious of it or not, a lot of the things disturbed patients talk to you about are the kinds of things you're likely to react to very strongly in a positive or negative way. . . . I mean, it's all very well to say you're not judging these people, for instance. But you can get annoyed as heck with some of them, or lose your sympathy even though you know they're psychoneurotic. . . .

To sum up: the fourth-year student is repeatedly impressed by the diagnostic and therapeutic uncertainties he encounters in dealing with patients during his semester in Comprehensive Care.

Some of these uncertainties, he realizes, result from his own lack of medical knowledge and some from the limitations of medicine itself. In this respect, they are no different from those he has met at earlier points in his training. However, the physician-like responsibilities ascribed to him by the Program, along with the continuing and holistic nature of his relationship to patients, magnify the problem of uncertainty for the student, and make it harder for him to deal with it in a dispassionate way. In turn, the student's emotional involvement increases the difficulty he has in distinguishing between those uncertainties that grow out of his personal ignorance and those that stem from the current limitations of medical science. It is particularly when he feels unsure about how to classify the ulcer-like symptoms of a Mr. T., or what to do about the obesity of a Mrs. H., that a student "doesn't know whether [his] uncertainty is a reflection of his lack of knowledge and technique or whether such cases would be perplexing" even to more experienced physicians. As we have seen, a student is at first more apt to blame himself, or by projection, the patient, than he is to attribute his uncertainty to gaps in medical science.

Coming to Terms with Uncertainty in Comprehensive Care

The student's increased awareness of uncertainties in medicine is of course not the chief by-product of his term in Comprehensive Care. The same experiences which lead to such awareness also enlarge his skills in the realms of diagnosis and patient management. From the absence of expected findings in a case like that presented by Mr. T., for example, he learns how to appraise conflicting evidence in arriving at a diagnosis. From the complex problems of Mrs. B. he learns something of the connection between emotional stress and physical illness and gains some experience in dealing with patients who are under such stress. When he leaves the Program the student, therefore, has considerably more confidence about his ability to cope with these problems than he did six months before.

Moreover, the fourth-year student finds ways of adjusting to his remaining uncertainties. The organization of the Comprehensive Care Program and some of its precepts help the student to recognize that he shares part of his uncertainty with fellow classmates and instructors. This enables him to meet his uncertainty with greater confidence and equipoise.[14]

In contrast to the many small groups into which the class is divided during the third year, half of the senior class is enrolled in Comprehensive Care at one time, spending a continuous six months together in the Program. This arrangement facilitates that kind of interchange between students which from the earliest days of medical school provided them with mutual aid and the supportive knowledge that "others feel the way [they] do."

> In the process of a routine physical, I performed a pelvic and rectal, and the glove specimen of the stool was strongly guaiac positive! And I didn't quite know what to do. The patient lives in upstate New York and can come to the City only when her husband drives in once a month. A decent GI workup would require her spending four full days at the Hospital. To further complicate matters, I wasn't sure of the significance of the positive test. I had rinsed my glove between pelvic and rectal, but the possibility of a positive test from blood in the vagina remains. . . . In the course of describing this experience at lunch . . . one of my classmates suggested that it was a crime to let her out of the building without a GI series, Ba. enema, and proctoscopy. He felt that even if subsequent stool examinations are negative, such a workup is obligatory. . . . This is the sort of decision I would prefer to force on someone else. I would feel foolish if such a workup showed nothing and subsequent stools were negative, but I'd feel worse if she showed up with an inoperable cancer a few months hence. . . . The lunch table of four was evenly divided on the question of what one should do if such a circumstance arose in general practice. . . . This problem is a real threat to the young physician. . . .

[14] An indication of the marked increase in confidence is contained in a simple statistical result. In May 1955, all four classes at Cornell were asked how capable they felt about dealing with a number of problems encountered by practicing physicians. One of these problems concerned "the uncertainties of diagnosis and therapy that one meets in practice." The class-by-class distribution of replies on this item was as follows:

	Percentage of each class			
Problem of "uncertainties"	First year	Second year	Third year	Fourth year
Quite sure I can deal with this	10	11	21	25
Fairly sure I can deal with this	52	61	60	72
Not sure I can deal with this	38	28	19	3
No. of students	(82)	(82)	(85)	(85)

Although uncertainties such as these are "threatening," the student can perhaps find some reassurance in the fact that his classmates experience the same difficulties in deciding on appropriate action.

The opportunity to work as coequal with the attending physicians of Comprehensive Care also gives the student a chance to see that, at times, expert doctors are no more facile than he in making a diagnosis or deciding upon a course of treatment:

> My second case was a three-year old girl with a swollen, red, warm left hand, which seemed to itch more than it hurt. No signs of infected wound—only history of a possible insect bite. I felt this was a contact dermatitis. The pediatrician felt it was obvious cellulitis, but insisted we call in a surgeon to confirm him. The surgeon leaned toward my diagnosis—and we called in a dermatologist who felt this was definitely infection—which was very amusing. . . .

Finally, the experimental milieu of the Program also furthers the student's realization that neither his classmates nor his instructors have sure and easy answers to some of the questions he finds puzzling. Because one of the primary aims of the Program is self-critically to develop a more comprehensive type of medical care, students and staff are continuously engaged in a process of inquiry. Conjoined by a living experiment, they openly express their feelings of doubt and uncertainty, and systematically try to resolve them. In one of the weekly Comprehensive Care conferences, for example, we can see this process taking place. A fourth-year student is presenting the history of the Gonzales family, whom he serves as general physician:

> The Gonzales family is a Puerto Rican family that has been in this country for sixteen months. It consists of eight members: Mr. Gonzales, a 38-year old unskilled laborer; Mrs. Gonzales, his 25-year old uneducated wife; and their six children. . . . They live in a three-room, unheated apartment on 60th Street. From the outset of our contact with this family, it was obvious that there were a number of interrelated sociological, economic, and medical problems, all of which could not be treated at the same time. We have tried to proceed in the most logical manner, but often our efforts have had to be side-tracked by the appearance of new problems. First, there was the real possibility of the family breaking up under the existing stresses. This immediate crisis passed. Then, there was the problem of tuberculosis with the diagnosis of Anna's active case, the question

of Mrs. Gonzales' status, and the necessity of evaluating other members of the family. Coincidental with this investigation was the series of upper respiratory infections, otitis medias, episodes of gastro-enteritis and pyelitis, Carlo's seizure disorder, and finally, Mr. Gonzales' admission to the Hospital. Many of the family are known to be anemic, so following our satisfaction that none of the other children had tuberculosis, it was agreed that the known parasitic infections should be next attacked. . . . It seems certain that poor nutrition is another contributing factor to the anemias, and we have taken steps along this line as well. . . . One of the family's food difficulties has been the inability to shop properly. Previous to our contact with them, they purchased all of their groceries from a store uptown where Spanish was spoken, and high prices asked. On our advice, Mr. Gonzales now does most of his shopping at the A & P. . . . The situation has been in a constant state of flux since we first came in contact with the family, and shows every evidence of continuing in the same state. . . . All our efforts still leave many of the major problems of the family unsolved. . . . We will welcome any suggestions and opinions you may have. . . .

A series of student comments followed upon this presentation, gradually crystallizing around one of the major ideas of the Program. ("There is consensus that adequate care must include preventive, emotional, environmental, and familial aspects if it is to offer the most that modern knowledge can supply in the management of those who are ill."[15] But it has not yet been determined how inclusive "adequate care" can and should be):

I was thinking as I sat there listening to the Gonzales case . . . is it or isn't it part of the doctor's job to be concerned with such things as where his patients buy their food?

Theoretically, I guess it's part of the doctor's job. . . . But from my own point of view, I'm afraid that if I had a family like this, all I'd want to do is throw up my hands completely. . . .

As far as the question of whether or not the doctor is obligated to look into such matters as the food people buy is concerned, I'd say yes . . . so long as those things pertain to medical illness. And in this particular family, it's especially important because they're all anemic. . . . But as for the social problems of this Puerto Rican family, they're beyond the scope of an everyday doctor to crack, in my opinion. . . .

[15] From a report of the Comprehensive Care and Teaching Program to the Commonwealth Fund, March 30, 1954.

What we have here is a group of Americans coming from highly sordid conditions to live in highly sordid conditions. . . . Well, I think it's part of our responsibility to do something about this problem. . . .

We had another case in a session on Thursday that bears on this. This is an Irish woman who's tied down with arthritis and who has a number of problems in addition. Among them is the fact that she lives in a one-room flat—dirty and with no heat. Well, the question arose as to whether it's the doctor's responsibility to get her another apartment and encourage her to move . . . or whether it's beyond the scope of the physician's work. . . .

The variety of opinion voiced in the course of such a conference provides a student with intimations that not only his classmates, but his instructors and physicians in general, are as perplexed as he is by questions about such matters as the boundaries of the doctor's professional task and the unsolved problems of patients like the Gonzales family. In the words of a faculty member who spoke up at the end of this conference:

These questions don't only concern students. . . . They concern doctors as well. . . . There just aren't many "ground rules" in this area. . . .

CONCLUSION

This paper reviews some experiences which acquaint the medical student with the different types of uncertainty he will encounter later as a practicing physician, and some of the ways in which he learns to deal with these uncertainties.

Because this is a preliminary description of what, it turns out, are rather complex processes, we have not organized the analysis around several basic distinctions that could be made. But it seems appropriate to introduce these now so that lines of a more systematic analysis can begin to emerge.

One basic type of uncertainty distinguished at the outset is that deriving from limitations in the current state of medical knowledge. Clearly, the different medical sciences vary in this respect. It has been indicated, for example, that limitations in a field like Pharmacology are now considerably greater than they are in, say, Anatomy. There are comparable differences among the clinical sciences. There would probably be general agreement that gaps in psychiatric knowledge are considerably greater than those in the field of Obstetrics and Gynecology. Such distinctions would provide a focus for further and more rigorous study of training for uncertainty. The different fields would be arranged according to the degree of uncertainty which characterizes them in order to see whether this ranking is paralleled by what the student learns from his different courses about the uncertainties of medicine. Are students made most aware of uncertainties when they are exposed to fields in which these uncertainties are greatest? More important, perhaps, is the question whether those fields in which limitations of knowledge are particularly prominent offer more or fewer means of coming to terms with uncertainty.

The second type of uncertainty, resulting from imperfect mastery of what is currently known in the various fields of medicine, was not analyzed in terms of its variability. We chose rather to concentrate on the "typical" or "modal" student at different phases of his medical school career. But, obviously, there are significant individual differences, and these could provide a second focus in a more systematic study of training for uncertainty. Students vary in the level of skill which they achieve at any particular stage of their training. For example, those who find it easy to memorize details may have an advantage over their classmates in the study of Anatomy; those whose manual dexterity is highly developed may not experience the same degree of personal inadequacy as the less adroit students when they begin to carry out surgical procedures; extroverted students may find it easier to get along with patients than introverted classmates. These variations in aptitudes, skill, and knowledge may lead to individual differences in the extent to which students experience the uncertainties which derive from limitations of skill and knowledge. Students probably differ also in awareness of their own limitations and in response to these limitations. Some may be more sensitive than others to their real or imagined lack of skill. Some may be more able than others to tolerate the uncertainties of which they are aware. As we have seen, distinctions such as these would have to be considered in a more precise investigation of training for uncertainty. Are relatively skilled students less likely than relatively unskilled students to become aware of those uncertainties that derive from limits on medical knowledge? Are students especially sensitive to the uncertainties which confront them better able than less sensitive classmates to cope with such uncertainties? Or, to raise a somewhat different sort of problem, do students with a low level of tolerance for such uncertainty perform less effectively in their medical studies than students who are able to accommodate themselves to uncertainty? The level of tolerance might also affect the choice of a career: for example, do students who find it difficult to accept the uncertainties which they encounter elect to go into fields of medicine in which there is less likelihood of meeting these uncertainties?

A third distinction involves the experiences through which the student becomes acquainted with the uncertainties of medicine. Some of them are directly comparable with those which a mature physician would encounter. For example, when he meets the tentative and experimental point of view of pharmacologists or when inconsistent findings make a definitive diagnosis problematic, the student is faced with exactly the same sort of unsurenesses met by a practicing physician. But other experiences seem to derive their elements of uncertainty from the teaching philosophies or curricular organization of the medical school. For instance, the uncertainties which a student experiences as a result of the avoidance of spoon feeding by the basic science faculty at Cornell or the atomistic division of his class in the third year are by-products of particular conditions in the medical school, although they may have their analogues in actual practice. This distinction would consequently have to be incorporated into a more detailed analysis of training for uncertainty. Which type of experience is more conducive to recognition of the uncertainties in medicine? Which is more easily handled by students? In view of the wide range of experiences in medical school which have a bearing on training for uncertainty, what is the relative balance between those experiences which are inherent in the role of physician and those which inhere in the role of student?

This concluding section is clearly not a summary of what has gone before. Instead, we have chosen this opportunity to make explicit some of the variables and distinctions which were only implicit in earlier pages in order to indicate further problems for the more systematic qualitative analysis of a process like training for uncertainty.

Part IV

Two Studies of the Cornell
Comprehensive Care and
Teaching Program

INTRODUCTION

Educational innovations like the Comprehensive Care and Teaching Program at Cornell University Medical College usually excite considerable research interest. Those who have introduced the innovation and who are concerned with its day-by-day activities are eager to assess how well the new program is fulfilling its stated objectives, to find out whether it has had any unanticipated consequences, and to evaluate alternative ways of proceeding. Other educators not directly connected with the innovation are often equally eager to find out how well the program is functioning so that they may consider the possibility of adapting it to their own teaching situations.

For reasons such as these, it can be expected that plans for a new teaching program like the C. C. & T. P. will usually provide for research. In his description of the origins and activities of the C. C. & T. P., Dr. Reader has already indicated that, from its very inception, self-evaluation and self-analysis were considered integral parts of the Program, and he has pointed to some of the specific lines of investigation which have been followed during the five years the program has been in operation.

The Comprehensive Care and Teaching Program affects many different groups within the medical center. It is a teaching program; it therefore involves medical students and their teachers. At the same time, it is a program of patient care; it therefore involves patients, on the one hand, and physicians, nurses, social workers, and related medical personnel, on the other. Because

245

it draws so many different groups within its orbit, the C. C. & T. P. can be studied from numerous points of view. This last section of our book is devoted to two examples from this large array of studies. They are intended as illustrations of the diverse problems to which research on the C. C. & T. P. can be addressed, and of the varied methods which may be used in carrying out such studies.

The first of these papers, by Mary E. W. Goss, is one of a class of studies which is becoming more frequent. Any innovation, be it educational or otherwise, undergoes change as its blueprint of intentions is translated into actual practice. There are various questions to be raised about such institutional change. How does the administrator responsible for the innovation come to recognize the need for changes? Are the required changes radical or minor in nature? What are some of the conditions facilitating, or hindering, both the recognition and the implementation of institutional change? These are exactly the sorts of questions to which Goss addressed herself. She started her investigation prior to the actual inception of the Comprehensive Care and Teaching Program, studying the statements of objectives and plans of organization, and discussing these documents with those people in the Medical Center who were most centrally responsible for introducing the Program. For a full year thereafter she made firsthand observations of activities in the Program, supplementing these observations, as she indicates, with other relevant data. The result is a description of some of the different sorts of changes which came about during that first year of operation, and an analysis of some of the processes making for such change.

The second paper, by Margaret Olencki, represents a very different type of study; it might best be described, as the author herself suggests, as a form of "social bookkeeping." Any change in the routine of medical students, such as that introduced by the Comprehensive Care and Teaching Program, is likely to be met with questions regarding the character of the experiences which students have in the new program. As Olencki points out, for example, some educators expressed fear that the plan to have fourth-year students spend six months in the General Medical Clinic, instead of shorter periods of time in each of a number of specialty clinics, might mean that the variety of patients seen by students would not be as great as formerly. Or, one might ask whether the plan to have students follow patients over a period of time actually works out in practice. The kind of statistics collected and analyzed by Olencki provide preliminary answers to these and related questions. Based on one-page Visit Reports which a group of C. C. & T. P. students were asked to fill out each time they had a contact with or about one of their patients, these statistics permit one to draw a rough description of the types of experiences gained in the Program, and they offer some basis for deciding whether or not such experiences are adequate. In this way they contribute to the over-all evaluation of the Program.

Both of these studies were confined to limited periods of time—Goss's to the first year of the Comprehensive Care and Teaching Program, Olencki's to the second semester, an even shorter segment of time. In both, therefore, are found statements about prevailing conditions and activities which would have to be modified in the light of subsequent changes in the Program. Goss, for example, elected to center her discussion of institutional change upon problems in the selection and treatment of Family Care groups; since her data were collected, however, the focus of the Program has shifted somewhat from the Family Care patients to Home Care patients. For this reason, also, the statistics reported by Olencki would be quite different had they been collected this year rather than four years ago.

In other words, these two papers are included in the present volume, not because they give an accurate description of the way the C. C. & T. P. looks now, but rather because each illustrates a particular type of problem and a particular set of methods which may be called upon in assessing an educational innovation.

Mary E. W. Goss

CHANGE IN THE CORNELL COMPREHENSIVE CARE AND TEACHING PROGRAM

When the Comprehensive Care and Teaching Program began full-scale operation in June 1952, there was little doubt that changes in the initial plan might eventually be required. The organization was new, and as in all untried endeavors, some alteration was expected. Because the Program was experimental as well, it was considered important to be aware of these changes. Program activities were, therefore, systematically studied during the first year so as to provide a record of the emerging character of the C. C. & T. P. and of the processes through which it came to develop. Data were obtained from many sources—from C. C. & T. P. documents, from informal interviews with staff members and students, from formal questionnaires filled out by students, and, most important, from notes recording firsthand observations of events in the Program.[1]

This paper deals with findings from that study of C. C. & T. P. changes and how they came about. But the part must stand for the whole; the data are too voluminous to present in full. Thus only a small fraction of the specific cases of modification which occurred are described. Through the use of examples, however, attention is focused on the various kinds of changes that took place in the original plan. And, since changes were generated

---

[1] During the period under analysis, the writer was allowed free access to virtually all of the events which took place in the Program, including staff meetings, student seminars, medical conferences, etc.

by problems encountered, these also simultaneously come under scrutiny. Finally, cases are analyzed to determine what, within the functioning organization, apparently facilitated the occurrence of change.

THREE CASES OF CHANGE: CRITERIA FOR SELECTION OF
FAMILY CARE PATIENTS

As part of his training in comprehensive medicine, each of the students participating in the Program was expected to serve as "family physician" to a particular patient and, if possible, to the patient's family as well. Although this task was to take proportionately little of the student's time, the administrators of the Program believed it should constitute a valuable learning experience for students.[2] Thus criteria for selection of these "comprehensive care patients"—or as they were later called, "Family Care patients"—were enumerated from the very beginning; they were not left to chance. An official C. C. & T. P. statement, issued in June 1952, lists these requirements. To be eligible for Family Care at that time, a patient was supposed to have: "(1) a chronic illness requiring continuous medical supervision, (2) residence in the New York Hospital district, (3) membership in a family unit, (4) desire to take part in the Comprehensive Care Program."[3]

When these criteria for patient selection were actually put into use, however, they were soon revised in the light of several problems which emerged. What kinds of changes occurred, and why?

"There Aren't Enough Families to Go Around"

One problem revolved about the fact that finding suitable families proved more difficult than had been anticipated. As the Social Service Coordinator—who was charged with securing and screening potential Family Care patients—stated the matter to the Program staff at a meeting in September 1952:

> We now have thirty-three Comprehensive Care families. Two students have two each, however, so *that leaves twelve students without*

[2] The rationale for providing experience in Family Care for medical students is described by George G. Reader in "The Cornell Comprehensive Care and Teaching Program," in this volume, p. 89.
[3] "Course in Comprehensive Medicine, Fourth Year" (mimeographed), p. 1.

families. . . . I have combed our files, and I just can't find any more families in the New York Hospital district who also fill the other requirements.

The difficulty encountered in recruiting families was, in itself, annoying to the Social Service Coordinator; a conscientious person, she wanted very much to perform her assigned tasks efficiently and well. More than that, it was a source of mounting concern, since the semester was progressing and over one-fourth of the students still had no families assigned to them.

Upon learning of the situation, other full-time staff members shared this concern. According to one of them, "So far there aren't enough families to go around, and that isn't good. We'll have to do something." In other words, as long as not all students had families, an organizational commitment remained unfulfilled.

The felt need to "do something" so that more families might be recruited was no doubt reinforced by student pressure; witness the comment of a student–representative. When asked by the Director of the Program if his constituents had any "gripes," he answered, "A few of the boys are complaining that they don't have any families yet. They want to know 'how come?' "

A possible solution to the problem was suggested by the Social Service Coordinator, who believed that if she were not restricted to finding families living in the district, filling the quota would be easier. For, she said, "I know of some other families, from *outside* the Hospital district, who seem like a good bet. Why can't we include them?" In view of the pressing need for families, this suggestion seemed feasible to those present at the staff meeting; the Director said he would discuss the proposed change in the selection criteria with the Chairman of the Advisory Committee. Subsequently, the Director announced that Family Care patients need not come from the district, though they should live within a reasonable distance of the Hospital.

"This Case Is Too Complicated for Anybody"

Since the residence requirement for Family Care patients apparently served as a bottleneck in obtaining patients, staff members were prepared to say that originally the plan had perhaps been too particular in this respect. Another problem of a different sort arose, however, which indicated that the outlined criteria apparently were not particular enough. In fact, to deal with the problem, an additional requirement was introduced.

As students and staff came to know individual families of patients, it became increasingly clear that some of the families had, along with their physical ills, more or less complex social problems, e.g., poverty, unemployment, juvenile delinquency, disorganization of family relationships. Usually the presence of these problems appeared to be connected, closely or remotely, with the general state of health manifested by family members. Thus, adequate care of a patient and his ailment might ideally require not only drugs, diet, etc., but alteration in the patient's social milieu as well: arranging for children to go to camp so that a sick mother might rest; finding a job for an unemployed, partly disabled father who has demoralized his whole family because of his illness.

In actual practice, however, the social problems encountered were not always easy to remedy; the sick mother might refuse to be parted from her children, a job might not be available for the disabled man. When confronted with these medically relevant but sometimes practically irremediable social difficulties in the lives of their Family Care patients, students tended to feel frustrated. The concept of comprehensive medical care required that the patient be considered as a person functioning within a family unit, not just as a disease entity. Yet, in a small but significant proportion of the families, ameliorative efforts on the personal level were unsuccessful. How was this to be handled?

One possibility was to reject the "comprehensive" approach, and attend solely to the "strictly medical" needs of the patient. As one student, who had been faced with management of a patient within a particularly complex family configuration concluded:

> It is not the responsibility of the physician to solve the social problems of his patients. Their solution is primarily the responsibility of his patients, and secondarily within the province of the social agencies.

Another student, expressing a somewhat more moderate view, stated:

> I think they [the social worker and the physician] should work as a team, and therefore the doctor should not wash his hands of the

[social] problem but should refer the patient to the social worker and *follow* the patient. . . .

Still a third reaction among student–physicians was to concentrate even harder and longer on ways of solving the patient's social problems. Thus, in presenting "his" family at a Comprehensive Care Conference, a student listed the organic and social ills he had noted in the family, and then went on to say:

> *The real problem is a family problem that exists in the tortured interrelationships among these people.* . . . The main problems are the ones involved in the fact that these children are growing up in an environment with no love. . . . Mrs. —— tries to be a good mother but she doesn't have the necessary skills . . . she presents a variety of chronic illnesses . . . she also has a severely psychoneurotic personality with some mental retardation. . . . Mrs. —— very much wants to help her children, but she can't do it.

> *In the past, most of our energies have been placed on Mrs. ——. . . . Yet we haven't gotten anywhere with her. Now what concrete measures can we put forth?* . . . We're going to have to work through Mr. ——, the husband. Also, we want to pull the children away from the home . . . to place them in camps, recreational organizations. . . .

Far from rejecting patients' social problems as out of his sphere of interest or competence, this student was determined to try to solve them, even though he recognized that "a lot of what should be done gets into the province of the social worker."

Faced with these varying student reactions to frustrating social problems presented by patients, staff members were led to re-examine their goals in connection with Family Care. On the one hand, they did not want to see medical students so involved in their patients' life situation that attention to classical medicine became secondary. But, on the other hand, neither did they believe the "comprehensive" approach need be condemned because, in a few cases, nothing constructive could be accomplished in the personal and social realm. For as one faculty member said, in commenting on the efforts of the last-quoted student:

> It has been said by some people that we have been giving you [students] too complicated cases. I think this case is too complicated for *anybody.*

Through staff discussions—mainly at History meetings and Intake meetings—a compromise solution to the dilemma was reached. To avoid extreme student anxiety and frustration, with its occasional consequence of over-reaction to very "complicated" social problems of patients, a new criterion for selection of Family Care patients was formulated: "that the social problems of the family not be overwhelmingly complex."[4] The reasoning of Program administrators recognized the fact that sooner or later physicians in practice may face patients with such "overwhelmingly" complex social problems. But, they held, exposure to overly complicated familial difficulties of patients had turned out to be more detrimental than helpful for certain students at the fourth-year level, allowing them to learn little of the possibilities of comprehensive care, but only of the limitations. Thus the additional requirement, which insured that students might more easily maintain perspective, was added.

"Families with Children Are Better for Teaching"

Still a third sort of change occurred in the selection criteria for Family Care patients. It differed somewhat from either of the preceding types, and consisted in making the original criterion that patients be "members of a family unit" more specific.

During the first few months of the Program, Family Care patients were selected without particular regard to the composition of their families. Some families in the initial group of patients had as many as six or eight children in the home; others had none. And, as it happened, students serving as physicians to the families with children generally had an opportunity to see their patients more often and to treat a greater variety of illness within the context of Family Care than did students who ministered to childless couples. Children, according to the Assistant Director of the Pediatric Clinic, "obligingly provide a variety of acute though minor clinical problems during the course of the time they are being followed."[5]

---

[4] Cited in George G. Reader, "Comprehensive Medical Care," *J. Med. Educ.*, 28:38, July 1953.

[5] Minutes of meeting of C. C. & T. P. Advisory Committee, November 20, 1952, p. 7.

Customarily students welcomed the opportunity to deal with such clinical problems, whether presented by children or adults. They were eager to learn and to help wherever possible. This motivation, the desire to face and handle challenging medical situations in the realm of Family Care above and beyond the chronic illness of one patient, was easy for C. C. & T. P. staff members to recognize; students were not particularly reticent in making it known to their instructors, in consultations over Family Care patients and elsewhere. As one medical student summed up his situation:

> *My family . . . has not made a unique contribution to my medical education.* I have followed the mother with no more revisits than I would have devoted to any patient with a chronic disease, namely, mitral stenosis. *There are no medical problems in the other members of the family.*

Nevertheless, he went on to say his case was not necessarily typical:

> *Other students, however, have had families with myriads of problems in many members of the family.* These students have spent a great deal of time on their families and have made many house calls. Several of these students have told me that *their Comprehensive Care Families have made a definitely unique contribution to their medical education. . . .*[6]

In the belief that medical problems are more likely to arise in families with children, staff members concluded—at an intake meeting, during one of their many discussions of Family Care patients—that preference in selection of these patients should be given to "families which include young children." For, according to one of the faculty members present, "we discovered that families with children are better for teaching."

Types of Changes

For later descriptive purposes, it is convenient to label the three types of changes which are manifest in the cases presented. In the first case of change in selection criteria, one residence requirement for Family Care patients was replaced by another, presum-

---

[6] Minutes of meeting of C. C. & T. P. Advisory Committee, November 20, 1952, p. 4.

ably better calculated to meet current organizational needs. This sort of alteration, wherein one item is eliminated from the whole and replaced by another item, may be called *substitution*. The second instance of change cited did not involve replacement of an already-existing requirement, but rather, introduction of a new and unanticipated criterion: "that the social problems of the family not be overwhelmingly complex." This kind of change can be designated *innovation*, with the understanding that more generally, it means addition of an entirely new and unforeseen item to a given whole. A third kind of change was evident in the final case described, for there the already-existing criterion that patients be "members of families" was elaborated to refer specifically to "families with children." The term *specification* covers this sort of change reasonably well; it may be taken to mean that hitherto implicit or vague implications of a given item are made explicit.[7] Obviously, accurate classification of a given change in the C. C. & T. P. as "substitution," "innovation," or "specification" requires knowledge of staff expectations as well as of initial formal arrangements.

CHANGES IN OTHER ASPECTS OF THE PROGRAM

Because particular alterations in criteria for selection of Family Care patients have been described in detail, it should not be assumed that change in the C. C. & T. P. was limited to this feature. Quite the contrary. Just as the beginning requirements for Family Care patients were modified in the face of experience, so also other areas of Program activity—home care, regular clinic patient care, student seminars, conferences and lectures, research commitments, administrative tasks—were changed in greater or less degree.

Specification of the Program's activities and regulations within each of these areas was by far the most common type of modification. Both innovation and substitution of one activity or rule for another were less in evidence. No major Program objective or activity was discarded; all of the broad goals which initially gave impetus to the organization of the Program were retained in the

[7] For a somewhat different yet related classification of types of organizational changes, see Peter M. Blau, *The Dynamics of Bureaucracy* (Chicago: University of Chicago Press, 1955), pp. 23–28.

following year. The dominant developmental trend, in other words, was toward making the original plan *more particular,* rather than in the direction of large-scale substitution or innovation in the blueprint.

The fact that the major activities and objectives of the C. C. & T. P. were continued for the following year suggests that these arrangements were in the process of becoming *institutionalized.* That is, initially novel sets of interlocking behaviors on the part of students, staff, and patients were becoming accepted as right and proper everyday activity, at least by C. C. & T. P. participants. Nevertheless, the occurrence of many minor changes—such as those described with respect to selection criteria for Family Care patients—furnishes evidence that *what* was being institutionalized was not so much the original plan, but a modified version, tempered and sharpened by experience.

CONDITIONS AND PROCESSES FACILITATING CHANGE

How did this modified version of the C. C. & T. P. come about? Thus far only part of the story has been made explicit, namely, certain situations arose within the organization, were defined as problems, and dealt with by altering arrangements believed responsible for the difficulties. But what motivated C. C. & T. P. participants to notice situations, to decide they were in need of change? And what, in the nature of the organizational set-up itself, facilitated such decisions?

Experimental Outlook

One reason the C. C. & T. P. staff members were "geared" to see problems was that they were well aware of the experimental nature of the Program. The Chairman of the C. C. & T. P. Advisory Committee had formally stated that "the enterprise as outlined must be regarded as an experiment in medical education,"[8] and this view was reinforced by the Director's informal interpretation: "We won't know whether the idea of comprehensive care is worthwhile unless we try it. If something turns out to be ineffi-

[8] David P. Barr, "The Teaching of Preventive Medicine," *J. Med. Educ.,* 28:55, March 1953.

cient or undesirable, we can always change it." Many times over
staff members heard statements such as this, emphasizing the trial
character of C. C. & T. P. aims and activities. There was definite
understanding, therefore, that beginning Program arrangements
were not considered fixed and immutable by those in charge, and
need not be so viewed by staff members.[9]

This meant, in practice, that no stigma attached to finding
"something wrong" with the Program; in fact, the Director welcomed knowledge of problems encountered, since such information allowed planning for the future on a more informed basis.
When, for example, the Social Service Coordinator reported that
despite her best efforts not enough families had been recruited,
the situation was cause for deliberation over which of the original
selection criteria might be at fault, rather than recrimination concerning a job not completed.

Responsibility for "Improvement"

Not only were C. C. & T. P. personnel prepared to see problems;
they were also ready to help solve them. This fact was, of course,
clearly evident in all three examples of change cited earlier. In
each case, attempting to eliminate the perceived difficulty was a
group process, rather than one in which a single individual wrestled
alone with a problem, or turned it over to the Director to handle.

The explanation of this group willingness to cope with problems
lies, at least in part, in the fact that responsibility for "improvement" of the Program was informally shared; it was not confined
to the Director or the C. C. & T. P. Advisory Committee. Thus
the regular duties of each person—doctor, nurse, or social worker
—included the unwritten obligation to assist in the ongoing
process of assessing "trouble-spots" and suggesting possible solutions. The Program's Nursing Coordinator, for instance, felt
she was doing no more than her duty when she reported to the
C. C. & T. P. staff that a few students who were caring for patients
requiring minor surgical dressings (in addition to other medical

[9] Through having its own budget, the Program was freed from the necessity of
following long-established departmental systems of priority in allotting funds for
specific projects. Funds allocated to the C. C. & T. P. by the Commonwealth Fund
were therefore undoubtedly influential in promoting and maintaining the experimental outlook described above.

attention) had complained to her that they could "hardly give comprehensive care in the Medical Clinic as we're supposed to when a patient has to leave the Clinic and make a special trip to the Minor Surgery Clinic just to have a little dressing changed!" She believed it well within the confines of her role to suggest at a staff meeting that "this situation could be remedied quite easily by the addition of a surgical dressing tray as standard equipment for the General Medical Clinic." Doing one's job well, then, *encompassed* participation in this process of adapting the organization to existing conditions; helping was not a gratuitous favor, extraneous to other duties.

Personal Involvement

Moreover, staff members frequently had an additional personal stake in seeing a particular condition changed. For, if the potential alteration involved some aspect of their own work, it generally meant that the task would subsequently go more smoothly. Early in the first semester, for example, the Obstetrical and Gynecological consultant to the Program found himself instructing students individually in matters of general office gynecology. Since this group of students had not yet spent their allotted two months in clinical Obstetrics and Gynecology, and were therefore unsure about some procedures, instruction by the Obstetrical consultant was necessary. But, the consultant reasoned, there was no need to repeat the same information many times; much of it could be communicated through lectures which all students might attend. By giving lectures to the group, that is, he would have more time available for consulting on special problems, he would avoid the dreary chore of repeating basic principles to each individual student, and he would be sure, nevertheless, that students obtained the requisite information. Consequently, he proposed giving a series of six one-half hour lectures on office gynecology, and the proposal was adopted.

Through this change, the consultant benefited personally—and, one may presume, so also did the Program as a whole. That he was motivated to suggest the alteration in the first place is not, therefore, surprising. Nor is this an isolated instance. Many times suggestions for changes came from the very people who were *experi-*

encing particular problems in the course of their work which, they felt, would be more satisfying or efficient if their proposed modification were adopted.

Not all of the groups who functioned in the Program, however, were as concerned with improving the organization. While full-time staff physicians, consultants, social service, nursing personnel, and—to some extent—students shared the general sort of responsibility which has been described, the part-time attending staff as a group was less involved. Most of these men were private practitioners who spent one or two half-days each week supervising students in the Comprehensive Care Clinics. Even though they were thus an integral part of the Program, they apparently had little time to become interested in assessing trouble-spots and suggesting solutions. When, for example, several of these physicians were asked whether they "would recommend any changes in the Program," the majority had no improvements to suggest. One part-time attending's answer typified the attitude of relative indifference which evidently prevailed in this group: "Change in the Program? I haven't really thought about it."

Administrative Approval

It has been noted that "while the medical school may have superb potentialities as an instrument of change, it is itself an institution with a rigid structure and powerful vested interests."[10] Traditional departmental prerogatives tend to be carefully guarded in such a setting, and even small departures from customary routine may be perceived as possible encroachment upon someone's long-standing rights. It is therefore relevant to ask why various modifications in the C. C. & T. P. met little resistance on higher administrative levels.

One part of the answer is the fact that many of the alterations in Program detail were formally presented to the C. C. & T. P. Advisory Committee for final approval only after they had been at least tentatively shown to be useful. Another lies in the *composition* of the Advisory Committee and the relationship of Pro-

---

[10] *The Commonwealth Fund Annual Report, 1952* (New York: The Commonwealth Fund, 1952), p. 2.

gram personnel to the members of that Committee. Representatives of all of the groups concerned with patient care in the hospital and in the medical college were included in the Advisory Committee; as the Program's Director has described the arrangement:

> Because administration of a comprehensive care program encompasses so many disciplines and crosses so many departmental lines, the planning group devised [the C. C. & T. P. as] a non-departmental organization responsible directly to the Joint Administrative Board of the Medical Center. The President of the Joint Administrative Board appointed first an Advisory Committee composed of the Chiefs of the Clinical Services, the Professor of Preventive Medicine, the Director of Social Service, the Chairman of the Out-Patient Department Committee, the Superintendent of the Hospital, the Dean of the Medical College, the Dean of the Nursing School, and himself. The Advisory Committee then designated an internist as Director of the Comprehensive Care and Teaching Program and Assistant Directors for Medicine and Pediatrics.[11]

Each of the groups working *within* the C. C. & T. P., therefore, had a counterpart on the Advisory Committee to whom they were unofficially responsible for the progress of Program activity within their particular domain. This meant, in practice, that potential plans for modification tended to be informally "cleared" with the appropriate department head or other administrator before they were put into operation. The Program's Social Service Coordinator, for example, gradually switched from mainly providing direct service to patients to acting primarily in an administrative and teaching capacity. Since the change required the services of additional social workers, she could not have done this without the approval and aid of her representative on the Advisory Committee (the Director of Social Service of New York Hospital).

In short, it was not simply an accident that Program modification met little organized administrative resistance. From the very beginning, the planners of the Program had taken into account the varied and perhaps diverse interests which would be included in the working personnel of the organization, and had accordingly devised an administrative body wherein all interests were repre-

[11] George G. Reader, "Organization and Development of a Comprehensive Care Program," *Amer. J. of Public Health*, 44:762, 1954.

sented.[12] Before given changes were adopted, therefore, consultation with the persons most likely to be concerned was possible. And, as suggested earlier, the approach of those in charge tended to be experimental in outlook.

Communication among C. C. & T. P. Personnel

All of the instances of change cited have indicated that problem-solving within the C. C. & T. P. was a group process—that, in fact, the organization *as a unit* was prepared to cope with whatever problems might arise. Obviously, this state of affairs could hardly have existed without channels of communication among C. C. & T. P. personnel, for staff ideas and suggestions concerning specific improvements would never have reached the Director, whose authorization was required to put the suggestion into effect. And, on the other hand, those originating with the Director would have met with but uncertain reception if their feasibility had not been discussed beforehand with the persons involved. In order for staff members to keep in touch with each other's activities, ideas, and complaints, therefore, certain regular communication devices were planned.

A monthly staff meeting to which all C. C. & T. P. personnel (excluding students) were invited constituted the main official medium of communication.[13] At these meetings general announcements were made and the Program's policies, progress, and problems were discussed—as well as frequently debated. The range of ideas and information interchanged at such meetings is perhaps best illustrated by listing the topics discussed at a fairly typical staff meeting:[14]

[12] In Selznick's terms, this situation wherein responsibility is shared represents the end-product of the process of "cooptation," which he defines as "the process of absorbing new elements into the leadership or policy-determining structure of an organization as a means of averting threats to its stability or existence," in *T.V.A. and the Grass Roots* (Berkeley: University of California Press, 1953), p. 259. It is an end-product in the case under discussion because, on the administrative level at least, all relevant power groups within the sphere of the Program were already represented in the original formal structure of the organization.

[13] Other official meetings were also held, but they dealt with topics of more specialized interest. See George G. Reader, "The Cornell Comprehensive Care and Teaching Program," in this volume, p. 87.

[14] Held April 6, 1953.

Student performance in general and with reference to a few students in particular.

Teaching problems, and how certain of these might be corrected for the following year.

Advisability of extending inpatient rounds (supervised visits to the bedside of former outpatients who are currently hospitalized) for students to include pediatric patients.

Family and Home Care patients, with reference to the current number as well as to policy regarding re-admission of Home Care patients to the hospital.

Rehabilitation patients and the policy to be followed in their selection.

Progress in revising the C. C. & T. P. Reading List.

Possible content of the final examination for students.

Current state of evaluation research activities.

Construction plans for offices in the General Medical Clinic.

Organization of the "Stat" Clinic, where patients with medically urgent problems are treated, with suggestions for making it more efficient.

Probable date student schedules for coming semester will be ready.

Psychiatric teaching in the General Medical Clinic and how students react to it.

Miscellaneous announcements and requests.

Customarily, the Director of the Program served as chairman, raising topics and asking group members for reports, comments, and suggestions regarding various features of the Program. Thus, at the meeting cited, the Assistant Director of the Medical Clinic was asked to report on inpatient rounds for C. C. & T. P. students. When he suggested that pediatric inpatients also be included in these rounds, the Director of the Pediatric Clinic commented that she saw no reason why this should not be done, and plans to schedule this new activity were begun. Interaction at the meetings was informal and friendly; when participants believed they had something to contribute they ordinarily spoke up without being asked, and humor was far from absent.

In addition to regularly scheduled meetings, informal conversations and discussions occurred frequently among staff personnel. Casual chats in someone's office or over afternoon coffee, or at lunch—all were significant occasions for the interchange of information and ideas concerning the progress of the Program. And since the Director of the Program was a regular participant in many of these informal gatherings, he received face-to-face accounts of problems encountered, along with occasional suggestions for their potential solution.

During this first year of the Program, part-time attending doctors, as a group, participated very little in either scheduled meetings or unplanned problem-solving sessions. This situation was a source of some concern to full-time C. C. & T. P. staff members, but the limited time these doctors had available, and the fact that they were never all in the Hospital simultaneously, seemed, temporarily at least, to preclude other arrangements.[15]

Student–Staff Communication

Students were also included in the communication network of the C. C. & T. P. In addition to announcements of general interest presented at the weekly Comprehensive Care Conference, regular weekly student–faculty luncheons were scheduled. These were attended by four elected student–representatives and the Program Director, with other staff members present on a rotating basis. At the luncheons, which were quite informal, faculty members learned from the students themselves how students felt about already-instituted Program activities. Typically, student–representatives were asked if their "constituents" had any complaints or comments on the "way things in the Program are going." Usually they did, and after the first few luncheons each semester, they seemed to feel free to express them.

It was, of course, initially necessary for faculty members to convince the representatives that they were really interested in knowing student reaction to the Program, rather than in receiving a standard answer such as "Everything's fine, sir." And, correlatively,

[15] Nevertheless, in the second year of the Program's operation, the formation of representative *committees* of attending doctors apparently decreased the communication gap described.

before students expressed themselves freely they apparently needed to know that criticisms they might make in their role as representatives would not call forth reprisals—that the faculty would not regard criticisms of the Program as either personal affronts or indications of student maladjustment. Thus, during one of the first few luncheons, students were assured, for example, that "we know not everything in the Program is going as smoothly as it could, and we want to improve where possible. *You can help us* by telling us how things look from the students' angle." And, during comparable early luncheons in the second semester, with representatives from the other half of the class,[16] students heard, "What, you don't have *any* gripes? You're very unusual—your colleagues of last semester were full of them." Through such statements, student–representatives came to realize that faculty members were indeed interested in their remarks concerning the Program, and that they were prepared to hear critical as well as favorable comments.

Further, they learned through actually venturing negative comments that no punishment accrued as a result. For instance, one student said:

> We're all feeling very rushed in the clinic. There doesn't seem to be enough time allowed for us to get everything done—I think maybe we're being given too many patients per clinic session.

A faculty member replied:

> This is not unusual; in the beginning students generally feel rushed. But giving you more patients than you *think* you can handle seems to be the only way to teach you to work faster.

Once student–representatives began to feel secure in the knowledge that their comments would not be held against them, they offered remarks and experiences which—in the opinion of faculty members—were frequently constructive. Thus, in connection with a current requirement that each student should make at least one

[16] The fourth-year class of medical students was divided into halves, with one half participating in the C. C. & T. P. while the other group took courses in Surgery, Obstetrics and Gynecology, and an elective subject. At the end of 22½ weeks, the activities of each of the groups were reversed. For elaboration of this arrangement, see George G. Reader, "The Cornell Comprehensive Care and Teaching Program," in this volume, p. 85.

house call on his Family Care patients, one representative reported that a member of his group had said:

> They've let us down. They promised us this wouldn't be like [a course we had last year] where we had to go to patients' homes for no good medical reason, and now that's exactly what we have to do.

He continued:

> Take my family, for instance. Dr. N. knows the case—she has no difficulty climbing the steps, she is being adequately treated in the clinic, and there's no reason in the world I can think up to go to see her. . . . Going to the home without a good medical reason makes us like students again, and I thought we were supposed to act like doctors.

A second representative commented:

> Well, after all, we are students. But even so, I agree with you.

But a third representative disagreed, on the basis of his own experience. He said:

> My patient used to break appointments regularly in the clinic. When I went to her home, I found out why. I had known she had six children, but to actually see them around the house is a different thing. Because of her children, she just couldn't leave the house. I think there's a lot to be gained by home visits; I think it's a wonderful, revealing, and worthwhile experience.

Unconvinced, the first representative replied:

> But you have a good medical indication for going into the house, which is a very different situation from some other members of the class!

For staff members present at the luncheon, this discussion clearly brought out a teaching problem which had been only dimly seen up to that point: whether it was feasible to request students to take on the role of "family physician," and yet at the same time, ask them to do something which in particular cases conflicted with that role—e.g., make a home visit when there was no medical indication. Subsequently, staff members discussed the problem privately, and concluded by revising the home visit requirement. Specifically, they decided that students should be expected to make the house call *unless* no medical indication existed; in these cases, students would have to justify their decision to a faculty member. In this situation, as in several others, a student's complaint led to faculty awareness of a problem, which in turn prompted a change in Program arrangements calculated to eliminate the source of difficulty.

Communication with student–representatives was not confined to complaints. In addition, their opinion and advice were sought on C. C. & T. P. problems which had been troubling staff members, on the feasibility of certain changes proposed. For example, a staff discussion of how to cut down the time doctors and students spent waiting for new patients in the General Medical Clinic —and the time patients spent waiting for doctors—resulted in the tentative proposal to change the system by assigning the first patients to arrive to the first doctors and students to arrive (instead of by name, which was the current arrangement). Student–representatives were then asked whether they thought this change would be "a good idea." The representatives deliberated, asked clarifying questions, and concluded the change was definitely "worth a try." For, as one representative said, "If it works we'll save a lot of time—and so will the patients." In this fashion students were, in some respects, treated as "junior partners" in attempts to improve the Program.

Sometimes, when representatives felt they did not actually know what their "constituents" would think about a given change, they were asked to find out, and report on their "poll" the following week. Thus, before many changes were formally made, the Program Director often knew in advance whether students would be dominantly positive, negative, or neutral regarding any given alteration. And even though student advice was not always followed, it was usually taken into account in assessing the wisdom of a particular course of action.

Between students and staff, then, as well as among staff members, there was considerable communication concerning the progress of the Program. To a large extent, this was made possible by the existence of regular, planned events—such as staff meetings and student–faculty luncheons—where information and opinion could circulate freely. Without such facilitation, it is doubtful whether the concept of sharing responsibility for Program improvement and change would have been particularly meaningful.

Special Information

Another aspect of the planned problem-solving format of the C. C. & T. P. consisted of the availability of special information. This information was the product of several ongoing research activities designed to furnish data which would aid in evaluating the progress and effect of the Program.[17] It contributed to Program alterations first, by providing suggestive evidence—independent of staff "impressions"—regarding conditions in the C. C. & T. P. which particularly concerned the staff.

Tabulation of anonymous student responses to a query[18] concerning the weekly Comprehensive Care Conference indicated, for example, that over half of the students (60 per cent) were prepared to say that attending these conferences had not been particularly worthwhile in contributing to their medical training. This information buttressed the reports of Preceptors and other staff members regarding student reactions to the conference, and thus gave additional impetus to attempts aimed at improving the conference.

Such information rarely constituted the only grounds for Program modification, however, since staff members tended to be aware—quite apart from such information—of conditions which might be improved. But, as in the case just cited, even elementary research findings frequently *documented* a condition about which there had previously been only vague or incomplete impressions, and in this fashion furnished additional incentive for change.

Sometimes the research data played a role in *maintaining* rather than changing arrangements, in that they pointed out areas of "success" as well as those of "failure" in achieving Program goals. For instance, information concerning student experience in providing continuous care for patients in the Program showed that students saw Family Care patients an average number of 4.4 times, and other patients an average of 1.8 times during the semester.[19]

[17] Detailed description of these research activities is presented by George G. Reader, "The Cornell Comprehensive Care and Teaching Program," in this volume, pp. 90–100.

[18] This question was one of many contained in a lengthy questionnaire first administered to C. C. & T. P. students in December 1952.

[19] See Margaret Olencki, "Range of Patient Contacts in the Comprehensive Care and Teaching Program," in this volume, p. 276.

These figures were seen as representing "good" continuity by the C. C. & T. P. staff, with the result that no alterations in arrangements relevant to this situation were considered necessary. Nevertheless, this stabilizing function of the information does not negate the role it played, from time to time, in stimulating change.

A second way in which the research studies played a part in Program alterations is implicit in the comment of one staff member, who said:

> *We want this to be a model program,* something that other medical schools can copy with profit. Everything isn't going exactly the way it should yet, but *we've made considerable headway and we have statistics to prove it.*

This kind of statement was made frequently by staff members; it suggests that precisely because the C. C. & T. P. was being studied, a certain amount of motivation to be alerted to problems and to try to correct them "for the final record" was engendered in C. C. & T. P. participants.

SUMMARY

Many specific problems were encountered in the C. C. & T. P. during its first year of full-scale operation. These problems were dealt with by changing, in one fashion or another, the arrangements believed responsible for the difficulty. Though extensive in number, the changes made were minor in the sense that no major objective or activity stipulated in the original plan was eliminated or altered beyond recognition.

Certain conditions and processes facilitated the occurrence of change in the organization. Setting the stage for change was the recognition that since the Program was experimental in character, no particular initial arrangement need be considered sacrosanct, but rather was to be judged on its demonstrated merit. This outlook permeated the attitude of C. C. & T. P. staff members toward their daily activities, and served as a motivating force in alerting these persons to the presence of problems. An even stronger incentive stemmed from the fact that the regular duties of full-time C. C. & T. P. staff members included unofficial responsibility for "improving" the Program; awareness of problems and suggestions for improvements were expected and rewarded by approval from peers and superiors. In addition, satisfaction frequently came from putting one's own suggestion into effect with apparently salutary results. Responsibility for the progress of the Program was officially shared among representatives of all of the groups concerned with patient care in the hospital and medical college. This situation made possible the practice of "clearing" plans for modification with the appropriate department head or other administrator on the C. C. & T. P. Advisory Committee before the plans were put into operation, and thereby reduced potential administrative resistance to change. Improving the Program was a group process and, as such, required regular channels of communication. Frequent scheduled meetings among staff members and between staff members and students served this purpose. Supplementing the information acquired through these communication devices were research findings designed to help in assessing the progress and effects of the Program.

In short, changes in the C. C. & T. P. occurred because staff members were motivated to think in terms of possible improvements in the Program, and because "machinery" for change—a problem-solving format—was built into the organization from the outset.

Margaret Olencki

RANGE OF PATIENT CONTACTS IN THE COMPREHENSIVE CARE AND TEACHING PROGRAM

Early in the development of the Comprehensive Care and Teaching Program a system of "bookkeeping" statistics was established to give a formal picture of the amount and type of experience students received in the clinics during their term in the Program. It aimed to give information both on the opportunities open to students, and on the use which they made of these opportunities. It was considered desirable to keep account of the number of patients students saw, the continuity of care they gave them, the range of diagnoses with which they were confronted, the degree of responsibility they were actually given in the care of patients, and the extent to which the various services and specialties were able to coordinate their activities in the care of patients.

Data were obtained from a one-page Visit Report which the students were asked to fill out each time they had a contact with a patient in any of the clinics in which they were working. (For these purposes, "contact" was broadly defined to include not only seeing the patient in the clinic, but also home visits, telephone conversations with the patient or members of his family, and consultations about the patient in the latter's absence.) This Report, in addition to giving brief personal data on the patient, distinguished Family Care from other patients; recorded the place and type of contact; indicated whether or not it was a first contact; listed the diagnoses, specifying those which were new and also those which received treatment on that visit; and indicated any consultations, conferences, or referrals which took place.[1]

After a pilot run of three weeks in the first semester of the Program, complete recording was carried out in the second semester, between December 1952 and June 1953. There were 41 students in the Program during that time, and about 6,500 Visit Reports were turned in. It was not feasible to analyze all of them; instead, all the reports for Family Care patients were coded, since they were few in number, and a 10 per cent random sample of the rest was selected.[2]

The resulting tabulations have been referred to as "bookkeeping" statistics because they show the frequency of various experiences but provide no standard of comparison by which to evaluate them. The Comprehensive Care and Teaching Program was initiated in July 1952 and from that date on all fourth-year medical students have participated in it. No statistics comparable with the Visit Reports were kept before the Program started, and whatever one wants to find out about that earlier period must be pieced together from the patients' charts and from the ordinary records of the hospital. Needless to say, these do not always provide what one wants to know. One must be content for the present to summarize the totals of various student activities without being dogmatic as to whether they represent good learning opportunity and good medical care rendered, or the reverse.

NUMBER OF PATIENTS AND VISITS

During the semester studied, December 1952 to June 1953, a student saw an average of 83 patients, with whom he averaged 159 contacts. Again talking in terms of averages, about 4 of these were Family Care patients, and they accounted for 16 of the contacts. In absolute figures, the number of patients seen by individual students ranged from 50 to 145, and the total number of contacts from 105 to 243.

The distribution of these average figures according to the clinics in which the patients were seen is shown in Table 29.

[1] Dr. Dorothy Beck designed the Visit Report and supervised its administration and the ensuing tabulations; the present writer succeeded her only when the study was at the stage of analysis.

[2] Every Report on which the patient's history number ended in 1 was taken.

TABLE 29. Average Case Load of Student, According to Clinic

Place patient seen	No. of patients	No. of contacts
General Medical Clinic	29	74
Pediatrics Clinic	19	29
Psychiatric Clinic	3	13
Other specialty clinics	31	42
Home	1	1
Total	83	159

About half of each student's patient contacts took place in the General Medical Clinic. In the specialty clinics, where the students worked on elective subjects, they made considerably fewer patient contacts than in the G.M.C., despite the fact that they spent about the same percentage of time in each; the apparent explanation is that some of these specialty clinics devote more time to didactic teaching, as opposed to working with patients, than is the case in the General Medical Clinic. The student spent only 11 weeks in Pediatrics and Psychiatry, compared with 22 in Comprehensive Medicine, so he naturally had fewer contacts in these clinics. The small number of visits in Psychiatry is presumably due to the fact that contact with a psychiatric patient ordinarily involves more time than with a medical patient.

CONTINUITY OF CARE

One of the basic aims of the Program, it will be remembered,[3] was to see that a patient returned to the same student–physician for as great a part as possible of the period in which he required continuing care. The Visit Reports provide information on how far this aim was carried out in the second semester of the Program. At first glance, the general picture may suggest lack of continuity: nearly two-thirds of all patients with whom students had contact during this semester were seen only once by the same student. There was wide variation among the clinics, however, and the low general average for continuity of care was largely due to the influence of the specialty electives which accounted for more than

[3] See George G. Reader, "The Cornell Comprehensive Care and Teaching Program," in this volume.

a third of the patients seen, but a much smaller proportion of total visits. These specialty clinics, which more or less lay outside the scope of the Comprehensive Care and Teaching Program, often aimed deliberately at providing a large number of different patients rather than encouraging follow-up of a smaller group. In the specialty clinics only 11 per cent of the patients were seen more than once by the same physician, and practically none was seen more than 4 times.

In General Medicine the picture is quite different. Two-thirds of the patients were seen more than once; more than one-fifth were seen 4 times or more; about fifteen patients, more than 10 times each; and one even made 22 visits with the same student.[4] The staff of the General Medical Clinic have expressed surprise that as many as one-third of the patients were seen only once by the same student;[5] it is their impression that very few patients are discharged, and not many referred elsewhere, after only one visit. It would be interesting, therefore, to find out how many of the "one-visit" patients were given appointments for a second visit and failed to keep them.

From the point of view of the student's learning, however, it is probably not so essential that he should see every single patient at least twice as that he should have some experience of following patients over a considerable length of time. This the Comprehensive Care and Teaching Program does seem to be providing. As far as one can gather from an impressionistic review of records kept by the General Medical Clinic before the Program got under way, students never saw a patient in the G.M.C. more than 4 times, and probably in only a few instances as many as 4. Since the Program started, it is fairly certain that all students carry some patients longer than that. This was so even in the semester under discussion, and since that time the growth of the Family

---

[4] Continuity figures refer to visits with the same student. Total visits for these patients would be slightly higher, since if a patient made a visit when his student–physician was sick or otherwise unavailable he would see another student or a staff member on that occasion.

[5] One must bear in mind that some of these were the new patients seen near the end of the semester, when there was no longer time for a revisit with the same student. A little earlier than this, there would be time for one revisit but not two; and so on. In other words, the time limit on the student's participation in the Program inevitably imposes a limitation on the continuity of his contacts with patients.

TABLE 30.   Continuity of Patient Care, According to Clinic

No. of times same patient seen by student	Percentage of patients in each clinic				
	Total, all clinics	General Medicine	Pediatrics	Psychiatry	Specialty clinics
1	62	35	65	30	89
2	18	27	23	7	7
3	9	17	7	5	2
4	4	9	3	5	1
5–10	6	11	2	47	1
11–23	1	1	—	6	—
Total no. of patients	(3,385)	(1,223)	(789)	(110)	(1,263)
Total no. of visits	6,516	3,206	1,218	585	1,507
Average no. of visits per patient	1.9	2.6	1.5	5.3	1.2

Care Program, and then the development of Home Care,[6] make this ever increasingly true. Moreover, before the Program was introduced, a patient seen twice quite probably made both visits in the same month. Now he may return four or five months later for his second visit, thus giving the student an opportunity to observe change in the patient's condition over a much longer period. This represents an improvement in learning experience, even when it involves no more visits than previously.

In Pediatrics the continuity was far less, partly because the student was there for only 11 weeks, and partly also because of the emphasis in that department on health promotion and well-baby care. In Psychiatry there were more visits with the same student than anywhere else; each student saw only two to four patients and followed them very intensively.

Up to this point in the discussion of continuity of care, no distinction has been drawn between the 151 Family Care patients and the rest; Table 30 combines them all. There is, however, a

[6] Home Care is not described in this paper, since it did not officially become a part of the C. C. & T. P. until May 1954, nearly a year after the end of the semester studied here; but it obviously deserves mention in the context of continuity of patient care. During 1954–1955, the first year of its full operation, 67 patients were carried for a total of 5,752 days. Half of the first group of students coming through the Program in that year cared for a Home Care patient at some time; all of the second group of students had this experience. They averaged 7.9 visits with the same patient, the range being 1 to 28. The duration of time individual patients were carried on Home Care varied from 5 days to 52 weeks. A monograph, giving full details of the Home Care Program, is now being prepared by Dr. Lawrence Sonkin.

considerable difference between the two groups. The average number of visits per Family Care patient is 4.4, compared with 1.8 for other patients; in Pediatrics it is 2.6, compared with 1.5 for other patients; in General Medicine, Family Care patients average 5.1 visits, compared with 2.4 for the rest. This difference is no doubt partly due to the fact that Family Care families were chosen because at least one of their members had a condition which would probably require continuing and intensive care. Nevertheless, it is probably fair to say that some of the difference is accounted for by a more intensive interest in, and study of, Family Care patients on the part of the students.[7] This view gains strength if we consider that occasional check-ups with healthy members of the family make the continuity average lower than it would be if only the visits with ill members of the family were counted.

RANGE OF DIAGNOSES

It has been suggested in criticism of Comprehensive Care that allowing students to follow particular patients over a fairly long period of time, and thus cutting down the number they can see, will restrict their experience of different diseases to an undesirable extent. It might be thought, too, that a longer time spent in the General Medical Clinic at the expense of the specialty clinics could reduce considerably the range of diagnoses encountered.

So far as the first point is concerned, one cannot be certain yet of the extent to which *individual* students had broad experience of different diseases. It was the policy of the staff assigning new patients to students to take into consideration the kinds of disease entities the student had already met, in an attempt to give him a well-rounded experience; but it is not yet known how successfully this worked out in practice. It is hoped that in a larger-scale follow-up study it will be possible to obtain accurate results for individual students. It can be shown from our data, however, that the range of diagnoses available to *all* students during the semester was wide, without undue concentration on any particular type of disease; this can be seen in the first column of Table 31.

[7] The frequent discussion and evaluation of Family Care families at history meetings and seminars must also have contributed to this closer scrutiny.

TABLE 31. Diagnoses, According to Clinic

Diagnosis	Percentage of patients in each clinic			
	Total, all clinics	General Medicine	Pediatrics	Specialty clinics
Cardiovascular disease	24	44	6	16
Respiratory disorders	22	17	35	20
Digestive disorders	21	31	14	17
Nervous system and sense organ disorders	16	19	15	14
Genito-urinary disorders	15	28	6	9
Endocrine and metabolic disorders	15	23	4	14
Mental disorders	14	16	3	18
Skin and cellular tissue disorders	13	9	13	16
Diseases of bones and organs of movement	12	14	10	11
Diseases of early infancy	—*	4	16	8
Healthy individual	9	4	30	1
Nervousness, vague headache	7	9	10	11
Neoplasms	5	6	3	6
Anemias, etc.	5	9	5	2
Infectious and parasitic diseases	5	5	3	6
Syphilis	5	2	—*	9
Tuberculosis	4	4	2	5
Allergy	4	3	5	3
Accidents, poisoning, violence	1	2	1	—*
Prenatal and postnatal care	1	2	—*	—*
Undetermined	2	5	—*	—*
Total no. of patients	(3,385)	(1,223)	(789)	(1,373)
Average no. of diagnoses per patient	2.1	2.6	1.8	1.8

* Less than 1 per cent.

The evidence indicates that there is little basis in fact for the second criticism mentioned above—that the General Medical Clinic may not provide the student with an adequate range of diagnoses without heavy supplementation from the specialty clinics. There are few cases in which a lower percentage of General Medical patients have a given diagnosis than the patients of all clinics taken together. In fact, most percentages are substantially higher, because General Medical patients average more diagnoses each than patients in other clinics—2.6 each compared with 1.8 elsewhere. A second reason for the richness of material in the

G.M.C. is the innovation of the Comprehensive Care and Teaching Program in bringing more of the new cases through the General Medical Clinic instead of sending them directly to the specialty clinics as was previously done. This was designed to give the students on the G.M.C. a wider range of patients, and to make sure of an ample supply of "new"[8] patients from whom to take medical histories and on whom to perform complete physical examinations. In fact, with two exceptions, all patients possibly destined for any of the Medical Specialty Clinics were supposed to be sent to the General Medical Clinic first. (The exceptions were patients with syphilis or with skin complaints; they were sent directly to the clinics concerned with those diseases. The Syphilis Clinic has since been made a part of the General Medical Clinic, adding still another area in which G.M.C. provides as wide a range as all clinics.) The other areas in which the percentage of General Medical patients with a given diagnosis is lower than that of all patients in the clinics considered here—respiratory disorders, diseases of early infancy, and healthy individuals—are amply compensated for in the Pediatrics Clinic, which is also a Comprehensive Care clinic.

One fact worth noting is that the figures from the specialty clinics are unstable in a way in which those from the Comprehensive Care clinics are not. The students have some choice as to which electives they will take, and therefore which specialty clinics they will work in. Their choices vary from semester to semester. If, for instance, many students elect Cardiac Clinic one semester and very few the next, this will greatly affect the number of cardiac patients seen in specialty clinics.

In this discussion of diagnoses, it is only the matter of range of diagnosis that is being considered. There is no intention of claiming that the Out-Patient Department necessarily shows disease in all the phases with which a physician should be familiar: ambulant patients, on the whole, only give experience with the less severe

---

[8] The student's patient load is made up of the "new" patients assigned to him, about one per clinic session, as well as the revisits with patients he has seen before. According to hospital policy, a "new" patient in the G.M.C. is one who has not attended the General Medical Clinic for over a year, and therefore needs a thorough examination; it need not mean that the patient has never been to New York Hospital before.

forms of various conditions. All that is suggested here is that there are ample opportunities for seeing many different diagnoses under Comprehensive Care.

From the standpoint of learning there is a great difference between passively observing a condition (or confirming, after reading the patient's chart, that it is still current) and actively making the diagnosis oneself. Comprehensive Care aims to give the student as much responsibility for the patient and as much opportunity for exercising clinical judgment as possible. To help measure how far this aim was being achieved, students were asked to distinguish on the Visit Reports the diagnoses they themselves made together with their instructors from those they merely observed or confirmed. In the course of the semester, the average student made 120 diagnoses and encountered another 51; that is, he took an active part in some 70 per cent of the diagnoses that were made. The percentage varied from clinic to clinic: in General Medicine it was 75 per cent, in Pediatrics 81 per cent, and in the specialty clinics 58 per cent. This relatively greater degree of active participation in General Medicine and Pediatrics is not wholly an innovation of the Comprehensive Care and Teaching Program; students working in these clinics have always been assigned to "new" patients, and, obviously, it is such new patients who present the student–physician with the greatest opportunity to take active part in the process of diagnosis. But the longer time spent in these clinics offering a more active role to students *is* of course an innovation; moreover, instructors may feel more inclined to allow students freedom of action when they see them gain in maturity and judgment over a longer period of time.

It should be noted in passing that the Family Care group, besides having more visits with the same physician, also had a higher average number of conditions diagnosed—in General Medicine it was 3.4 each, compared with 2.5 each for non-Family Care patients; in Pediatrics it was 2.7 compared with 1.8 for the others. As with the greater number of visits for this group, the difference probably reflects in part an objective difference in the patients; but it also suggests that the student was led to scrutinize them more closely than his other patients and thus to make more complete diagnoses.

COORDINATION OF SERVICES—CONSULTATIONS AND
REFERRALS

Comprehensive Care aims to bring to the patient all the different
kinds of service he may need, often transcending that which can
be supplied by one physician alone (or, in a teaching situation,
by the student–physician and his instructor). Under the Program,
students were encouraged to consult medical specialists and to
confer with nurses and social workers whenever they deemed it
necessary. It is difficult to measure the result with respect to conferences, since students definitely underreported these.[9] The more
nearly complete figures reported by Social Service and the Public Health Nurse indicate that there was an average of 4.3 conferences per student with Social Service, and 2.1 per student with
the Public Health Nurse. Some conferences were also held with
other nurses, with the dietician, speech therapist, and others; so
the general average for conferences is probably around 8 per
student.

The consultation system was initiated to help coordinate patient
care within the general clinic, and to reduce the number of referrals that needed to be made from one clinic to another. The patient thus benefits from more continuous and convenient care,
while the student learns to work as a member of a team, and has
a chance to follow interesting cases which would have been lost
to him under the earlier system of referring patients to other
clinics.

As an alternative to referrals, the consultation system does not
at first glance seem to have been very successful—at least in the
semester under review. Students had an average of 12 consultations,[10] but referred patients to other clinics on an average of
27[11] occasions. From the point of view of the patient, about 1 in
10 received a consultation, while about 3 in 10 were referred to
other clinics. Here again the Family Care group received more

[9] In a sense this is a compliment to the way conferences were organized. The
Public Health Nurse, for instance, was so easily available that students would chat
with her informally about their patients and forget to enter a conference on the
Visit Report.
[10] Ten were in the General Medical Clinic or Pediatrics, 2 in specialty clinics.
[11] Twenty-three were from the General Medical Clinic or Pediatrics to specialty
clinics; 4 were from specialty clinics to General Medical Clinic or Pediatrics.

attention. Consultations were requested for 7 out of 10 of them, compared with 1 out of 10 for other patients, constituting a remarkable difference. Referrals were about the same in the two groups.

However, the matter is not as clear-cut as these figures may suggest. In some instances, it would not have been desirable, and no attempt was made, to replace referrals by consultations. In others, it would have been desirable to establish a consultation system, but it was not possible to arrange it with the department concerned.

It is to be expected that the system of consultations would be most successful in those cases requiring aid from departments which had a part-time consultant in the General Medical Clinic, i.e., Surgery, Obstetrics and Gynecology, and Psychiatry; and the figures indicate that, by and large, this was the case. Table 32, which bears on this point, lists the cases seen in either the General Medical Clinic or the Pediatric Clinic for which the student and his instructor sought assistance, according to the department from which aid was solicited; it also indicates how these cases were handled, that is, whether by consultation, by temporary referral, or by permanent referral. (The bases for the percentages in Table 32 are, in each case, the total requiring the aid of a particular specialty clinic.)

As has already been suggested, the data of Table 32 show that consultations were most likely to result when aid was sought from departments which had consultants working within the General Medical Clinic. For example, in 157 surgical cases not handled alone by the student and his instructor, 80 per cent were dealt with in the General Medical Clinic by the consultant in surgery, and only 20 per cent were referred to another clinic (8 per cent temporarily and 12 per cent permanently). This might be contrasted with cases requiring assistance from the Ear, Nose, and Throat Department, which had neither a consultant in the General Medical Clinic nor any particular arrangements for consultation. In 182 ear, nose, and throat cases not handled by the student alone, only 1 per cent ever had a consultation; the other 99 per cent were referred to the Ear, Nose, and Throat Clinic, 46 per cent temporarily and 53 per cent permanently.

TABLE 32.   Consultations and Referrals in Comprehensive Care Clinics, According to Assisting Departments

Assisting department	Percentage of patients			No. of cases not handled by student alone
	Consul-tations	Temporary referrals	Permanent referrals	
1. Departments with consultants:				
Surgery	80	8	12	(157)
Obstetrics-Gynecology	64	18	18	(137)
Psychiatry	60	11	29	(45)
Average percentage of patients	68	12	20	
2. Departments without consultants:				
Ear, Nose, Throat	1	46	53	(182)
Neurology	11	35	54	(102)
Eye	—	53	47	(94)
Orthopedic	16	33	51	(82)
Cardiac	38	18	44	(77)
Dermatology	28	39	33	(64)
Allergy	17	25	58	(60)
Urology	25	38	37	(52)
Dental	29	47	24	(38)
Hematology	26	26	48	(34)
Pulmonary	7	45	48	(29)
Endocrine	—	56	44	(25)
Arthritis	—	28	72	(18)
Minor Surgery	—	75	25	(16)
Gastrointestinal	7	29	64	(14)
Other	48	18	34	(142)
Average percentage of patients	16	38	46	
No. of patients	(426)	(412)	(530)	(1,368)

The extent to which consultations replaced referrals in the other two departments sending part-time consultants to the General Medical Clinic was not as notable as in the case of Surgery, but was still considerable. In nearly two-thirds of the cases requiring attention from the Department of Obstetrics and Gynecology, consultations were held; in Psychiatry 60 per cent of the cases were handled by the consultant.[12] The number of cardiac consulta-

[12] The percentage may in fact have been higher, since some of the referrals may actually have been made by the consultant himself, on the grounds that only the specialty clinic had the necessary equipment, in the case of Obstetrics-Gynecology, or that the patient was too seriously disturbed to be dealt with in a general clinic, in the case of Psychiatry.

tions is higher than might be expected with no consultant in the General Medical Clinic; this probably reflects the fact that one of the residents in Cardiology was particularly interested in Comprehensive Care and went out of his way to make consultations possible.

Table 32 has been considered so far in terms of the percentage of cases requiring specialized attention which were handled through consultations, and the percentage which were referred to specialty clinics. It can also be considered in terms of the total number of cases of various kinds in which there was recourse to specialists, for this may suggest the areas in which consultations may be most needed. E.N.T. heads the list with 182 cases. Some people have made this a case for urging the introduction of an Ear, Nose, and Throat consultant into the General Medical Clinic. The other school of thought maintains that E.N.T. conditions are usually fairly easily diagnosed, the treatment clear-cut, and that they often occur in patients who have no other complaint, so that referring them to the E.N.T. Clinic does not deprive the student of a particularly valuable opportunity for learning and does not usually subject the patient to the inconvenience of being followed in two clinics at once. They would prefer, if a choice had to be made, to have a consultant from the Department of Neurology, from whom expert advice was sought in 102 cases. These 102 cases probably represent a large proportion of the total number of neurological cases seen in the General Medical Clinic;[13] in other words, it seems that very few neurological cases are handled by the student and his instructor unaided. Moreover, it is argued, neurology is intimately related to Internal Medicine, is an interesting and difficult specialty, and one in which it would be rewarding for students to gain more experience. Thus any arrangement which would allow more of these cases to be followed by students in the General Medical Clinic, instead of being referred to the Neurology Clinic would seem to be desirable as far as Comprehensive Care is concerned.[14]

Neurological cases offer an instance in which expert advice is

[13] It is hard to know exactly how many cases should be so classified, but it is probably in the neighborhood of 150.

[14] Of course, other considerations, such as the needs and attitudes of the Neurology Clinic, must be taken into account.

frequently sought; cardiac cases provide an example of the opposite kind. It is true that there were 77 cases who received specialized attention from cardiologists; but this is surprisingly few in view of the large number of cardiac cases encountered in the General Medical Clinic (44 per cent of all General Medical patients seen by students exhibit some form of cardiovascular disease). This probably reflects the particular interests of the Comprehensive Care staff, among whom, it so happens, there have always been one or more doctors who have specialized to some extent in Cardiology.

SUMMARY

These tabulations have permitted us to obtain a preliminary picture of the clinical experiences which one group of fourth-year students had during the term in Comprehensive Medicine. On the whole, the results seem to indicate a wide range of experience and activity. They also suggest that, at least during the semester studied, the goals of the Comprehensive Care and Teaching Program were rather successfully met.

Appendices

Appendix A

SOCIALIZATION:
A TERMINOLOGICAL NOTE

Ratified by more than two generations of use in psychology and sociology, the technical term socialization designates the processes by which people selectively acquire the values and attitudes, the interests, skills, and knowledge—in short, the culture—current in the groups of which they are, or seek to become, a member. It refers to the learning of social roles. In its application to the medical student, socialization refers to the processes through which he develops his professional self, with its characteristic values, attitudes, knowledge, and skills, fusing these into a more or less consistent set of dispositions which govern his behavior in a wide variety of professional (and extraprofessional) situations. Socialization takes place primarily through social interaction with people who are significant for the individual—in the medical school, probably with faculty members above most others, but importantly also with fellow-students, with the complement of associated personnel (nurses, technicians, caseworkers, etc.), and with patients. Since the patterns of social interaction of medical students with these others are only similar and not identical, the variations result in different kinds of medical men emerging from what may at first seem to be the "same" social environment of the medical school.

The *fact* that socialization occurs, that people tend to acquire the culture and subculture of the groups with which they are affiliated, has been noticed for so long that the memory of man

287

runneth not to the contrary. But the social and psychological processes through which this comes about, so that different individuals in the same group variously assimilate the established culture have become, only in recent years, the object of methodical and sustained inquiry.[1] Just as everyone, even Macaulay's schoolboy, knows by the repeated evidence of his own eyes that objects fall when they lack support and knows this without recourse to the law of inertia, so everyone knows without recourse to sociology and psychology, that individuals brought up in a Japanese, or American, or Bantu culture tend to acquire the speech, values, and ways of life current in their culture. As attention shifts to less commonplace, less gross, matters of socialization, however, even the unexplained *facts* may not be easily available. Is it the case, for example, that as they move through successive years of medical school, students acquire a greater, or a diminishing, preference for patients who express their appreciation of the physician's services? Does the value placed upon such responses by patients vary in the cultural climates of different schools? Familiarity with some of the gross events is of course only a specious substitute for more detailed knowledge of the processes through which socialization comes about or fails to occur in determinate respects. In considering the "socialization of the medical student," then, we consider the processes by which neophytes come to acquire, in patterned but selective fashion, the attitudes and values, skills, knowledge, and ways of life established in the professional subculture.

In our studies we return, repeatedly and in various connections, to the sociological and psychological concept of socialization,

[1] The annals of science—physical, biological, and social—are crowded with instances of the premature suspension of curiosity because a commonsense knowledge of gross phenomena had precluded interest in the mechanisms through which these phenomena came to be. Out of this indefinitely large class of cases, one example will perhaps suffice: as Köhler has pointed out, everyone knows that we come to forget many experiences, and many take it for granted that this decay of memory is simply the result of passage of time. Yet recent experimental work in psychology has shown how much more complex are the processes which make for faulty memory; that forgetting is less a case of old experience fading from memory than of "the interference, inhibition, or obliteration of the old by the new." It might also be said that it is the office of systematic study to question the "self-evident" commonplaces of human experience and to show, often if not invariably, that these are not what they seem. On this general issue, see Wolfgang Köhler, *Dynamics in Psychology* (New York: Liveright Publishing Corporation, 1940), pp. 30–31.

which is central to the inquiry into the making of the medical man. Here, however, we want to distinguish *this* concept of socialization—hopefully, once and for all, so far as this particular study is concerned—from the concept of *socialization* as it is understood in economics and politics and, derivatively, in the vernacular. The *economic* and *political* usage of the word socialization stems from the doctrine which advocates the ownership and control of the apparatus of production by the community as a whole, and its administration by political agencies of the community. Loosely speaking, it refers to the "nationalization" of industry, business, or professional services. It is this sense of the word, of course, which is current in medical circles in the form of the stock phrase, "the socialization of medicine." In the course of generations of controversy—at least since the days of Bismarck in Germany, Lloyd George in England, and Wilson, if not Theodore Roosevelt, in the United States—the words, "socialized medicine," have become fighting words. Indeed, "socialized medicine" has become so much the stereotyped phrase that, in some quarters, the first word almost invariably produces the second, both among those who oppose and those who support certain kinds of arrangements for the distribution of medical care by physicians. To recognize this tendency in the use of language may perhaps be enough to nullify it—or, less optimistically, to put it in question. When we say that "the medical student is being socialized" in the professional culture, we plainly do not mean that he is being "nationalized" or imbued with a belief in the virtues of socialism. For it should be clear, by now, that the technical term *socialization* as employed for half a century and more in sociology and psychology has nothing whatever to do with the technical term *socialization* as employed in economics and politics since the middle of the last century.

In the context of sociology and psychology, "to socialize" means to render *social*, to shape individuals into members of groups (whatever they may be—familial, religious, or professional); in the context of economics and politics, "to socialize" means to render *socialistic*, to modify political or economic systems according to the doctrines of socialism. The first of these is a wholly descriptive concept, devoid of implicit or explicit preferences; the second is often an optative concept, advocating or rejecting as well as describing. The one is generally confined to use as a technical term, neutral and emotionally unexciting; the other is frequently extended into an invective, a signal for attack or support. In psychological and sociological usage, *socialization* refers to ways in which *individuals* are shaped by their culture; in economic and political usage, it refers to ways in which an *organization* of human activities is shaped into a designated kind of structure. In short, all that the two words now have in common is their spelling.[2]

All this is simply a reminder that *socialization* is a member of that large class of words which are called homonyms. In spite of their superficial family resemblance and their common etymological ancestor in the distant past, *socialization₁* and *socialization₂* are semantically neither kith nor kin. This kind of case is familiar enough: the vocabularies of science have a large stock of homonyms, quite distinct words which happen to be, as Fowler puts it, "like in look but unlike in sense." A few examples must stand for the many that make up the imposingly long list of technical homonyms that turn up in the various branches of science. The bacteriologist, come of age since the days of Koch and Pasteur, does not hesitate to use the term *culture* simply because the anthropologist, from the days of Tylor and Kidd, has utilized *culture* in quite another sense. Nor, rightly enough, does the anthropologist hesitate to speak of *material culture,* by which he means generally the physical artifacts produced by man-in-society, for fear that this might be confused, in the minds of some, with a *bacterial culture.* The parallelism, which is not apparently the result of borrowing, indeed runs to specialized formations of the basic homonym: both bacteriologist and anthropologist, for example, speak, in their several ways, of *subcultures.* And neither

[2] And a common etymological lineage. It is idle, of course, to debate matters of priority or "correct" usage when the same collocation of letters happens to have quite distinct and unrelated meanings. In some contexts, the psychological and sociological meaning of socialization is appropriate; in others, the economic and political meaning. To assert that one, rather than the other, meaning is correct would be to legislate in a realm where laws which collide with the folkways are notoriously ineffective; to confuse the two meanings would border on the grotesque. But it is of passing interest that such an established repository of word meanings as the *Oxford English Dictionary* first cites the psychological and sociological sense of the term socialize, and only then turns to its economic and political sense.

denies himself the term because "culture" is colloquially still understood as fastidious self-cultivation or, after the fashion of Matthew Arnold, as the "disinterested search for sweetness and light." As is generally the case with language, the context aptly enough shows which meaning of the homonym is intended and, in a language shot through with homonymous constructions, words of the same outward appearance are bound to appear in quite unrelated fields of inquiry.[3]

Perhaps a closer parallel to the case of *socialization* is the case of *rationalization*. Economists use the term to refer to "the 'scientific' organization of industry to ensure minimum waste of labor, standardizing of production and, presumably, a resulting maintenance of prices at a constant level" even though Ernest Jones had introduced the term into psychoanalysis to signify those morally or rationally elevated explanations of one's conduct which are plausible and unwittingly false. And again, the homonym rationalization,[4] firmly rooted in both economics and psychology, is anything but misleading, except to those who are bent on misunderstanding. The report that "Smith is rationalizing his own inadequacy as a supervisor when he describes his staff as uncooperative" is not likely to be understood as an oblique allusion to Smith's plans for industrial reorganization, even by those trained wholly in economics and untutored in the intricacies of psychoanalysis.

And so it goes with a multitude of homonyms, scientific and colloquial. As is evident, homonyms may lead more than a double

---

[3] That the same technical word with*in* a discipline may come in the course of events to have several related meanings is a fact which has nothing to do with scientific homonyms. See the extensive monograph on such a case of multiple meanings by A. L. Kroeber and Clyde Kluckhohn, *Culture: A Critical Review of Concepts and Definitions* (Cambridge: Peabody Museum of American Archaeology and Ethnology, 1952).

Kroeber and Kluckhohn observe that "the word culture with its modern technical or anthropological meaning was established in English by Tylor in 1871, though it seems not to have penetrated to any general or 'complete' British dictionary until more than fifty years later—a piece of cultural lag that may help to keep anthropologists humble in estimating the tempo of their influence on even the avowedly literate segment of their society." (p. 9). By the same token, the degree of humility due from psychologists and sociologists is profound beyond measure: the word socialization in its technical sense has yet to find its way into general dictionaries.

[4] It is perhaps best to say nothing here of the use of the word *rationalization* in mathematics to refer to the process of clearing from irrational quantities.

life. The physician uses *percussion* diagnostically; the musician, esthetically; the gunman, destructively. A *section* is one thing for the surgeon and anatomist, another for the botanist, and still a third for the mathematician; just as the geologist, printer, military man, college teaching assistant, real estate broker, and railwayman have each their own technical meaning for this versatile word. *Remission* may denote a decrease in the violence of a disease in pathology and relief of quite another kind in theology. The word *mass* takes on distinct and severally useful meanings in physics, politics, and pharmacy, in mining, fine arts, military science, and Catholic ritual. *Force* carries lightly the burden of its varied significance as "unlawful violence" in the sphere of law and as a collective term in the vernacular for the policemen engaged in maintaining law and order, just as it stands for quite different matters in physics, ethics, and literary accounts of love-making.

If only on the basis of ample precedent, it would seem that the widespread currency of the economic and political meanings of *socialization* in debates over appropriate arrangements for distributing medical services need not rule out the use of the psychological and sociological homonym, as in the phrase "socialization of the medical student," to refer to the processes through which he is being inducted into the professional culture of medicine. This review of usages would be unnecessary were it not for two things.

First, the "socialization of medicine" is a matter of great and acrimonious controversy, which for many is charged with intense feeling and passion. Such affect-laden words seem to have a way of driving their affectively-neutral and therefore dull homonyms out of circulation.[5] It is therefore necessary to emphasize the particular technical sense in which we employ the term socialization throughout these sociological studies of medical education.

Second, technical homonyms seldom result in misunderstandings since the readers of writings containing these terms are ordinarily themselves at work in the same technical field, and con-

---

[5] This would be somewhat akin to the process, noted by students of language, through which words "go to the bad" ("pejoration"). For example, the modern English word "silly" stems from the Middle English word *seli*. This originally

sequently share a common universe of discourse. Readers in the same field at once supply the appropriate, rather than the extraneous, meanings of the homonym, since they are socially insulated from the like-appearing word of quite different meaning. But when, as in the present instance, a technical term, such as *socialization,* comes to the attention of those in other fields, quite the contrary is apt to occur. Readers will naturally enough supply the meaning with which they are most familiar, and some may actively resist the thought that it may have an equally well-established though different meaning in the technical field previously unknown to them. And since "the socialization of medicine" has entered as a stock phrase into the vernacular, it is likely that the psychological and sociological meaning of socialization will be repeatedly subordinated to its economic and political meaning, unless this tendency is countered in advance.

That is why it has been emphasized throughout this volume and in other papers reporting our studies that the terms *socialization, socialize,* and *socialized* are employed almost without exception in their psychological and sociological sense.

---

meant "blessed" (Anglo-Saxon *soelig,* Modern German, *selig,* etc.). But "since 'the children of this world are in their generation wiser than the children of light,' and since the good will not stoop to the tricks of the evil, the latter regard them as lacking intelligence and as mere fools to have such scruples. . . ." For this and other examples of pejoration, see Louis H. Gray, *Foundations of Language* (New York: The Macmillan Company, 1939), p. 259 ff.

Just as there are cultural patterns of change in the meanings of words, so there are psychological patterns of supplying one, rather than another, meaning to homonyms, depending on temperamental characteristics of the individual. Thus, L. L. Thurstone has developed a "homonyms test" in which subjects are asked to respond with a synonym or definition to each word in a list of forty. The words have at least two common associations, one of these being physical and literal, the other more nearly human and emotional. For examples: lead, fire, taste, strike, slight, exhaust, push, revolution, nerve, pull. The responses of subjects, who are of course unaware of the nature or purpose of the test, are classified and counted to find out the ratio of emotional connotations to physical or literal connotations. This yields an objective score which is then related to other known temperamental characteristics of the subject. See L. L. Thurstone, *A Factorial Study of Perception* (Chicago: University of Chicago Press, 1944), p. 78 ff.

Patterns of associations with homonyms would presumably relate not only to psychological characteristics, such as temperament, but also to social characteristics, such as occupation. It is assumed in our discussion that, in a test, most physicians would spontaneously supply the economic and political meaning to the homonym *socialization,* and most sociologists, the psychological and sociological meaning.

Appendix B

RESEARCH IN PROGRESS

The papers in this volume are based on a small part of the data assembled in the course of these introductory studies in the sociology of medical education. A series of five monographs, dealing with a variety of interrelated problems, is now in preparation. Four of these studies deal with the relations of the medical student to groups significant to him: (1) to the faculty, (2) to fellow-students, (3) to patients, and (4) to his own family. The fifth deals, in effect, with the development of attitudes toward himself, i.e., his self-image and self-evaluation. Throughout, these are related to the process of socialization and professionalization of the student.

The monographs and the authors of each are as follows:
 1. *Reciprocal Relations of Medical Students and Faculty Members:* David Caplovitz

During the course of our research, we have obtained repeated data from students about their images of the values held by the faculty. Clinical students at Cornell University Medical College have also been asked to designate the faculty members whom they take as role models—the men whom they especially admire as physicians and those for whom they have particular respect as teachers. With data of this kind, it becomes possible to discover, for instance, how the selection of role models differs with the capacity or interests of the student or with the relative position of the faculty member in the school hierarchy. But if we are to understand the effects of the social environment provided by the faculty, we must have *independent* data *on the values actually held by the faculty.* For this purpose, Caplovitz developed a schedule of questions which were answered by nearly 500 members of the clinical faculty at Cornell. Comparable data are thus available for both faculty and students. (Within the limits of our knowledge, such reciprocal materials have not been collected before in any professional school; quite apart from their specific relevance to the sociology of medical education, they provide a benchmark for a study design in the investigation of educational institutions generally.) With these two sets of data, he is proceeding to locate the kinds and frequency of perceptions of one another's values by students and faculty alike. What are the images of the promising student as seen by faculty members in different departments? To what extent do the values of students resemble those actually held by their role models among the faculty? The parallel information on attitudes and values of both faculty and students, as well as the perceptions of each group by the other, provides a promising and extensive field for inquiry.

   2. *Social Relations among Medical Students and Attitudinal Learning:* William Nicholls, II

Nicholls is investigating the ways in which friendship and alienation among medical students come about and the consequences of these for maintaining or modifying professional interests, attitudes, and values. This is of more than casual significance for an understanding of processes of learning in medical school. As we have already found, the interaction among students importantly affects their professional socialization, and it is precisely this unorganized and unplanned aspect of the educational process which has tended to be a matter of anecdote and conjecture, rather than of methodical inquiry.

   Three consecutive sets of panel data make it possible to trace the concomitant changes of attitudes and values among each pair of student-friends. With material such as this, the role of student friendships can be assessed by noting the extent to which friends come to have similar professional values. Since not all such friendships are uniformly important, it becomes necessary to study *types* of friendships in their bearing upon attitudes and values. For example, do students with friends further along in medical school acquire new attitudes earlier? Are friendships carried over from pre-medical school days an aid or a hindrance to attitudinal learning? Unlike the asymmetrical relation of student and teacher, the symmetrical relation between friends affords no antecedent grounds for assuming which member of the pair is more influential. Does the academic standing or the relative popularity of students determine which direction the influence will take? Another type of problem has to do with the bases on which these friendships are formed. How do these shift in the course of time? It has been found that many friendships are broken and new ones formed, particularly in the period between the second and third years of medical school. Is this the result of new interests, or do new situations make it difficult to maintain previous friendships? What are the consequences of this turnover in friendships for the morale and the socialization of students? In short, this monograph is directed toward searching out the significance of peer-relations for professional learning.

3. *Medical Students and Patients: A Study in the Formation of a Professional Role:* William Martin

A substantial body of data concerns the relationship between the student-physician and the patients he is called upon to see during the course of his undergraduate training in medicine. The school provides a value-environment within which students learn the types of attitudes and behavior in relation to patients which are judged normatively correct. This monograph examines the types of norms and experiences with patients to which students are exposed in succeeding phases of their training and the bearing of these on the development of attitudes toward patients.

Some preliminary evidence suggests that the meaning of contact with patients differs substantially for second-year and for fourth-year students, the former centering on the opportunity to acquire knowledge and the latter on the opportunity to test professional competence. Since contacts with patients serve distinct and differing functions, attention is being devoted to characteristic changes in orientations toward patients on the part of students as they move through medical school. The study focuses upon the patterned situations in medical school which facilitate or hinder the efforts of students to conform to the professionally defined norms of behavior and attitudes toward patients. For example, which students tend to react to the necessity for speedy though effective examination of the patient by placing less emphasis upon investigating social and psychological factors in his illness, even when both faculty and student recognize these factors as important for the understanding and treatment of the illness? What social mechanisms make for conformity or for nonconformity to the standards of appropriate behavior and attitudes toward patients?

In sum, this study deals with: (1) the orientations of students toward patients, (2) the norms governing professional behavior and attitudes toward patients, (3) the conditions making for greater or less conformity to these norms, and (4) the consequences of conformity or nonconformity for effective learning of the role of the physician. These are being examined at several stages of the student's undergraduate training.

4. *Social Status of Medical Students and Their Professionalization:* E. David Nasatir

Little is now known about the influence of family background upon the attitudes, performance, and career orientations of medical students. This study compares students who are the children of physicians and students coming from other types of occupational backgrounds. There is some preliminary evidence that initial differences between the sons of physicians and other students tend to diminish as students advance through medical school. Another line of inquiry relates the attitudes and behavior of the student to the type of practice of the physician-parent. Do variations in the professional status of the parent have any bearing on the degree of influence which he exerts upon the student-physician?

The study thus considers students as they are involved in the two social systems of the family and the medical school. It examines compatibilities and incompatibilities of expectations of students deriving from these two sources and traces out consequences for adaptation and learning by students.

5. *Self-Images and Self-Appraisals of Medical Students:* Mary
Jean Huntington

Since the writings of George Mead were published a generation
ago, there has gradually developed a socio-psychological theory
of the sources and consequences of self-images and self-appraisals.
But only recently has there developed a body of inquiry which
empirically tests and develops the implications of this theory, say,
within the sphere of formal education. Yet it would seem important to learn how students arrive at self-appraisals, the standards
they use in evaluating themselves, and the consequences of all
this for professional development.

We have in hand an abundance of data on these matters—for
example, on the standards used by students in judging their level
of competence in various aspects of the professional role. Students
of the same degree of ability in selected respects rate themselves
quite differently depending upon their choice of reference groups,
i.e., whether they compare themselves with classmates, faculty
members, practicing physicians, or interns and residents. What
kinds of students, then, choose different reference groups for
self-appraisal and how do these cumulatively affect their self-
images? The data also make it possible to trace out the implications of the idea that self-images are formed through social interaction—specifically, that medical students tend to live up to
the expectations which designated others have of them and to
appraise themselves accordingly. Finally, it is possible to examine
the consequences of students' self-evaluations. Some students, for
example, who by objective measure have considerable ability may
nevertheless judge themselves as lacking in needed competence.
How does this affect their subsequent performance when they are
called upon to exhibit their ability under the stress of examinations? Similarly, other students judge their trained abilities as
greater than they objectively are; how does this affect their acquisition of requisite skills which they mistakenly feel they already possess?

Appendix C

NOTE ON SIGNIFICANCE TESTS

The reader will find that no traditional significance tests have been reported in connection with the statistical results in this volume. This is intentional policy rather than accidental oversight. It is a policy, furthermore, which the Bureau of Applied Social Research has always adhered to in reporting the results of exploratory studies such as are presented in this volume. Some of the reasons for this decision may be described as follows.

To begin with, traditional tests of significance have been developed to study the probable correctness or incorrectness of *single, isolated* statements, for example, that Drug A is more likely than Drug B to cause nausea. But it is an essential feature of these exploratory studies in medical education, and of many other empirical investigations in the social sciences, that there is no single hypothesis which can be viewed independently of other hypotheses. Instead, there is a series of loosely interrelated hypotheses which must be looked at in combination. For example, we may hypothesize that medical students will respond more favorably to some features of an educational innovation than they do to others. But a corollary hypothesis, which must be borne in mind when this first one is stated, is that those aspects of the innovation which are reacted to negatively may have as much—or more—impact on student attitudes and self-images as those which are

Editors' note: Dr. James Coleman and Dr. Hanan C. Selvin contributed to the formulation of some of these points while they were members of the Bureau staff.

301

better liked. In other words, it can be misleading to focus attention on one hypothesis without taking into consideration other related hypotheses. In a situation such as this it does not help to apply significance tests as standard procedure, for this assumes that each result is isolated from and independent of every other. Perhaps the solution is to consider the probability of the joint occurrence of the several results; but this has the shortcoming of assuming that we know, quite explicitly, which of the hypotheses are related, and in what manner.

Another reason for feeling that traditional significance tests are not appropriate relates to the purposes of our studies. These tests are designed to keep one from making statements about percentage differences (or other differences) when there is too little evidence to justify the statement. In order to do this, in order to avoid making unjustified claims about the magnitude and importance of an observed difference, one sets a rather high level of significance; one says, in other words, that if there is more likelihood than 1 in 100 (or 5 in 100) that the observed difference could have come about by chance, one must conclude that it is not a "real" difference. But in the effort to avoid mistaken decisions that an observed difference is significant, one runs the danger of making another kind of error. By insisting on a high level of significance (a low probability that there is no real difference) one increases the possibility of rejecting as insignificant differences which actually do exist. And this is a serious error in exploratory studies of the kind which we have been conducting. At this early stage of thinking about the processes of medical education it would seem desirable to assemble a wide array of evidence, even if some of it is not conclusive. We want to gather together as much information as we can about the relations between experiences in medical school and the development of particular attitudes and values. Later on, some of the hypotheses which we set up before starting the research, and others which have emerged during the course of our investigation, can be submitted to more definitive and rigorous test. Until that time, however, we do not want to cut short possibly productive lines of investigation by insisting now that our preliminary results prove themselves significant. We do not want to say now that, because some of our early results do not meet stringent criteria of significance, they should be disregarded, or discounted, or not reported.

There are still other reasons why we believe that the routine application of significance tests to our data is not fully justified. For one, these tests presuppose that the units being studied were sampled randomly from the populations to which they belong. We have administered our questionnaires to the total student bodies of three medical schools; in no sense can these groups be considered random samples, or even, for that matter, samples. There is a real question, therefore, whether there would be any justification at all for making use of traditional tests of significance.

Moreover, there is a distinction to be made between the importance of a result and its statistical significance. Reliance on tests of significance generally carries with it an obligation to report only those results which meet the criteria of the tests; where a significant difference is not found the result is not presented. But this can often be quite misleading in social research. In this field some of the most important results are those in which an expected relationship is not revealed by the data. Statistically, such results are not significant; conceptually, they have great significance. For example, we should expect students in the lower half of their class to be more likely than top students to favor a system of anonymous examinations in medical school. We would consider it highly significant if they did not, if in other words, there were no relationship between class standing and preferences for an examination system in which the students' anonymity is preserved.

These are the most important reasons why we have intentionally refrained from applying traditional tests of significance to our findings. This is not to say, of course, that we have been indiscriminate in our presentation of statistical results. We have established criteria of significance for ourselves, even though these do not involve the usual and more familiar tests. Essentially, these criteria involve two related types of *consistency*.

The first criterion is that, to be considered significant, results must be *internally* consistent. That is, a finding with regard to one question is held to be valid only if it also holds true in connection with a closely related question. For example, we may find that, as they advance through medical school, students become increasingly likely to say that they want to know their patients only on a doctor–patient basis, and not also as friend to friend. We attach significance to this finding only when we uncover other evidence that preferences for such detached relations are progressively learned; if we find, for instance, that advanced students are more likely than their junior colleagues to say that it is important for the physician to control his affective reactions in the doctor–patient relationship.

The second criterion is that results must be *replicatively* consistent if they are to be considered significant. That is, a finding in one group must also hold true in a second independent group, if the same general conditions prevail in both. The groups in which such consistency is studied may be comparable classes in two or more medical schools, different classes at comparable stages of their training within one medical school, or particular subgroups of the classes. The only requirement is that they be independent of each other. In these instances, according to this criterion of consistency, results found in one group should be repeated in others. For example, we may find in one medical school that, as the students move from one stage to another in their training, they become progressively more likely to say that they view their contact with patients as an opportunity both to learn medicine and to help patients, rather than just to learn medicine. We consider this a valid result only if the same pattern is observed in a second medical school, or in the same medical school at different times.

There is, of course, one type of situation where the criterion of replicative consistency must be modified. If two medical schools differ markedly in their organization or curriculum, then we should not expect to find that attitudes or preferences affected by these organizational features will be replicated from one school to the other. For example, in a school where students do not have substantial contact with patients until their third or fourth years, we may find that first-year students worry more about their performance in their medical studies than they do about their competence to deal with patients. In a second school, where first-year students have considerable contact with patients, we may find exactly the reverse—namely, that first-year students in this school worry more about their adequacy in dealing with patients than they do about their performance in their studies. Because this discrepancy can be related to significant differences in the organization of medical studies in the two schools, we consider both findings valid. Or, if two classes within the same school are very differently composed, we do not expect that attitudes or behavior affected by these differences will be replicated from one class to the other. For example, one entering class may contain a relatively large number of married students, while the class entering the next year contains relatively few. Under these conditions, we expect very different findings with regard to such matters as the way in which friendships are formed, the extent to which friends function as significant points of reference, and patterns of leisure-time activity.

Appendix D

QUESTIONNAIRE ON ATTITUDES AND EXPERIENCES OF MEDICAL STUDENTS

TIMING OF THE QUESTIONNAIRES

In May 1952, the first questionnaire developed for this research was administered to the entire student body of Cornell University Medical College. All save the graduating class thus began their participation in the "panel" of medical students—i.e., students whose attitudes and experiences were to be traced through the later years of their school career. In 1953, the four classes then studying at the medical schools of the University of Pennsylvania and of Western Reserve University were questioned for the first time. In all, there have been 9 panel waves of questionnaires at Cornell, 7 at Pennsylvania, and 6 at Western Reserve. The time schedule has been as follows:

Medical school	Date	Student classes
Cornell	May 1952	First through fourth year
	Dec. 1952	Fourth year only
	May 1953	First through fourth year
	Dec. 1953	Fourth year only
	May 1954	First through fourth year
	Dec. 1954	Fourth year only
	May 1955	First through fourth year
	Dec. 1955	Fourth year only
	May 1956	First through fourth year

307

Medical school	Date	Student classes
Western Reserve	Sept. 1953	Entering first year
	Nov. 1953	Second through fourth year
	May 1954	First through fourth year
	Sept. 1954	Entering first year
	May 1955	First through fourth year
	May 1956	First through fourth year
Pennsylvania	August 1953	Entering first year
	Dec. 1953	Second through fourth year
	May 1954	First through fourth year
	August 1954	Entering first year
	May 1955	First through fourth year
	August 1955	Entering first year
	May 1956	First through fourth year

In December of each year, half of the fourth-year class at Cornell completes its six months of training in the Comprehensive Care and Teaching Program, while the other half is about to enter the Program (after spending six months in Surgery, Obstetrics and Gynecology, and an elective subject). The December Cornell questionnaires therefore serve as a means of assessing the effects of the Comprehensive Care and Teaching Program on students' attitudes, relative to the effects of other fourth-year experiences.

Questionnaires given to students about to begin their first year of medical school at the University of Pennsylvania were mailed to the students' homes before their arrival on campus. In all other cases, students reported to a classroom at a prearranged time and filled out the schedules under the supervision of a representative of the Bureau of Applied Social Research.

A slightly different procedure was followed with entering students at Western Reserve, who filled out their initial questionnaire during the first morning of the orientation program preceding classes.

A summary of questionnaire data now available is shown in Table 33. Each row in the table indicates the number of classes (and the number of students) of a given status in medical school from whom data were collected. For example, the first row shows that data are available on 5 classes of students about to enter their first year (a total of some 525 persons). Each column indicates the

TABLE 33. Outline of Questionnaire Administrations

	MEDICAL SCHOOL																			
	Cornell								Western Reserve						Pennsylvania					
Status in medical school	Class of:								Class of:						Class of:					
	'52	'53	'54	'55	'56	'57	'58	'59	'54	'55	'56	'57	'58	'59	'54	'55	'56	'57	'58	'59
Entering first year				x	x	x	x	x				x	x	x					x	x
End of first year			x	x	x	x	x				x	x	x					x	x	x
Beginning of second year				x							x						x			
End of second year			x	x	x	x					x	x	x				x	x		
Beginning of third year				x	x					x						x				
End of third year		x	x	x	x					x	x	x				x	x	x		
Beginning of fourth year	x								x						x					
Middle of fourth year			x																	
End of fourth year	x	x	x	x					x	x	x				x	x	x			
No. of students in the class*	82	84	78	85	84	81	83	84	87	87	78	78	77	80	127	130	117	119	126	125

* The size of each class varies slightly from year to year as students drop out, drop behind, or transfer from other schools; the cited figures are the minimum for each class.

number of panel waves administered to a given class as it moved through medical school. Thus, the Class of 1955 at Cornell was questioned 5 times: at the end of its first, second, and third years, and at the midpoint and end of its fourth year.

The response rate has been uniformly high at every administration. In most instances, 100 per cent of the class completed questionnaires; the largest number of students in a class ever missed was 7, representing a minimum response rate of 94 per cent.

CONSTRUCTING THE QUESTIONNAIRES

The development of the first questionnaire began in the spring of 1952. As a preliminary step, a number of fourth-year students at Cornell Medical College were intensively interviewed about their experiences in medical school, their attitudes toward patients, their plans for later medical practice, and so on. In addition, staff members of the Medical College were asked to furnish factual information about the science and practice of medicine around which questionnaire items might be constructed. Gradually, tentative questions began to take shape, and they were subjected to vigorous discussion in a group which included both sociologists and physicians. The purpose of these discussions was twofold: first, to improve the wording of the questions so that they were as simple and direct as possible, and second, to make sure that there was a rationale for including any particular item. Following each of these discussions, some questions were deleted from the draft of the schedule, others were newly formulated, and others, already drafted but not considered entirely satisfactory, were revised.

> For example, the first draft of the questionnaire included the following item: "In your opinion, are medical students at Cornell given too little, enough, or too much responsibility for diagnosis and care of patients?" In the course of our discussion of this question we decided that, if the item were allowed to remain in this form, students might answer in terms of a vague "other student." We therefore revised the question so that it referred specifically to the student's own experience: "With respect to responsibility for diagnosis and care of patients, would you say that at Cornell you have had too little responsibility, enough responsibility or too much responsibility?" (The question was further modified, after this first administration, so that responsibility for diagnosis and care of patients was separated. See Question 30, p. 333.)

Similarly, the first draft included this question: "Assuming that you have correctly diagnosed (and treated) a certain condition in a patient, do you think you would get more personal gratification from knowing that the patient appreciated what you have done for him or from knowing that you have done what is medically sound, regardless of whether or not the patient appreciates it?" In this form, it was feared, the dilemma between the patient's appreciation, on the one hand, and gratification from sound performance, on the other, was not stated forcefully enough. Consequently, the question was revised as follows: "Do you think you would get more personal gratification from successfully solving a relatively simple medical problem for a patient who expresses great appreciation or from successfully solving a very complicated medical problem for a patient who expresses no appreciation whatever?"

In all, this first questionnaire went through four drafts, and consequent revisions, before it was considered ready to be administered.

At least some modification has been introduced at each administration of questionnaires. At the same time, a substantial core of items has remained constant over the four years in order to maximize the possibility of studying social processes through panel analysis. Any variation between questionnaires is traceable to one or several of the following sources.

1. Better understanding of medical school experiences. From earlier questionnaire analysis, from field notes and student journals have come sharper formulation of old questions as well as ideas for items not previously included. For example, students were first asked if they felt they had been given enough responsibility for the "diagnosis and care" of patients they had seen. We then learned that this wording covered up an important distinction in the minds of students; by separating the one question into two, the insight was confirmed that third-year students felt more satisfied with the amount of responsibility they were given in *treating* patients than in *diagnosing* them, while fourth-year students were happier with the responsibility they enjoyed in diagnosing than in treating patients.

2. Growing awareness of experiences unique to each year in medical school. The first questionnaire reflects a conception of medical school as being "all of a piece," except for the obvious change from preclinical to clinical years. Subsequent versions have become increasingly differentiated; specific batteries of items have

been developed to deal with the entering student, the student at the end of his first year, the preclinical vs. the clinical student, and the student at the middle and at the end of his fourth and last year.

3. Institutional variations among medical schools. Special programs are in operation at each of the schools: the Comprehensive Care and Teaching Program for fourth-year students at Cornell; the Family Health Advisor Service at the University of Pennsylvania, an optional program in which entering students are assigned to families known to the clinic; and, finally, the complete revamping of the entire curriculum at Western Reserve. Students who participate in each of these special programs are asked a number of questions about their experiences in and reactions to them. Interestingly enough, as our knowledge of these innovations has grown, each has been seen to have some elements in common with the others. Where appropriate, items developed for one school have therefore been used at others as well. Because the questions dealing with these programs would require lengthy explanations of the particular contexts, they are omitted here.

Since limitations of space preclude the publication of all questions ever asked, what follows is a synthesis, stressing those parts considered of most value and interest.[1] The items are presented in two sections. Part A consists of a sampling of the questions asked of students about to enter their first year; advance knowledge and expectations of medical school are dealt with, as is the process by which medicine was selected as a career. Part B gives a selection of items asked of students in all four years of medical school. Although many of the questions were worded differently for students in different years (e.g., anticipatory vs. retrospective formulations) only one wording is presented here to conserve space. Part B is, in turn, divided into five sections, as follows:

    I.   Experience in medical school
   II. Views on the medical profession and on medical care
  III. Career plans
  IV. Self-ratings
   V. Background data

[1] Copies of all forms of the questionnaires are on file at the Bureau of Applied Social Research.

INSTRUCTIONS TO MEDICAL STUDENTS

This questionnaire is another part of a continuing study being conducted by the Bureau of Applied Social Research of Columbia University in collaboration with your medical school and other leading medical schools. As before, it is designed to find out what you, as a medical student, think about various aspects of medical training and practice. The information which you provide will be helpful in clarifying certain problems of medical education.

As you will notice, you have answered some of the questions before. Your cooperation in answering these questions again—on the basis of your *present* feelings—is essential to the study.

We recognize that many of the questions deal with complex issues, and that the check-list alternatives do not always express the subtleties of your opinions. But the purpose of a questionnaire like this one is to obtain an overall picture of the attitudes held by medical students. Other procedures are being used to explore more detailed opinions.

There are a few points which you should bear in mind while filling out this questionnaire:

(1) *The questionnaire is not a "test"*—there is no "grade" or other mark. The only "right" answers to the questions are those which best express *your* feelings, *your* opinions, and *your* experiences.

(2) *Your individual identity will not be revealed and your personal answers will be kept confidential.* The information provided by your class will be tabulated by the Bureau of Applied Social Research and will be made available to the faculty *only* in the form of statistical summaries.

(3) Read every question or statement carefully before answering. Please answer *every* question in accordance with the directions.

Thank you for your cooperation in this study.

PART A

Prospective Medical Students' Expectations and Advance Knowledge

1.* (a) At what age did you *first think* of becoming a doctor? (Check one)

.... Before the age of 10
.... Between 10 and 13 years of age
.... At 14 or 15 years of age
.... At 16 or 17 years of age
.... Since the age of 18

(b) At what age did you *definitely decide* to study medicine? (Check one)

.... Before the age of 14
.... At 14 or 15 years of age
.... At 16 or 17 years of age
.... Between 18 and 20 years of age
.... Since the age of 21

2. Before deciding on medicine, did you ever seriously consider any other occupation or profession? Yes........ No........

IF YES:* Which occupations or professions did you consider? (Check as many as apply)

.... Elementary or high school teaching
.... College or university teaching (What field? ....)
.... Scientific research (What field? ....)
.... Engineering, architecture
.... Law
.... Ministry
.... Business
.... Other (Which? ....)

3. Which *one* of the following statements *best* describes the way you feel about a career in medicine? (Check one)

.... It's the only career that could really satisfy me
.... It's one of several careers which I could find almost equally satisfying
.... It's not the most satisfying career I can think of, everything considered
.... A career I decided on without considering whether I would find it the most satisfying

*Questions marked with an asterisk (*) were initially asked in open-ended form. Students were not provided with a check list of categories from which to select, but responded to the questions in their own terms. Codes were then constructed and used as response categories in the later questionnaires.

4. (a) How important was each of the following in your decision to enter the medical profession? (Answer for each)

	Very important	Fairly important	Of minor importance	Not at all important
(1) Mother	....	....	....	....
(2) Father	....	....	....	....
(3) Other relatives	....	....	....	....
(4) Friends who are not in medicine	....	....	....	....
(5) Physicians you know personally	....	....	....	....
(6) Physicians you have heard or read about	....	....	....	....
(7) Medical students you know	....	....	....	....
(8) Undergraduate teacher	....	....	....	....
(9) Books, movies or plays (Give titles ....)	....	....	....	....
(10) Other (What? ....)	....	....	....	....

(b) Which *two* of these were of most importance in your decision to become a doctor? (List the appropriate numbers) #........ and #........

5. Since you made the decision, how much have the following members of your family encouraged you to become a doctor? (Answer for each)

	Strong encour- agement	Slight encour- agement	Expressed no opinion	Slight opposi- tion	Strong opposi- tion	Doesn't apply
Mother	....	....	....	....	....	....
Father	....	....	....	....	....	....
Wife or husband	....	....	....	....	....	....
Brother or sister	....	....	....	....	....	....
Other relatives	....	....	....	....	....	....

6. Once you made up your mind to become a doctor, did you ever have any doubts that this was the right decision for you? (Check one)

.... Yes, serious doubts
.... Yes, slight doubts
.... No, no doubts at all

7. All things considered, about how much do you know about what you can expect in medical school? (Check one)

.... A great deal
.... A fair amount
.... Only a little
.... Practically nothing

8. (a) How important has each of the following been in helping you to form a picture of what medical school is like? (Answer for each)

	Very important	Fairly important	Of minor importance	Not at all important
Medical school bulletins	....	....	....	....
Medical students at (your) school	....	....	....	....
Medical students at other schools	....	....	....	....
Members of your family who are doctors	....	....	....	....
Your family physician	....	....	....	....
Other physicians who are friends	....	....	....	....
Medical school faculty	....	....	....	....
College faculty	....	....	....	....
Books, movies, plays (Give titles ....)	....	....	....	....
	....	....	....	....
Other (What? ....)	....	....	....	....
	....	....	....	....

9. (a)* Have you any friends who are members of upper classes in (your) medical school? (Check one)

.... No
.... Yes, one
.... Yes, two
.... Yes, three or four
.... Yes, five or more

(b) What kinds of things have you discussed *in some detail* with them? (Check as many as apply)

.... Course work (Which courses? ....)
.... Research projects
.... Individual faculty members
.... The faculty as a whole
.... The grading system
.... Competition among students
.... Cooperation among students
.... Fraternities
.... Work with patients on clinics and wards
.... Other (What? ....)

10. (a)* What are the *major kinds* of adjustment you will probably have to make during your first year of medical school? (Check as many as apply)

.... I will have to improve my study habits
.... I will have to improve my memory
.... I will have to learn to work with less guidance from instructors
.... I will have to take on a more mature attitude and become a more responsible person
.... I will have to adjust to less free time for leisure and personal interests
.... Other (What? ....)

(b) *How difficult* do you expect to find these adjustments? (Check one)

.... Very difficult
.... Quite difficult
.... Not so difficult
.... Not at all difficult

11. All things considered, how do you think medical training compares with each of the following kinds of training? Are medical studies more difficult, less difficult, or about the same? (Answer for each)

	MEDICAL TRAINING IS				
	Much more difficult than	Somewhat more difficult than	About the same as	Less difficult than	Don't know
Studying to be a lawyer	....	....	....	....	....
Studying to be an engineer	....	....	....	....	....
Studying to be a dentist	....	....	....	....	....
Training to be an Army officer	....	....	....	....	....
Studying for a Ph.D. in physics	....	....	....	....	....
Studying for a Ph.D. in psychology	....	....	....	....	....

12. Which of the following statements comes *closest* to describing the way you feel about medical school? (Check one)

.... Basically, it's going to be a tough, four year grind, but I'll manage to enjoy it somehow
.... Basically, it's going to be an enjoyable experience, even though it will mean very hard work at times

13. Do you think that, as you move from the first to the fourth year of medical school, your studies will become more difficult for you, less difficult, or do you think they will remain relatively unchanged in this respect? (Check one)

.... Will become more difficult
.... Will become less difficult
.... Will remain about the same
.... Don't know

14. (a) Compared to your undergraduate courses, how much time do you think your first year courses in medical school are going to take? Will you have to spend more time, less time, or the same amount of time on them? (Check one)

.... I think I am going to have to spend more time on my studies in medical school
.... I think I can spend less time on them
.... I think I'll have to spend about the same amount of time on them
.... Don't know

(b)* In addition to attending lectures and working in the labs, about how many hours a week do you plan to study during your first year of medical school? (Check one)

.... 10 hours or less
.... 11–15 hours
.... 16–20 hours
.... 21–25 hours
.... 26–30 hours
.... 31–35 hours
.... 36 or more hours

15. (a) Do you expect to have to develop *new study habits* during your first year of medical school? Yes........ No........

(b) Do you expect to have to develop *new skills* during your first year of medical school? Yes........ No........

16. In your opinion, how important is each of the following for a student to get the most out of the first year of medical school? (Answer for each)

	Very important	Fairly important	Of minor importance	Not at all important	Haven't thought about it
Manual dexterity (with instruments, tools, machines, etc.)	....	....	....	....	....
Ability to memorize	....	....	....	....	....
Ability to cope with theoretical material	....	....	....	....	....
Previous knowledge of physical science	....	....	....	....	....
Ability to put aside almost everything for your studies	....	....	....	....	....
Previous knowledge of social science	....	....	....	....	....
Getting along with other students	....	....	....	....	....
Ability to remain relaxed, rather than overly tense and nervous about your work	....	....	....	....	....

Learning as many medical facts as possible	....	....	....	....	....
Making up your own mind about what to emphasize in your studying	....	....	....	....	....
Getting along with the medical faculty	....	....	....	....	....
Ability to carry out research	....	....	....	....	....

17. What is your realistic appraisal of how well you will do in your first year courses compared with the other members of your class? (Check one)

.... I expect to do considerably better than average
.... I expect to do somewhat better than average
.... I expect to be about average
.... I expect to be below average
.... Don't know

18.° How difficult do you think each of the following will be for you in your first year of medical school? (Answer for each)

	Very difficult	Fairly difficult	Not very difficult	Not at all difficult
Making friends in your class	....	....	....	....
Keeping up with other students	....	....	....	....
Learning what is expected of you	....	....	....	....
Adjusting to the sights and smells of the anatomy lab	....	....	....	....
Learning to think for yourself	....	....	....	....
Getting to know faculty members	....	....	....	....
Not allowing yourself to become overly tense or nervous about your work	....	....	....	....

19. How much contact with each of the following groups do you think you will have during your first year in medical school? (Answer for each)

	More than enough	The right amount	Not enough	Don't know	Haven't thought about it
Members of other classes in medical school	....	....	....	....	....
Patients	....	....	....	....	....
Basic science faculty	....	....	....	....	....
Full time clinical faculty	....	....	....	....	....
Practicing physicians	....	....	....	....	....
Administrators of the medical school	....	....	....	....	....
Medical specialists	....	....	....	....	....
Friends outside of school	....	....	....	....	....
Members of your family	....	....	....	....	....
Faculty heads of departments	....	....	....	....	....

20. (a) How much do you feel you already know about faculty members at (your) medical school? (Check one)

.... A great deal
.... A fair amount
.... Only a little
.... Nothing at all

(b) From what sources have you obtained this information? (Check as many as apply)

.... From students in (your) medical school
.... From students at other medical schools
.... From faculty members at undergraduate schools
.... From relatives who are physicians
.... From friends who are physicians
.... From the writings of the faculty members
.... From personal contact with faculty members
.... From other sources (What? ....)

21. (a) How much contact do you expect to have with faculty members during your first year of medical school? (Check one)

.... A great deal
.... A fair amount
.... Only a little
.... Don't know

(b) On the whole, do you expect that your contacts with the medical school faculty during your first year will be more formal, less formal, or about the same as your contacts with your undergraduate professors? (Check one)

.... Contacts in medical school will be *more* formal
.... They will be *less* formal
.... They will be about the same
.... Don't know

22. During your first year of medical school, about how many hours a week, on the average, do you expect to spend with your classmates in each of the following situations? (Answer for each)

	HOURS PER WEEK			
	One or two	Three or four	Five to seven	Eight or more
Informal discussion groups in connection with your courses	....	....	....	....
Bull sessions about life in general	....	....	....	....
Discussions about the medical profession in general	....	....	....	....
Participating in leisure time activities together	....	....	....	....

23. To what extent do you think the first year medical students will try to help each other? (Check one)

.... They will try to help each other a great deal
.... They will try to help each other a fair amount
.... They will try to help each other only a little
.... They will not try to help each other at all

24. When would you *like* to have your first substantial amount of contact with patients? (Check one)

.... I would like to have my first substantial contact in my first year
.... I would like to have it in my second year
.... I would like to have it in my third year
.... I would like to have it in my fourth year
.... I would like to have it during my internship
.... Don't know

25. In which year of training do you *expect* to have your first substantial amount of contact with patients? (Check one)

.... I expect to have my first substantial contact in my first year
.... I expect to have it in my second year
.... I expect to have it in my third year
.... I expect to have it in my fourth year
.... I expect to have it during my internship
.... Don't know

26. When do you expect that you will *first* come to think of yourself as a doctor? (Check one)

.... During my first year in medical school
.... During my second year
.... During my third year
.... During my fourth year
.... During my internship
.... During my residency
.... Haven't given it any thought

27. Although as an entering medical student you are not likely to know medical terms and expressions, you may have become familiar with some of them.

(a) How familiar do you feel you are with medical terminology? (Check one)

.... Very familiar
.... Fairly familiar
.... Only slightly familiar

(b) For which of the following diseases can you *now* describe one major symptom? (Check those you can now describe)

.... Peptic ulcer
.... Keratitis
.... Migraine
.... Pellagra
.... Angina pectoris
.... Conversion hysteria
.... Herpes zoster
.... Menopausal syndrome
.... Hansen's Disease
.... Kidney stone
.... Acute pyelonephritis
.... Diabetes mellitus

(c) What are the main sources from which you have learned the medical information which you already have? (Check as many as apply)

.... Relatives or friends in medicine or medical school
.... Undergraduate studies
.... Reading not connected with undergraduate work
.... Personal experience in medically related fields (hospital, lab work, etc.)
.... Other (What? ....)

28.* What things do you think you will like best about being a doctor? (Check as many as apply)

.... Being able to deal directly with people
.... Being able to help other people
.... The fact that medicine is a highly respected profession
.... Having interesting and intelligent people for colleagues
.... Doing work involving scientific method and research
.... Being my own boss
.... Being sure of earning a good income
.... The challenging and stimulating nature of the work
.... Other (What? ....)

29. (a) In your opinion, how well does each of the following phrases describe the medical profession? (Answer for each)

		Very good description	Fair description	Poor description
(1)	A profession which has high standing in the community	....	....	....
(2)	A profession of service to the community	....	....	....
(3)	A profession which is secure and lucrative	....	....	....
(4)	A profession which helps individuals directly	....	....	....
(5)	A profession in which real ability is recognized by one's colleagues	....	....	....
(6)	A profession requiring harder work than others	....	....	....

(b) In your opinion, which *one* of the above phrases *best* describes the medical profession? (List the appropriate number) ....

PART B

Medical Students'
Experiences and Opinions

I. THIS SECTION OF THE QUESTIONNAIRE DEALS WITH YOUR EXPERI-
ENCES IN MEDICAL SCHOOL AND WITH YOUR FEELINGS ABOUT THE
KIND OF TRAINING A MEDICAL STUDENT OUGHT TO RECEIVE.

1. Many medical students seem to feel that they do not always have
enough time to do all the things they want to. How do you feel in this
respect—do you feel that you have enough time for each of the following activities? (Answer for each)

	Ample time	Just about enough time	Not quite enough time	Not nearly enough time
Learning all that you are expected to know in medical school	....	....	....	....
Following the latest medical advances in books and journals	....	....	....	....
Spending time with your family and friends	....	....	....	....
Following up your own interests in the field of medicine	....	....	....	....
Reading the newspaper, and keeping up with current affairs	....	....	....	....
Working up patients in the clinics or on the wards	....	....	....	....

2. Compared to the other students in your class, how hard would you
say that you have worked in your studies during the current semester?
(Check one)

.... Considerably harder than average
.... Somewhat harder than average
.... About average
.... Somewhat less than average
.... Considerably less than average

3. (a) Which phase of your medical training do you think will be
most important for your later career in medicine? (Check one)

.... First two years of medical school
.... Last two years of medical school
.... Internship
.... Residency
.... Don't know

(b) Which phase of your medical training do you expect to find
most difficult? (Check one)

.... First two years of medical school
.... Last two years of medical school
.... Internship
.... Residency
.... Don't know

4. Everyone knows that medical students are given much more factual information than they can possibly assimilate. In general, do you think that the faculty gives medical students enough direction in what to emphasize in their studying? (Check one)

.... Faculty gives too little direction
.... Faculty gives about the right amount of direction
.... Faculty gives more than enough direction

5. (a) What is your realistic appraisal of how well you are doing in your courses compared with the other members of your class? (Check one)

.... Considerably better than average
.... Somewhat better than average
.... About average
.... Below average
.... Don't know

(b) How sure are you about how well you are doing? (Check one)

.... Completely sure
.... Quite sure
.... Not sure

(c) Rank the following according to their importance to you in deciding how well you are doing at the present time. (Rank all three, placing a *1* before the most important, and so on)

.... Comments of your fellow students
.... Information given you by the faculty
.... Your own personal self-evaluation

6. To what extent are you concerned about how well you are doing in comparison with the other students in your class? (Check one)

.... Deeply concerned
.... Quite a bit concerned
.... Little concerned
.... Not at all concerned

7. How do you feel about competing with other people, especially when the stakes are high? My feeling about competitive situations is that (Check one)

.... I dislike them and prefer to avoid them completely
.... I dislike them somewhat
.... I have neutral feelings about them
.... I enjoy them somewhat
.... I get a kick out of them and sometimes seek them out

8. How much competitiveness have you found among your classmates in medical school? (Check one)

.... A great deal of competitiveness
.... A fair amount of competitiveness
.... Only a little competitiveness
.... No competitiveness at all

9. Below are some statements about medical students and physicians. How true do you consider each one? (Answer for each)

	Definitely true	Probably true	Probably untrue	Definitely untrue
"A man may not be able to do original work but if he has a good memory for facts he'll do all right in medical school."	....	....	....	....
"Every doctor should, at some time, have been a patient."	....	....	....	....
"The student who feels uneasy in meeting people should not consider practicing medicine."	....	....	....	....
"An instructor ought to show the same kind of respect for students as a doctor for patients."	....	....	....	....
"A student who does well in medical school should feel obligated to go into specialty practice or research."	....	....	....	....

NOTE: Although the five items in Question 9 lent themselves to a similar "True-False" design, they are not intended to be used as a battery dealing with the same content area. Each item refers to a distinct attitude, and is therefore subject to separate analysis, or to combination with items appearing elsewhere in the questionnaire.

10. One can't help being annoyed occasionally by the behavior of fellow students. As you think back, which of these experiences in medical school have you found particularly annoying? (Answer for each)

	Very annoyed	Fairly annoyed	Not especially annoyed	Not at all annoyed	Have not met this situation
When you felt that a fellow student was not carrying his full share of work	....	....	....	....	....
When a student was discourteous to a faculty member	....	....	....	....	....
When a student asked questions just for effect	....	....	....	....	....
When a student was inconsiderate of a patient's feelings	....	....	....	....	....
When a student seemed to regard medicine just as a means of income	....	....	....	....	....
When a student seemed to get by on personality rather than on medical knowledge	....	....	....	....	....

11. How much importance do you personally attach to each of the following when judging how good, as medical students, your classmates are? (Answer for each)

	Great importance	Moderate importance	Minor importance	No importance
Extensive knowledge of medical facts	....	....	....	....
Ability to get along with other medical students	....	....	....	....
Ability to get along with the faculty	....	....	....	....
Ability to put aside everything but medical studies	....	....	....	....
Ability to carry out research	....	....	....	....
Skill in the realm of diagnosis	....	....	....	....
Ability to establish rapport with patients	....	....	....	....
Knowledge of therapy	....	....	....	....
Skill in dealing with the social and psychological problems of patients	....	....	....	....

12. (a)* How many members of the medical school faculty know you by name? (Check one)
- .... No more than 5 or 6
- .... About 10
- .... About 20 or 25
- .... More than 25

(b) What about *other* students—do you think that more, fewer, or about as many faculty members know *them* by name? (Check one)
- .... More faculty members
- .... Fewer faculty members
- .... About as many faculty members

13. The friendships which students form in medical school are undoubtedly a very important part of their experience. Below are some questions about the friendships which you have formed. (We would like to emphasize once more that the information you give will be held in strictest confidence, and will not be seen by anyone connected with [your] medical school.)

(a) Would you please name your three best friends now in *medical school*. (Answer below)

(b) When did you *first meet* each of these people—that is, in what year and in approximately what month? (Answer below)

(c) How, specifically, did you happen to meet each of your friends? For example, did you meet him in a class, where you lived, in a fraternity house, or in some other way? (Answer below)

(d) During the course of an average week this past semester, about *how many hours* did you spend with each of these friends in the following activities?

(1) Working together at the same lab table (Answer below in column #1)

(2) Working together on wards or in clinics (Answer below in column #2)

(3) Listening to lectures in the same class room (Answer below in column #3)

(4) Studying together outside of class (Answer below in column #4)

(5) Recreational activities, like movies or sports (Answer below in column #5)

(6) Lunches and bull sessions (Answer below in column #6)

(a) Name of friend	(b) Date first met	(c) Circumstances of meeting	(d) HOURS SPENT TOGETHER					
			#1	#2	#3	#4	#5	#6
....	....	....	......	......	......	......	......	......
....	....	....	......	......	......	......	......	......
....	....	....	......	......	......	......	......	......

14. (a) From what you have observed, would you say that your *instructors* are generally more skilled in the realm of physical diagnosis and treatment than they are in handling the interpersonal aspects of patient care, less skilled, or are they generally about equally skilled in both? (Check one)

.... Generally more skilled in the realm of physical diagnosis and treatment
.... Generally more skilled in interpersonal aspects of patient care
.... Equally skilled in both respects

(b) How do you feel about *yourself*—would you say that you are more skilled in the realm of physical diagnosis and treatment than you are in handling the interpersonal aspects of patient care, less skilled, or are you equally skilled in both? (Check one)

.... More skilled in the realm of physical diagnosis and treatment
.... More skilled in interpersonal aspects of patient care
.... Equally skilled in both respects

(c) Obviously, a medical student gains most from working with an instructor who is skilled both in the realm of physical diagnosis and treatment *and* in handling the interpersonal aspects of patient care. But in actuality, some physicians are more skilled in one respect than they are in the other. At this stage in your training, do you get more out of working with (Check one)

.... An instructor whose special ability lies more in the realm of physical diagnosis and treatment, and less in the interpersonal aspects of patient care

.... An instructor whose special ability lies more in the realm of the interpersonal aspects of patient care, and less in physical diagnosis and treatment

15. Do you look upon your contact with patients while in medical school (Check one)

.... Primarily as an opportunity to learn medicine

.... Primarily as an opportunity to help patients

.... As presenting equal opportunities to learn medicine and to help patients

16. Now we would like to ask you about the kinds of patients with whom you would *like to deal.*

(a) Would you rather be assigned a patient with (Check one)

.... Positive physical findings who is beyond medical help

.... Negative physical findings who can be helped

.... It makes no difference

(b) Would you prefer (Check one)

.... A new patient who presents a diagnostic challenge

.... An old patient where the problem for the physician gradually unfolds in the course of many contacts

.... It makes no difference

(c) Would you prefer a patient who is (Check one)

.... A close personal friend

.... A casual acquaintance

.... A complete stranger

.... It makes no difference

(d) Would you prefer a patient who (Check one)

.... Asks for detailed explanations

.... Accepts the explanations you give him without further question

.... It makes no difference

(e) Would you prefer a patient who (Check one)

.... Wants to know you only on a doctor–patient basis

.... Wants to know you also on a friend-to-friend basis

.... It makes no difference

(f) Would you prefer a patient (Check one)

.... Whose illness is entirely physical
.... Whose illness is chiefly emotional in origin
.... It makes no difference

17. (a) In your judgment, what proportion of patients makes a serious effort to follow the doctor's advice? (Check one)

.... Almost all
.... A majority
.... About half
.... Less than half

(b) Which *one* of the following would you say is the major reason for the inability of a patient to follow his doctor's advice? (Check one)

.... Not being able to understand the doctor's orders
.... Being in so difficult and complex a life situation that he cannot handle any of his problems
.... Not having enough confidence in the doctor
.... Getting so much gratification from his illness that he really does not want to regain his health
.... Showing as little initiative in following the doctor's orders as he does in anything else
.... Other (What? ....)

18. (a) As a *medical student,* do you think you would get more satisfaction from (Check one)

.... Successfully solving a relatively simple medical problem for a patient who expresses great appreciation
.... Successfully solving a very complicated problem for a patient who expresses no appreciation whatever

(b) As a *practicing physician,* do you think you will get more personal satisfaction from (Check one)

.... Successfully solving a relatively simple medical problem for a patient who expresses great appreciation
.... Successfully solving a very complicated problem for a patient who expresses no appreciation whatever

19. On the whole, would you prefer to (Check one)

.... Work at some interesting research problem that does not involve any contact with patients
.... Work directly with patients, even though your tasks are relatively routine
.... It makes no difference

20. (a) Below is a list of problems and situations which many medical students meet in their dealings with patients. How confident do you feel about your ability to deal with each of these problems *at the present time?* (Answer for each)

	Completely confident	Fairly confident	Not really confident	Completely lacking in confidence
(1) When a patient has an emotional outburst of some kind	....	....	....	....
(2) Preventing a patient from becoming embarrassed during a pelvic examination	....	....	....	....
(3) Having to do a painful procedure on a sick child	....	....	....	....
(4) Having to tell a patient that the tests performed on him do not reveal the cause of his problems	....	....	....	....
(5) Deciding what to tell a patient who has a serious and irremediable illness	....	....	....	....
(6) Knowing what to do in an emergency	....	....	....	....
(7) Being able to do a venipuncture without any difficulty	....	....	....	....
(8) Having a doctor as one of your patients	....	....	....	....
(9) Being able to make a diagnosis in a difficult case	....	....	....	....
(10) Deciding on appropriate medication and dosage	....	....	....	....
(11) Handling a patient who refuses to accept what you tell him	....	....	....	....

(b) About which of these problems do you expect to feel *more confident* once you have become an *experienced practitioner?* (Indicate the appropriate numbers from the list above ....)

(For fourth-year students only:)

21. Below is a line representing the distance between the third-year medical student and the House Officer

```
1           2           3           4           5           6
|_____|_____|_____|_____|_____|
Third-year                                              House
Student                                                 Officer
```

(a) Using one of the numbers on this line, where would you place yourself with respect to the *technical medical knowledge* you now have? ....

(b) Which point on the line is closest to your present *skill in handling patients?* ....

(c) It is often difficult to remember the opinions you held some time ago. But, looking back to last year, when you were a third-year student, where, on this same line, did you then rate fourth-year students with respect to the technical medical knowledge you felt they generally had? ....

(d) When you were a third-year student, how did you rate fourth-year students with respect to their skill in handling patients? ....

22. Although you are not yet a doctor officially, many people probably think of you as one.

(a) How do you feel about yourself in this respect? (Answer for each below)

	HAVE THOUGHT OF YOURSELF:	
	Primarily as a DOCTOR rather than as a student	Primarily as a STUDENT rather than as a doctor
In the most recent dealings you have had with *patients,* how have you tended to think of yourself?	....	....
What about when you have talked with your *classmates* in recent weeks?	....	....
When you have had contacts with your *instructors* in recent weeks?	....	....
When you had contacts with *nurses* in clinics or on the wards in the past month or so?	....	....
Finally, when you spent time recently with your *family and friends?*	....	....

(b) In your opinion, how have these different people thought of you in this respect? (Answer for each below)

	HAVE BEEN THOUGHT OF:	
	Primarily as a DOCTOR rather than as a student	Primarily as a STUDENT rather than as a doctor
In your recent dealings with *patients,* how have they thought of you, by and large?	....	....
How about the *classmates* with whom you have talked in recent weeks?	....	....
And the *instructors* with whom you have come in contact recently?	....	....
The *nurses* in clinics or on the wards in the past month or so?	....	....
Finally, how have your *family and friends* thought of you recently?	....	....

23. How much satisfaction have you derived from the physician–patient relationships you have had during the current semester? (Check one)

.... A great deal
.... A fair amount
.... Only a little
.... None at all

24. To what extent have you worried that patients with whom you were dealing would lose respect for you if they learned that you were a student? (Check one)

.... A great deal
.... Quite a bit
.... Not very much
.... Not at all

25. (a) How nervous were you *just before* your *first personal* contact with a patient? (Check one)

.... Extremely
.... Somewhat
.... Only a little
.... Not at all

(b) How about when you started *actually* working with your *first* patient—how nervous were you then? (Check one)

.... Extremely
.... Somewhat
.... Only a little
.... Not at all

26. As you look back on it, how well did the faculty instruct you about the kinds of problems you might meet in handling patients? (Check one)

.... Very well
.... Fairly well
.... Not especially well
.... Not at all well

27. Listed below are a number of statements about students' relationships with their patients. Indicate whether, *in your own experience,* each statement is true or false. (Answer for each)

	True	False	Have no basis for saying
I looked on most of my patients practically as friends	....	....	....
I often felt frustrated that I was *not competent* to do more for my patients along medical lines	....	....	....

I often felt dissatisfied that I was *not* allowed to do more for my patients along medical lines	....	....	....
There were times when I wanted to help my patients by buying things they needed	....	....	....
I sometimes became very irritated with patients who were uncooperative	....	....	....
I couldn't help feeling a sense of blame that there wasn't anything I could do for a patient who was incurably ill	....	....	....

28. From your own experience, how much difficulty would you say you have in handling patients? (Check one)

.... Considerable difficulty
.... A fair amount of difficulty
.... Only a little difficulty
.... No difficulty

29. (a) By and large, have patients generally been discussed with you as individual persons or as disease entities? (Check one)

.... As individual persons
.... As disease entities

(b) How have *you personally* thought of the patients you have seen—as persons or as disease entities? (Check one)

.... As individual persons
.... As disease entities

30. (a) With respect to responsibility for the *diagnosis* of patients, would you say that during the current semester you have had (Check one)

.... too little responsibility
.... enough responsibility
.... too much responsibility

(b) How about responsibility for *treating* patients—would you say that during the current semester you have had (Check one)

.... too little responsibility
.... enough responsibility
.... too much responsibility

31. Are there some kinds of sick people to whom you feel especially drawn or toward whom you feel particularly sympathetic? Yes........ No........

    IF YES:

    (a)* Toward which of the following types of patients are you most sympathetic? (Check as many as apply)
    .... Young people
    .... People with terminal illnesses
    .... People who are "down and out"
    .... Articulate people
    .... People who are optimistic about their illness
    .... People who have clear-cut physical illnesses
    .... People who have confidence in the doctor
    .... Other (Which? ....)

    (b) In your own experience, does this kind of involvement with a sick person have any bearing on how you manage him as a patient? (Check as many as apply)
    .... So far as I know, it makes no difference
    .... It *helps* me, because I am willing to spend a lot of time with patients whom I like especially
    .... It *helps* me, because I am more willing to talk about the various kinds of problems which are troubling them
    .... It *interferes* with my management, because I am especially hesitant to order painful or expensive diagnostic tests or therapeutic measures in cases like this
    .... It *interferes* with my management, because I sometimes overestimate the amount I can do for them
    .... Other (What? ....)

    (c) What do you think you should do when you find yourself positively drawn to a patient? (Check one)
    .... I'd try to control these feelings, and regain my sense of objectivity
    .... I'd take advantage of these feelings to try to draw the patient closer to me
    .... I wouldn't try to change my feelings at all
    .... Other (What? ....)

32. Are there some kinds of sick people toward whom you find yourself reacting negatively? Yes........ No........

    IF YES:

    (a)* Toward which of the following types of patients do you react negatively? (Check as many as apply)
    .... Old people
    .... People who think they know as much about medicine as the doctor
    .... Inarticulate people
    .... People who have nothing but psychogenic symptoms

.... People who feel sorry for themselves
.... People who have physiologically improbable symptoms
.... People who make no real effort to get well
.... Other (Which? ....)

(b) In your own experience, does this kind of negative reaction to a sick person have any bearing on your management of him as a patient? (Check as many as apply)

.... As far as I know, it makes no difference
.... It *helps* me manage the patient, because I am not likely to hesitate about performing or ordering unpleasant procedures which might benefit the patient
.... It *interferes* with my management of the patient, because I am less willing to spend a lot of time with him
.... It *interferes* with my management of the patient, because I am more likely to underestimate the extent to which I can help him
.... Other (What? ....)

(c) What do you think you should do when you find yourself reacting negatively to a patient? (Check one)

.... For the sake of the patient himself, I should turn his case over to another doctor
.... I'd keep him, as a challenge to myself in dealing with patients of this kind
.... I'd keep him, because I'm sure that my feelings would make no difference in the way I managed his case
.... Other (What? ....)

33. How would *most of your instructors* in medical school feel if you or your classmates were to do the following? (Answer for each)

	Would disapprove strongly	Would disapprove to some extent	Would not care	Would approve mildly	Would approve strongly
Express a desire to discharge a patient who has a functional problem	....	....	....	....	....
Question an instructor's judgment with respect to a clinical problem	....	....	....	....	....
Spend a lot of time exploring social and emotional factors when taking a history	....	....	....	....	....
Show little or no interest in patients with routine medical problems	....	....	....	....	....
Spend more than an hour-and-a-half working up a patient	....	....	....	....	....

Admit uncertainties
   with respect to a
   diagnostic problem ....
Wait for the instruc-
   tor to set up the plan
   of treatment for a
   patient ....
Always do more than is
   required for your cases ....
Make a diagnosis of
   psychoneurosis, with-
   out first ordering
   all possible tests
   to rule out organic
   factors ....
Admit to being moved
   by a particular
   patient ....

NOTE: This battery was repeated, asking the student to indicate how *he himself* would feel about any of his classmates who behaved in these ways.

34. With which of these groups of people do you generally compare yourself when you evaluate your own standing in the following respects? (Answer for each)

	Your class-mates	Full-time faculty	Part-time faculty	Other practicing physicians	Interns and residents
Physical diagnosis	....	....	....	....	....
Handling personal problems of patients	....	....	....	....	....
Medical knowledge	....	....	....	....	....
Carrying out clinical tests	....	....	....	....	....
Your standards of medical care	....	....	....	....	....

35. Below are some types of experiences you are likely to have had during your years in medical school. Which *two* of these types of experiences have afforded you the greatest amount of *personal satisfaction?* (Check two)

.... Being able to perform experiments of importance to medical science
.... Acquiring a detailed understanding of substances, such as epinephrine, insulin, etc., at a cellular and enzymatic level
.... Developing skill in the techniques of percussion, auscultation, and palpation
.... Understanding the processes of differential diagnosis
.... Having the opportunity to know, and perhaps to work with, a full-time faculty member

.... Understanding the complexity of the physician–patient relationship
.... Being able to see the patient as a person with emotional and social problems in addition to an organic illness
.... Other (What? ....)

II. THIS SECTION DEALS WITH THE MEDICAL PROFESSION IN GENERAL AND WITH STANDARDS OF MEDICAL CARE.

36. (a) In your opinion, how important is each of the following characteristics in making a good physician? (Answer for each)

		Very important	Fairly important	Of minor importance	Not at all important
(1)	Good appearance	....	....	....	....
(2)	Warm and pleasing personality	....	....	....	....
(3)	Dedication to medicine	....	....	....	....
(4)	High intelligence	....	....	....	....
(5)	Skillful management of time	....	....	....	....
(6)	Scientific curiosity	....	....	....	....
(7)	Integrity	....	....	....	....
(8)	Ability to think in an organized way	....	....	....	....
(9)	Research ability	....	....	....	....
(10)	Ability to get along with people	....	....	....	....
(11)	Recognition of own limitations	....	....	....	....
(12)	Getting real enjoyment out of medicine	....	....	....	....

(b) In your opinion, which two of these characteristics are *most important* in making a good physician? (List the appropriate numbers.) #........ and #........

(c) In your opinion, which of these are more important to *medicine* than to *other professions?* #........ and #........

37. How important is each of the following types of social behavior to the success of a physician? (Answer for each)

	Very important	Fairly important	Not at all important
To maintain a restrained and dignified manner	....	....	....
To wear conservative clothing	....	....	....
To participate in community activities	....	....	....
To be a good conversationalist	....	....	....
To have a degree from a top medical school	....	....	....
To maintain an air of confidence (even when he is not *feeling* confident)	....	....	....

38. Dr. G. is in his middle 40's and has had a successful career. He
serves as an instructor in the medical clinic of a large teaching hospital
in the mornings; in the afternoons he sees his many private patients;
and in the evenings he generally spends some time working on papers
for medical journals and meetings. All in all, he often works about 16
hours a day. When you read this brief characterization of Dr. G's day,
what are your main reactions? (Check as many as are appropriate)

.... Admiration for the full professional life which Dr. G. leads
.... Doubt that I would be able to keep up a pace like that
.... A strong conviction that a man should not let his professional career
              interfere with his family life to such an extent
.... Doubt that a man who divides himself in so many directions could
              do real justice to any of his activities
.... A feeling of pride that I am on my way to becoming a member of
              the profession which includes people like Dr. G.
.... A feeling of deep regret that the demands of the profession leave
              physicians so little time for their personal life
.... Other (What? ....)

39. (a) Do you think that an internist owes it to his patients to be on
call regularly 7 days a week, 24 hours a day? (Check one)

.... Yes, an internist should be available whenever any patients, *even
              new ones,* feel they need him
.... It depends; an internist should be available whenever his regular
              patients feel that they need him, but he is not obligated to new
              patients
.... No, an internist is entitled to have some time for himself, provided he
              makes sure that another doctor is available to his patients
.... No, an internist is entitled to regular hours just like anyone else

(b) How about a general practitioner—do you think that a general practitioner owes it to patients to be on call regularly 7 days
a week, 24 hours a day? (Check one)

.... Yes, a g.p. should be available whenever any patients, *even new ones,*
              feel that they need him
.... It depends; a g.p. should be available whenever his regular patients
              feel that they need him, but he is not obligated to new patients
.... No, a g.p. is entitled to have some time for himself, provided he
              makes sure that another doctor is available to his patients
.... No, a g.p. is entitled to regular hours just like anyone else

40. Below is a list of problems which practicing physicians sometimes
meet.

(a) To what extent have you thought about each of these problems? (Answer below)

(b) Do you feel that you are now able to deal with these problems? (Answer below)

Check one for each problem   *Check one for each problem*

(a) HAVE THOUGHT   (b) CAN DEAL WITH

Quite a lot	Little bit	Not at all		Quite sure I can deal with this	Fairly sure I can deal with this	Not sure I can deal with this
......	......	......	The uncertainties of diagnosis and therapy that one meets in practice	....	....	....
......	......	......	The difficulty of maintaining the proper degree of detachment from patients	....	....	....
......	......	......	The problem of employing necessary therapy which may have serious adverse side-effects on the patient	....	....	....
......	......	......	The difficulties of providing high quality medical care and still making a decent living in practice	....	....	....
......	......	......	The problem of ordering valuable diagnostic tests which are painful or unpleasant	....	....	....
......	......	......	The difficulty of feeling the proper degree of concern for all patients	....	....	....
......	......	......	The problem of "individual variability" in the signs, symptoms and response to treatment of patients	....	....	....
......	......	......	The fact that functional illness is a large part of the physician's practice	....	....	....

41. The various specialties within the medical profession present different opportunities, and correspond to different sorts of interests and talents among doctors. What is your judgment about the following specialties in the respects listed below? Please indicate to what extent

each of the following is a *good description* of the specialties listed. (If you think the statement is *very appropriate* to the specialty, please put a *1* on the corresponding line. If you think it is *fairly appropriate*, please put a *2*. If you think it is *not very appropriate*, please put a *3*. If you think it is *inappropriate*, please put a *4*.)

(Please put a number for *each* specialty on *every* statement.)

	Sur- gery	Medi- cine	Psy- chiatry	Pedi- atrics	Ob.-Gyn.	General Practice
A field where one can establish his own hours of work	....	....	....	....	....	....
A field in which patients are highly appreciative of what is done for them	....	....	....	....	....	....
A field where diag- nostic problems are especially challenging	....	....	....	....	....	....
A field where rela- tionships with col- leagues in the same specialty are particularly enjoyable	....	....	....	....	....	....
A field which is very likely to yield a good income	....	....	....	....	....	....
A field which pre- sents opportuni- ties for knowing patients well	....	....	....	....	....	....
A field which has high prestige within the medi- cal profession	....	....	....	....	....	....

42. In which one of the following categories would you say that the *average* yearly income of the specialist and of the general practitioner fall? (Check one in each group)

	SPECIALIST		GENERAL PRACTITIONER
....	Under $5,000	....	Under $5,000
....	$ 5,000 up to $10,000	....	$ 5,000 up to $10,000
....	$10,000 up to $15,000	....	$10,000 up to $15,000
....	$15,000 up to $20,000	....	$15,000 up to $20,000
....	$20,000 up to $25,000	....	$20,000 up to $25,000
....	$25,000 up to $35,000	....	$25,000 up to $35,000

III. THIS SECTION DEALS WITH YOUR PROFESSIONAL PLANS AND AMBI-
TIONS FOR THE FUTURE. EVEN THOUGH YOU MAY NOT BE CERTAIN
OF YOUR PLANS, PLEASE ANSWER THE QUESTIONS ON THE BASIS OF
YOUR PRESENT HOPES OR PREFERENCES.

43. How much have you thought about the kind of medical career you
would like to have? (Check one)
.... A great deal
.... A fair amount
.... Only a little
.... Not at all

44. (a) What kind of internship do you plan to obtain? Even though
you may not have decided definitely yet, please indicate your first *two
choices* in order of your preference. (Check one in each group)

First choice
.... Rotating
.... Straight medical
.... Straight surgical
.... Straight pathology
.... Mixed medical and surgical
.... Obstetrics and gynecology
.... Straight pediatrics
.... Other (What? ....)

Second choice
.... Rotating
.... Straight medical
.... Straight surgical
.... Straight pathology
.... Mixed medical and surgical
.... Obstetrics and gynecology
.... Straight pediatrics
.... Other (What? ....)

(b) How certain are you about your first choice of internship in
Question (a) above? (Check one)
.... Very certain
.... Fairly certain
.... Not at all certain

(c) In what kind of hospital would you like to intern? (Check
one)
.... Hospital in a small community
.... Hospital in a large city (not closely connected with a university)
.... Teaching hospital in a large city
.... Teaching hospital in a small city
.... Other (What? ....)

45. (a) Do you intend to take a residency in some specialty? (Check one)

.... Yes
.... No
.... Don't know
.... Have never thought about it

(b) How certain do you feel about this intention? (Check one)

.... Very certain
.... Fairly certain
.... Not at all certain

(c) (FOR STUDENTS WHO INTEND OR HOPE TO TAKE A RESIDENCY) In what specialty do you intend to take your residency? Even though you may not have decided definitely yet, please indicate your first *two* choices in the order of your preference. (Check one in each group)

First choice

.... Medicine
.... Surgery
.... Obstetrics and gynecology
.... Pediatrics
.... Pathology
.... Psychiatry
.... Other (What? ....)

Second choice

.... Medicine
.... Surgery
.... Obstetrics and gynecology
.... Pediatrics
.... Pathology
.... Psychiatry
.... Other (What? ....)

(d) (FOR STUDENTS WHO INTEND OR HOPE TO TAKE A RESIDENCY) How certain are you of your first choice? (Check one)

.... Very certain
.... Fairly certain
.... Not at all certain

46. Which field of medicine would you *least* like to enter? (Check one)

.... Medicine
.... Surgery
.... Obstetrics and gynecology
.... Pediatrics
.... Pathology
.... Psychiatry
.... Orthopedics
.... Dermatology
.... Ear, nose and throat
.... Other (What? ....)

47. *When you have finished your formal medical training (including work beyond your M.D.):*

(a) To what type of professional activity in the list below would you *prefer* to give most of your working time? Please indicate your first two choices in the order of your preference. (Check one in each group)

First choice
.... General practice
.... Specialty practice (Which specialty? ....)
.... Teaching some medical specialty
          (Which specialty? ....)
.... Doing research
.... Other (What? ....)

Second choice
.... General practice
.... Specialty practice (Which specialty? ....)
.... Teaching some medical specialty
          (Which specialty? ....)
.... Doing research
.... Other (What? ....)

(b) Apart from what you would like, to what type of professional activity in the list below do you *expect* to give *most* of your working time? (Check one)
.... General practice
.... Specialty practice
.... Teaching some medical specialty
.... Doing research
.... Other (What? ....)

(c) How certain are you about your choice of professional activity in Question (b) above? (Check one)
.... Very certain
.... Fairly certain
.... Not at all certain

48. (a) (FOR STUDENTS WHO HAVE DECIDED ON A PARTICULAR FIELD OF SPECIALIZATION OR WHO DEFINITELY PLAN TO GO INTO GENERAL PRACTICE) When did you make this decision? (Check one)
.... Before coming to medical school
.... In the pre-clinical years
.... In the third year of medical school
.... In the fourth year of medical school
.... Don't know

(b) (FOR STUDENTS WHO HAVE NOT YET COME TO ANY DECISION ON THIS) At what point in your medical training do you think you will make this decision? (Check one)

.... In the pre-clinical years
.... In the third year of medical school
.... In the fourth year of medical school
.... In the internship
.... Don't know

(c) In your opinion, when do the faculty members feel a medical student *should* make up his mind about his future career plans? (Check one)

.... Before coming to medical school
.... In the pre-clinical years
.... In the third year of medical school
.... In the fourth year of medical school
.... In the internship

49. If you could arrange it, in which *one* of the following situations would you plan to carry out the professional activity you said you prefer most? (Check one)

.... Own professional office with hospital affiliation
.... Own professional office without hospital affiliation
.... Large private clinic or hospital
.... Small group clinic
.... Medical school
.... Other (What? ....)

50. (a) For the student who does exceptionally well in medical school, how would you rank the following five career plans in order of their desirability? (Rank all five, placing a *1* before the most desirable, and so on)

.... Residency, followed by general practice
.... Advanced training, followed by a research career
.... Residency, followed by specialty practice
.... No residency, followed by general practice
.... Advanced training, followed by full-time teaching in medical school

(b) How do you think the *faculty* as a whole would rate these career plans for the student who does exceptionally well? (Rank all five)

.... Residency, followed by general practice
.... Advanced training, followed by a research career
.... Residency, followed by specialty practice
.... No residency, followed by general practice
.... Advanced training, followed by full-time teaching in a medical school

51. What yearly income do you think you might *realistically expect*

(a) Ten years after medical school? (Check one)
.... Under $5,000
.... $ 5,000 up to $10,000
.... $10,000 up to $15,000
.... $15,000 up to $20,000
.... $20,000 up to $25,000
.... $25,000 or over

(b) At the peak of your career? (Check one)
.... Under $5,000
.... $ 5,000 up to $10,000
.... $10,000 up to $15,000
.... $15,000 up to $20,000
.... $20,000 up to $25,000
.... $25,000 or over

How satisfied will you be with the yearly income you think you might *realistically expect*

(c) Ten years after medical school? (Check one)
.... Very satisfied
.... Fairly satisfied
.... Dissatisfied

(d) At the peak of your career? (Check one)
.... Very satisfied
.... Fairly satisfied
.... Dissatisfied

52. To what extent have you worried that you may not be able to have the kind of medical career you want? (Check one)
.... A great deal
.... A fair amount
.... Only a little
.... Not at all

53. Once you have received a license to practice medicine, to what extent do you expect to continue your medical education by each of the following routes? (Answer for each)

	Regularly	Occa-sionally	Never	Unsure
Reading medical journals	....	....	....	....
Reading medical textbooks	....	....	....	....
Attending local medical society meetings	....	....	....	....
Supplementing your practice with research activities	....	....	....	....
Teaching full-time in a medical school	....	....	....	....
Teaching part-time in a medical school	....	....	....	....
Serving in an out-patient clinic	....	....	....	....

Taking post-graduate and summer
    specialty courses   ....
Examination of publications of
    pharmaceutical houses   ....
By contacts with consultants
    on your cases   ....

54. (a) What *two* things or activities in the list below do you expect
will give *you* the most satisfaction? (Check one in each column under
"a")

   (b) In your opinion what two things or activities in the list below give *doctors in practice* the most satisfaction? (Check one in
   each column under "b")

	(a)		(b)	
	Most satis- fying to YOU	Next most satisfying to YOU	Most satis- fying to DOCTORS	Next most satisfying to DOCTORS
Working toward national or international betterment	....	....	....	....
Leisure time activities	....	....	....	....
Professional career	....	....	....	....
Participating in community activities	....	....	....	....
Family relationships	....	....	....	....
Religious beliefs or activities	....	....	....	....

55. Below are some considerations that might enter into your selection
of a specialty or of general practice in medicine. Which *two* are most
important to you as you think about your career? Which two are least
important? (Check two in each column)

	Most important	Least important
Having the opportunity to know your patients well	....	....
Being able to establish your own hours of work	....	....
Meeting diagnostic problems that are particularly challenging	....	....
Having enjoyable relationships with colleagues	....	....
Making a good income	....	....
Having patients who will appreciate your efforts	....	....
Having prestige within the medical profession	....	....

IV. IT IS A MATTER OF GENERAL KNOWLEDGE THAT PEOPLE DIFFER IN
    THEIR INTERESTS AND CAPACITIES. EVERYONE HAS HIS STRONG AND
    HIS WEAK POINTS. THE QUESTIONS THAT FOLLOW ARE DESIGNED
    TO ENABLE YOU TO MAKE ROUGH COMPARISONS BETWEEN YOUR
    OWN INTERESTS AND QUALITIES AND THOSE OF OTHER PEOPLE.

56. Compared with *other students in your class year*, how would you
say you stand in each of the following respects? (Assign yourself from

1 to 7 points for each item, in terms of the following meaning of the points.)

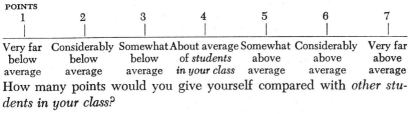

How many points would you give yourself compared with *other students in your class?*

POINTS
(use whole
numbers)

....	1.	Ability to memorize details
....	2.	Ability to cope with theoretical problems
....	3.	Ability to cope with practical problems
....	4.	Interest in politics and world affairs
....	5.	Interest in emotional problems of people
....	6.	Ability to put everything aside for your studies
....	7.	Manual dexterity (with instruments, tools, machines, etc.)
....	8.	Desire to help people
....	9.	Knowledge of physical science
....	10.	Knowledge of social science
....	11.	Getting the most possible out of your four years of medical school
....	12.	Ability to get along with the faculty
....	13.	Ability to remain relaxed, rather than overly tense and nervous about your work
....	14.	Ability to get good grades
....	15.	Readiness to assume responsibility

57. Compared with *physicians now in practice,* how well do you expect to do in the following respects when you are in practice? As before, assign yourself from 1 to 7 points for each item, in terms of the following meaning of the points:

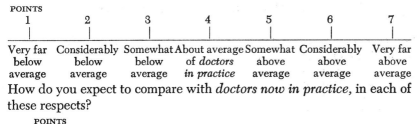

How do you expect to compare with *doctors now in practice,* in each of these respects?

POINTS
(use whole
numbers)

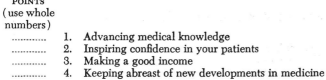

....	1.	Advancing medical knowledge
....	2.	Inspiring confidence in your patients
....	3.	Making a good income
....	4.	Keeping abreast of new developments in medicine

.... 5. Helping to keep fee-splitting and ghost surgery from your community
.... 6. Providing equally good care for all your patients
.... 7. Willingness to try new medicines and techniques
.... 8. Participating in national medical societies
.... 9. Recognizing your own limitations as a physician
.... 10. Developing your diagnostic skills
.... 11. Ability to remain sufficiently detached from patients to perform your medical tasks
.... 12. Getting along with nurses and other medical personnel
.... 13. Willingness to have your private life interrupted by your patients' needs
.... 14. Respecting the dignity of patients as individuals
.... 15. Being considerate of your patients' economic means

V. THIS FINAL SECTION DEALS WITH YOUR BACKGROUND AND YOUR IN-TERESTS. THE INFORMATION YOU PROVIDE HERE WILL PERMIT A COMPARISON OF THE OPINIONS, PLANS, AND EXPERIENCES OF STU-DENTS WITH DIFFERENT KINDS OF BACKGROUNDS.

58. Exact Date of Birth: Month................. Day................. Year.................

59. Sex: Male................. Female.................

60. Marital status:
.... Single
.... Married
.... Engaged
.... Divorced, separated, widowed
If engaged: When do you plan to marry?

61. If married: (a) How long have you been married? .... Years
                  (b) How many children do you have? ....

62. How much have you worried that you might not be happy in a medical career? (Check one)
.... A great deal
.... Somewhat
.... Only a little
.... Not at all

63. (a) How difficult is it for you to finance your medical education? (Check one)
.... Very difficult
.... Fairly difficult
.... Not very difficult
.... Not at all difficult

(b)* (FOR STUDENTS WHO DEPEND ON PARENTS FOR SOME OR ALL OF THEIR SUPPORT) How do your parents feel about having you depend on them for financial aid while you are in medical school? (Check one)

.... They are not happy about it
.... They are willing, although it is difficult for them
.... They are willing to do it
.... They are very glad to do it
.... Other (What? ....)

64. How much have you worried about the problems of supporting yourself (and your family): (Check one)

(a) While you are in medical school?
.... A great deal
.... Quite a bit
.... Not very much
.... Not at all

(b) During your internship? (Check one)
.... A great deal
.... Quite a bit
.... Not very much
.... Not at all

(c) During your residency? (Check one)
.... A great deal
.... Quite a bit
.... Not very much
.... Not at all
.... Do not plan to take residency

(d) During your early years in practice? (Check one)
.... A great deal
.... Quite a bit
.... Not very much
.... Not at all

65. Have you had a job for pay during the *current semester?* Yes........ No........

IF YES: On the average, how many hours a week have you worked? (Check one)
.... 10 or less
.... 11–20
.... 21–30
.... 31 or more

66. During the coming summer, do you plan to work (Check one)
.... full-time
.... part-time
.... not at all

IF "FULL-TIME" OR "PART-TIME":
Is this work related to medicine? Yes........ No........
Will you get paid for this work? Yes........ No........

67. (a) What are your favorite leisure time activities? (Check 2 or 3 favorites)

.... Going to the movies
.... Reading serious books and magazines
.... Listening to music
.... Attending sports events as a spectator
.... Participating in sports events
.... Going out on dates
.... Talking with friends
.... Working at special hobbies (What? ....)
.... Other (What? ....)

(b) During the last year, about how many hours a week, on the average, did you spend on activities of this kind? (Check one)

.... 10 hours or less
.... 11–15 hours
.... 16–20 hours
.... 21–25 hours
.... 26 or more hours

(c) How about the coming year—how many hours a week do you think you will be able to spend on leisure time activities? (Check one)

.... 10 hours or less
.... 11–15 hours
.... 16–20 hours
.... 21–25 hours
.... 26 or more hours

68. What is your father's occupation?

....

69. Name the community in which you lived longest before going to college.

....

70. What undergraduate college did you attend?

....

71. (a) In what field did you major as an undergraduate?

....

(b) If you had it to do over again in what would you major in undergraduate college?

....

72. Do you have any relatives who are in any of the following professions? (If yes, what is their relationship to you?)

	No	Yes	Parent	Other close relative	Other relative
M.D.'s?	....	....	....	....	....
Lawyers?	....	....	....	....	....
Dentists?	....	....	....	....	....
Clergymen?	....	....	....	....	....
Teachers?	....	....	....	....	....
Nurses?	....	....	....	....	....
Engineers?	....	....	....	....	....
Other professionals? (What? ....)	....	....	....	....	....

Index

INDEX

Ambulatory patients, care of, 82–85, 90
American Medical Association, *Principles of Medical Ethics*, 189
Appel, Kenneth E., ix
Arensberg, Conrad M., 39
Ashford, Mahlon, 31
Association of American Medical Colleges, 72
Atchley, Dana, 3
Ausubel, D. P., 67

Bachrach, Paul, 59–60
Barr, David P., ix, 3, 81–82, 90, 257
Bartlett, Sir Frederick, 60–61
Basowitz, Harold, 62, 67
Beck, Dorothy, 272
Bendix, Reinhard, 134
Berelson, Bernard, 105, 119, 169
Berry, George Packer, 33
Berson, Robert C., 35, 153, 155
Bidder, T. George, ix
Blau, Peter M., 39, 256
Bloom, Samuel, 43, 51, 70
Booth, Charles, 50
Borgatta, Edgar, 48
Brody, Irwin, 109–110
Bruner, Jerome S., 67
Bryson, Lyman, 18
Bureaucracy, definition, 39

Caplovitz, David, 295–296
Caplow, Theodore, 36

Career decisions
    age when decision made, 114–119, 131–137
    ambivalence about, 116–119, 121
    comparison of medical and law students, 115–116, 131–152
    degree of satisfaction with, 122–124, 139–143
    first consideration, 111–114
    influence of contact with profession, 132, 136
    influence of prestige of professions, 136–137
    of medical students, 68–71, 109–129
    role of institutional requirements in, 115–116, 132–134
    role of peers in, 125–127
    role of relatives in, 111–114, 116–119, 122–127, 134–136
Caughey, John L., ix, 34
Cecil, Russell L., 223
Child, Irwin L., 41
Class in medical school
    clinical years, 84, 165–174, 180, 190–205, 221–239
    entering students, 109–129, 131–152, 183–184
    inter-class comparisons, 153–165
    preclinical years, 180–187, 209–221
Cohen, Sir Henry, 27
Coleman, James S., 39, 301
Columbia University, Bureau of Applied Social Research, 34, 92, 95, 98, 160

355

Commonwealth Fund, ix, 83, 92, 258, 260
Competition
  between departments in medical school, 22–24
  law school compared with medical school, 143–151
  legal profession compared with medical profession, 147–149
Comprehensive medical care, 252
  definition of, 81, 85–87, 89–90
Conant, James B., 33, 207
Consultations with medical specialists, 84, 272, 280–284
Continuity of patient care, 82–87, 89, 94, 101, 271, 273–276
Cook, Stuart W., 42
Cooke, W. R., 78
Cooley, Charles H., 181
Coordination of services to patients, 86–87, 90, 271, 280–284
Cornell University Comprehensive Care and Teaching Program, 35, 228–239
  aims, 84–85
  changes in, 90, 249–270
  conditions and processes facilitating change, 257–270
  origin and plan, 81–84
  specification of plans, 85–90
  staff of, 89
Cornell University Medical College, 15, 34, 40, 72, 81, 83–85, 89–90, 93, 155, 170, 173, 174, 180, 190, 207
Cowen, E. L., 67
"Crock," 234
Curriculum
  graded sequences in, 13–14
  innovations in, 85–89, 180
  organization of, 209–210, 222–223, 228–229, 236
  time-budget of, 22–23
Cushing, Harvey, 118–119

Definition of the situation, 45, 183
Deitrick, John E., 35, 153, 155
Detached concern, 74, 161
Deutsch, Morton, 42
Diagnosis, range seen by students, 86, 271, 276–279
Dickson, William, 39
Diethelm, O., 67
Differential diagnosis, logic of, 233–234
Dollard, John, 40
Drill, Victor, 212

Dublin, Thomas D., 31

Eliot, Charles W., 16
Eliot, George, 26
Empiricism, reduction of in medicine, 33

Fabricant, Noah, 109
Faculty–student relations
  colleagueship, 88
  reciprocal relations, 295–296
Faculty of medical school, study of opinion, 98
Family Care, 86, 89, 99, 250–256, 263, 268, 271–272, 274–276, 279
Family physician, 82, 89, 154, 250, 266
Festinger, Leon, 42
Fishbein, Morris, 28
Fiske, Marjorie, 46
Fleming, Donald, 119
Flexner, Abraham, 8, 16–19, 53
Fox, Renée C., 43, 46
Francis, R. G., 39
Fulton, John F., 8, 24, 118–119

Garrison, F. H., 17
General Medical Clinic, 82, 259, 263, 267, 273–284
Gillin, John, 54
Ginzberg, Eli, 110, 115
Goldman, M., 67
Goode, William J., 37, 42
Goss, Mary E. W., 31, 43, 90
Gottheil, Edward, 59–61
Gouldner, Alvin W., 39
Grace, William J., 83
Grades of medical students, 50–51, 59–61, 65, 67–68, 95, 209–210
  related to self-evaluations, 203–204
  self-appraisals of performance, 171–172
Gray, Louis H., 293
Gregg, Alan, 72, 115
Grinker, R. R., 62
Guion, Connie M., 82
Guthrie, William S., 145

Hall, Oswald, 112
Ham, Thomas Hale, ix, 34
Hammond, Kenneth R., 34
Hanlon, Lawrence W., 209
Hatt, Paul K., 42, 137
Hawthorne experiments, 93
Health Information Foundation, 38
Henderson, L. J., 25, 29
Hinsey, Joseph C., ix

Homans, George C., 39
Home Care, 82, 85, 89–90, 275
Home visits, 265–267
Horowitz, Milton J., 43
Hospitalization, 82, 86, 89
Hubbard, John, ix, 29
Hughes, Everett C., 36, 40
Huntington, Mary Jean, 37, 299

Illness, social and emotional aspects of,
191–196, 200–201
related to uncertainty, 230–235,
237–239
Institutionalization of Comprehensive
Care and Teaching Program, 257
Internship assignments, 158, 160,
164–165, 174
influence of faculty members, 165,
171–174
relation to grades, 166, 168, 170–171,
174
relation to preferences, 160–165,
169–170
Internship preferences
changes in, 157–159, 173–174
postponement of decision, 155,
161–162, 174
relation to grades, 166, 173
rotating internships, 155–156,
158–162, 165–166, 168–170, 173
specialized internships, 155, 157–160,
165–166, 168–170, 173
stage of training as determinant, 157
Interviews, 44–47

Jackson, F. W., 31
Jahoda, Marie, 42
Jefferson, Sir Geoffrey, 26
Johns Hopkins Medical School, 16
Jones, Ernest, 291
Jones, M. R., 67

Katz, Daniel, 42
Katz, Elihu, 105
Kendall, Patricia L., 46
Kennedy, William B., ix
Kern, Fred, Jr., 34
Kluckhohn, Clyde, 291
Köhler, Wolfgang, 288
Kolb, William L., 137
Korchin, S. J., 62
Korsch, Barbara M., 83–84
Kroeber, A. L., 291
Kuhn, Adam, 15
Kutner, Bernard, 40

Lazarsfeld, Paul F., 18, 42, 47, 105,
110, 119, 169
Learning
attitudinal, 44, 72, 77, 91–93
cognitive, 44, 76, 91
psychology of, 9
sociology of, 9, 63
LePlay, Frederic, 50
Levine, Gene N., 72
Levine, Samuel, 83
Lincoln, Abraham, 137
Lindzey, Gardner, 41, 48
Lipset, S. M., 39, 134
Llewellyn, Karl N., 149
Locke, John, 25
Loeb, Robert, 223
Luckey, E. Hugh, ix
Lynd, Robert S., ix

McClelland, David C., 62
McPhee, William N., 105, 119, 169
Madge, John, 42
Malinowski, Bronislaw, 17
Mallick, S. M. K., 26
Martin, William, 297–298
Mayo Clinic, 83
Mayo, Elton, 25–26, 39
Mead, George Herbert, 181
Medical education
division of labor in, 11–13
experiments in, 14, 33–35, 66, 81–82,
90, 94, 100. *See also* Curriculum,
innovations in
forces for change in, 6, 8, 20–21, 24
historical perspectives, 7–21
resistance to change in, 6, 14–15, 24
Medical practice, choice of
general *vs.* specialty practice,
154–156, 164, 172–173
relation to internship preferences, 159
Medical practice, division of labor in,
10–11. *See also* Specialization
Medical school
as social environment, 63–65, 67, 287
as value-environment, 71–79
functions of, 5–7
social structure of, 38
university affiliation of, 16–17
Medical specialties
student attitudes toward, 233–234
supposed personality types in, 69
Medical students
admission of, 61, 64
compared with law students,
143–145
motivations of, 65–68

Medical students (cont.)
  psychological studies of, 57–58
  social relations of, 49, 64, 66. *See also* Peer group relations
  sociological studies of, 57–58
Medical team, 86
Medicine
  advances in, 21–22, 211, 212, 233
  as social institution, 4–5
  social functions of, 4
Merton, Robert K., 18, 37, 46, 51, 70, 77, 92, 181
Methods of social research
  cross-sectional analyses, 157
  diaries, 44–46, 98, 207
  documentary records, 49–51, 94, 98
  intensive interviews, 94–96, 207, 249
  observation, 42–44, 94–95, 98, 207, 249
  panel techniques, 47–48, 97, 106, 157, 160, 168–169
  questionnaires, 95–99, 268
    composite schedule, 307–351
  sociometry, 48–49
Michael, Carmen Miller, 59–61
Mitchell, John McK., ix
Moreno, Jacob L., 48
Morgan, John, 8–16, 19, 52–53
Motives, 12

Nasatir, E. David, 298
Nehnevajsa, Jiri, 47
Newcomb, Theodore M., 54
New York Hospital, 81, 83–84, 172–173, 251, 278
  Out-Patient Department, 81–86, 89, 273
Nicholls, William, II, 49, 64, 296–297
Norms
  factors affecting conformity to, 189–190, 194, 205
  of medical practice, 18, 71–79
  of medical students, 23, 220–221, 223, 236–239
North, Cecil C., 137
Norwood, W. F., 8

Observability, 17–18, 77–78
Organization, social, 39–40, 56, 77
Organizational change
  conditions and processes facilitating, 257–270
  types of, 255–257
    innovation, 256–257
    specification, 256
    substitution, 256–257

Osler, Sir William, 16, 19, 199

Park, Robert E., 36
Parsons, Talcott, 36, 39, 41, 54
Patient
  attitudes of, 227, 229–230, 231
  emotionally disturbed, 192, 194–196, 201
  environment of, 27
  index of preferential attitudes toward, 190–191
  number seen by students, 271–273
  rediscovery as person, 25
  satisfactions in working with, 198–199
  social problems of, 252–254
  students' preferences for, 189–205
  types of, 190–191
  uncooperative, 199–202
Patient–doctor relationship, 25–26, 78–79
  responsibility for patients, 154, 173
Patterson, John W., ix, 34
Peabody, Francis Weld, 25
Peer group relations, effects on attitudinal learning, 296–297
Pepper, William, 16
Persky, Harold, 62
Physical findings
  positive or negative, 191
  relation to uncertainty, 214–215, 217–219, 229–231, 236–237
Pitts, Robert F., 209
Postman, Leo, 67
Pratt, Lois, 181
Professional identity, 7. *See also* Self-image
Professional role, 41
  and personality, 69–70
Professions, social status of, 37
Psychology, general orientations of, 54–57
Puschmann, Theodor, 8

Querido, A., 27–28

Rappleye, Willard C., 29
Reader, George G., 29, 31, 34, 81, 84, 85, 90, 254, 261
Referrals to specialty clinics, 272, 274, 280–283
Rehabilitation, 81, 89
Rennie, Thomas A. C., 31
Residency training, 153, 155, 173
Responsibility for patients, relation to uncertainty, 224–226, 228–229

Riesman, David, 40
Roethlisberger, Fritz J., 39
Rogoff, Natalie, 51, 70, 134
Rohrer, John H., 39
Role models, 154, 173
  law student compared with medical
    student, 137–139
Role performance, 194
Role set of medical student, 180–181
  relation to self-image, 180–183, 186
Roper, Elmo, 160
Rosenberg, Morris, 42, 47
Rush, Benjamin, 15
Russell Sage Foundation, 37

Schiff, H. M., 67
Schwartz, Doris, 199
Schwartz, M. S., 39
Self-confidence
  and emotional involvement of stu-
    dents with patients, 201–202
  and students' grades, 203–204
  index of, 196–197
  of students working with patients,
    194–205
Self-images, 46, 73–74, 179, 204, 299
  as reflection of others' expectations,
    181–184, 187
  changes in, 179–180
  development of, 179–187
  expected, 183–184
  in relationships with classmates,
    181–182
  in relationships with faculty, 181–182
  in relationships with nurses, 181–183
  in relationships with patients,
    180–181, 183–187
  unstable, 181
Selvin, Hanan C., 301
Selznick, Philip, 39, 262
Sherif, Muzafer, 39
Shippen, William, 15
Shryock, Richard H., 17, 21, 30
Sigerist, Henry E., 29
Significance, tests of, 301–305
Simmons, Leo W., 38
Simon, Herbert A., 39
Smigel, Ernest O., 36
Smith, Adam, 10
Smith, Reginald Heber, 147
Socialization, 40–42, 53, 78, 287–293
Sociology
  general orientations of, 54–57
  images of among physicians, 27–33
  of occupations, 36–37, 52, 111

Sonkin, Lawrence, 275
Sons of physicians, 116–119, 298
Specialization, 11, 153–154, 158–159,
    164–165, 167, 172, 174
  trend toward, 153–174
  value in modern medicine, 173
"Spoon-feeding," 209–210
Stalnaker, John M., 145
Stanton, A. H., 39
Status-sequences, 56
Stone, R. C., 39
Straus, Robert, 38
Student–patient relationship, 189–205
  attitudes of patient toward, 181, 204
  continuity of, 200, 226, 229–231
  effect on student's self-image,
    183–187
  emotional involvement of student,
    198–202, 232–234
  formation of professional role,
    297–298
  interpersonal aspects of, 192, 194–195
  orientation toward patients, 127–128
  responsibility for patients, 87–88
  student's difficulty in, 186–187
  student's obligations in, 182, 184–185
Super, Donald E., 59–60

Taylor, Howard C., Jr., 31
Therapy, discrimination in application,
    86
Thomas, William I., 183
Thurstone, L. L., 293
Trow, M., 39

Uncertainty
  coping with, 218–221, 225–228,
    235–239
  relation to experimental viewpoint,
    213–214, 237–239
  types of, 208–218, 221–224, 229
Uncertainty, training for, 207–241
  contribution of
    autopsy, 216–218
    gross anatomy, 211
    pharmacology, 212
    physical diagnosis, 214–216
  role of faculty–student relations in,
    217–222, 226–227, 233, 234, 237
  role of peer group relations in,
    220–221, 224, 236–237
University of Colorado School of
    Medicine, 34, 40
University of Illinois Medical School,
    111, 114

University of Kansas Medical School, 40
University of Pennsylvania School of
  Medicine, 15, 34, 40, 72, 110, 131,
  133, 144, 156, 180, 190

Vanderbilt, Arthur T., 132
Visit reports, 271–273, 279

Watson, Sir Thomas, 189
Wearn, Joseph T., ix, 34
Webb, Beatrice, 43
Webb, Sidney, 43
Welch, William H., 19, 119
Wells, Joseph A., 212

Western Reserve University School of
  Medicine, 15, 34, 40, 51, 72, 111,
  114, 156, 180–187, 190
  Family Clinic, 182, 184–185
Whitehead, T. N., 93
Whyte, William F., 39
Williams, Josephine, 111, 114, 120
Wilson, Logan, 137
Wolf, George A., 84
Wolf, Stewart G., 83
Wolff, Harold G., 38, 67, 83
Women physicians, 120
Wood, Barry, 22

Znaniecki, Florian, 183